Biomedical Signal Processing

Iyad Obeid • Ivan Selesnick • Joseph Picone
Editors

Biomedical Signal Processing

Innovation and Applications

Springer

Editors
Iyad Obeid
ECE Department
Temple University
Philadelphia, PA, USA

Ivan Selesnick
Tandon School of Engineering
New York University
Brooklyn, NY, USA

Joseph Picone
ECE Department
Temple University
Philadelphia, PA, USA

ISBN 978-3-030-67493-9 ISBN 978-3-030-67494-6 (eBook)
https://doi.org/10.1007/978-3-030-67494-6

This Springer imprint is published by the registered company Springer Nature Switzerland AG
The registered company address is: Gewerbestrasse 11, 6330 Cham, Switzerland

Preface

This edited volume consists of the expanded versions of the exceptional papers presented at the 2019 IEEE Signal Processing in Medicine and Biology Symposium (IEEE SPMB) held at Temple University in Philadelphia, Pennsylvania, USA. IEEE SPMB promotes interdisciplinary papers across a wide range of topics, including analysis of biomedical signals and images, machine learning, data, and educational resources. The symposium was first held in 2011 at New York University Polytechnic (now known as NYU Tandon School of Engineering). Since 2014, it has been hosted by the Neural Engineering Data Consortium at Temple University as part of a broader mission to promote machine learning and big data applications in bioengineering. The symposium typically consists of 18 highly competitive full paper submissions that include oral presentations and 12 to 18 single-page abstracts that are presented as posters. Two plenary lectures are included – one focused on research and the other focused on emerging technology. The symposium provides a stimulating environment where multidisciplinary research in the life sciences is presented. More information about the symposium can be found at www.ieeespmb.org.

Biomedical engineering bridges the gap between biological science, medicine, and engineering. Innovative hardware solutions enabled by compact wireless devices are changing the way we can monitor and understand biological systems. Machine learning plays an integral role in real-time control and classification of signals collected by these devices. These rapid advances in hardware and software are paving the way for a new generation of technological developments in the health sciences.

The papers represented in this volume as chapters can be classified into three areas: (1) classification and control of biological signals, (2) improved transduction and processing of biological signals, and (3) enhanced infrastructure for electroencephalograms (EEGs). Algorithms and data play a key role in all these chapters, reinforcing the emphasis on data science we see across many engineering fields.

The first two chapters, titled "Multi-Class fNIRS Classification of Motor Execution Tasks with Application to Brain Computer Interfaces" and "A Comparative Study of End-To-End Discriminative Deep Learning Models for Knee Joint Kinematic Time Series Classification," address issues in motor control of the human body. The first chapter applies functional Near Infrared Spectroscopy (fNIRS) to the problem of classification of motor execution tasks. The second chapter addresses classification of knee kinematic signals using deep learning with a goal to improve diagnosis of knee joint pathologies.

The next group of four chapters focus more on acquisition and understanding of biological signals using novel signal processing techniques. The first chapter in this group, titled "Nonlinear Smoothing of Core Body Temperature Data with Random Gaps and Outliers (DRAGO)," proposes new ways to smooth core body temperature estimates acquired from an ingestible pill. The second chapter, titled "An Adaptive Search Algorithm for Detecting Respiratory Artifacts Using a Wireless Passive Wearable Device," proposes a new way to measure respiratory activity using smart fabrics. The third chapter, titled "The Spatial Distribution of a Seismocardiographic Signal," explores new ways to measure chest surface vibrations resulting from cardiac activity. The fourth chapter in this group, titled "Determination of Vascular Access Stenosis Location and Severity by Multi-Domain Analysis of Blood Sounds," analyzes blood sounds (bruits) using phonoangiography and classifies signals by the degree of stenosis. These chapters are good examples of how co-design of sensor technology and signal processing algorithms can result in significant improvement in performance.

The final two chapters deal with encephalography, which has been a popular focus for the symposium. The first chapter, titled "Fast Automatic Artifact Annotator for EEG Signals Using Deep Learning," introduces three deep learning methods for the classification of artifacts in EEG signals. The second chapter, titled "Objective Evaluation Metrics for Automatic Classification of EEG Events," promotes the use of industry-standard, open source evaluation paradigms to calibrate and advance technology development. These chapters deal with a problem known as sequential decoding, which involves identification of the onset and offset of an event in an EEG signal in addition to classification of the type of event. Standardization of scoring is an important step towards promoting community-wide collaboration on technology development.

We are indebted to all of our authors who contributed to making IEEE SPMB 2019 a great success. The authors represented in this volume worked very diligently to provide excellent expanded chapters of their conference papers, making this volume a unique contribution. In 2020, IEEE SPMB will celebrate its 10th anniversary and will include a special session on an industry-wide competition for classification of seizures in EEG signals.

Philadelphia, PA, USA Iyad Obeid
Brooklyn, NY, USA Ivan Selesnick
Philadelphia, PA, USA Joseph Picone

Contents

Chapter 1
Multi-class fNIRS Classification of Motor Execution Tasks with Application to Brain-Computer Interfaces

Foroogh Shamsi and Laleh Najafizadeh

1.1 Introduction

1.1.1 fNIRS

functional near-infrared spectroscopy (fNIRS) is a noninvasive brain imaging technique, which measures local changes in the cerebral concentration of oxygenated hemoglobin ([ΔHbO_2]) and deoxygenated hemoglobin ([ΔHbR]) associated with the underlying brain activities (Ferrari and Quaresima 2012). The continuous-wave (CW) fNIRS takes advantage of the principle that oxygenated and deoxygenated hemoglobin have different extinction coefficients in the near-infrared range (Ardeshirpour et al. 2013). In CW-fNIRS, light transmitters (sources), placed over the surface of the head, emit light at two different near-infrared wavelengths into the scalp. By measuring changes in the received light intensities as measured by the light detectors, at the two different near-infrared wavelengths, [ΔHbO_2] and [ΔHbR], can be quantified using the modified Beer-Lambert law (Ardeshirpour et al. 2013).

Although fNIRS is a relatively new neuroimaging tool for monitoring brain activities, it has been widely used in various neuroscience research studies, due to its advantages comparing to other noninvasive neuroimaging techniques such as electroencephalogram (EEG), functional magnetic resonance imaging (fMRI), and magnetoencephalogram (MEG). fNIRS offers a better spatial resolution than EEG and a better temporal resolution than fMRI (Ardeshirpour et al. 2013). Moreover, unlike fMRI and MEG, it is not vulnerable to electromagnetic environment, which makes it suitable for patients with metallic implants. fNIRS is known to have a low

F. Shamsi · L. Najafizadeh (✉)
Integrated Systems and Neuroimaging Laboratory, Departments of Electrical and Computer Engineering, Rutgers University, Piscataway, NJ, USA
e-mail: laleh.najafizadeh@rutgers.edu

I. Obeid et al. (eds.), *Biomedical Signal Processing*,
https://doi.org/10.1007/978-3-030-67494-6_1

sensitivity to motion artifacts which makes it ideal for monitoring brain activities associated with tasks that involve movements. Additionally, its portability and ease of use provide a comfortable setting for monitoring and recording brain activities in various patient groups (Amyot et al. 2012; Liu et al. 2019; Perpetuini et al. 2017).

In clinical studies, fNIRS have been used to detect abnormal activities associated with several psychiatric and neurological disorders such as schizophrenia (Hosomi et al. 2019; Song et al. 2017), depression (Baik et al. 2019; Nishizawa et al. 2019; Rosenbaum et al. 2017), and post-traumatic stress disorder (Gramlich et al. 2017; Tian et al. 2014; Yennu et al. 2016). Due to its ease of use and robustness to motion artifacts, fNIRS has been extensively used in studies related to infants and young children. For example, it has been used to investigate development of cognitive skills in children for educational purposes (Aslin et al. 2015; Soltanlou et al. 2018). fNIRS has also been extensively employed for identifying neurodevelopmental disorders such as autism spectrum disorder (ASD) (Mazzoni et al. 2019; Zhang and Roeyers 2019) and attention deficit hyperactivity disorder (ADHD) (Gu et al. 2018; Gu et al. 2017) in infants and children. Another clinical application of fNIRS includes neurorehabilitation (Mihara and Miyai 2016), where fNIRS has been utilized in studying the neural correlates of motor dysfunction induced by traumatic brain injuries (TBI), or stroke (Cao et al. 2015; Kato et al. 2002; Takeda et al. 2007). Furthermore, it has been used in understanding the underlying neural mechanisms of motor learning (Hatakenaka et al. 2007; Hatakenaka et al. 2012), gait, balance, and posture control (Hatakenaka et al. 2012; Koenraadt et al. 2014; Mahoney et al. 2016; Maidan et al. 2015; Rea et al. 2014a, b; Takakura et al. 2015). fNIRS has also been used as a therapeutic tool as neurofeedback in the treatments of disabilities and psychiatric disorders (Ehlis et al. 2018; Lapborisuth et al. 2017; Marx et al. 2015; Mihara et al. 2013; Naseer and Hong 2015b). Another major application of fNIRS is in brain-computer interfaces (BCIs), where it is employed for recording brain activities related to intended tasks performed by the user. fNIRS-based BCIs are described in more details in the following section.

1.1.2 fNIRS-Based BCIs

One major application of fNIRS is in BCIs. A BCI directly translates brain activities into commands to control external devices. BCIs can be integrated with assistive technologies to aid patients with severe motor disabilities such as individuals with high spinal cord injury (SCI), stroke, or amyotrophic lateral sclerosis (ALS) with their daily activities. BCIs have also been employed in rehabilitation and therapies (Ang and Guan 2013; Bamdad et al. 2015).

Compared to noninvasive techniques, the use of invasive neuroimaging techniques such as electrocorticographic (ECoG) (Schalk and Leuthardt 2011) for BCIs offers advantages including achieving high degree of spatial resolution and high signal-to-noise ratio (SNR) recordings. However, due to the required invasive procedures, invasive BCIs have been only used either in animal studies or in specific groups of patients (e.g., severely paralyzed patients or those with epilepsy) and are not currently applicable to the general population. Invasive BCIs also face other technical challenges. For example, the implants should be biologically compatible and able to function reliably for a long period of time. Additionally, implanted electrodes may become encapsulated by fibrous tissue, resulting in degradation in the quality of the recorded data (Nicolas-Alonso and Gomez-Gil 2012). As such, noninvasive neuroimaging modalities such as EEG (Lotte et al. 2018; McFarland and Wolpaw 2017) and fNIRS (Naseer and Hong 2015a) have received considerable attention in BCIs. The major problems with noninvasive techniques are that compared to their invasive counterparts, they provide signals with lower SNR and have relatively lower spatial resolution (Steyrl et al. 2016; Waldert 2016). For example, EEG is sensitive to muscle, eye, and movement artifacts and requires extensive noise and artifact removal analysis before the classification can take place (Gajbhiye et al. 2019; Lai et al. 2018; Minguillon et al. 2017; Singh and Wagatsuma 2017). Compared to EEG, fNIRS is less sensitive to movement artifacts comparing (Naseer and Hong 2015a) and has less setup preparation time. fMRI and MEG as other major noninvasive neuroimaging techniques are not generally well-suited choices for BCIs due to lack of the essential properties of portability and low cost.

During the past decade, several studies have employed fNIRS in developing BCIs (Abibullaev et al. 2013; Hennrich et al. 2015; Herff et al. 2013; Hong et al. 2015; Janani and Sasikala 2018; Naseer and Hong 2013a, c; Noori et al. 2016, 2017; Peifer et al. 2014; Rea et al. 2014a; Shamsi and Najafizadeh 2019; Shamsi and Najafizadeh 2020; Shin and Im 2020; Yin et al. 2015a, c; Zafar et al. 2019; Zephaniah and Kim 2014; Zhang et al. 2017). Moreover, in order to increase the classification accuracy and number of commands, it has been suggested to integrate fNIRS with EEG, forming hybrid EEG-fNIRS BCIs (Ahn and Jun 2017; Buccino et al. 2016; Chiarelli et al. 2018; Ge et al. 2017; Hong et al. 2018a, b; Koo et al. 2015; Li et al. 2017; Noori et al. 2017; Shin et al. 2018; Yin et al. 2015b). While using both modalities offers higher accuracy results, these hybrid BCIs have longer setup times and require more data processing steps.

In this chapter, we will focus on fNIRS-based BCIs only and present an overview of challenges associated with data acquisition and data analysis in these BCIs and discuss approaches for improving their performance and efficiency.

1.1.2.1 Data Acquisition

The first step of data acquisition deals with selecting the right set of tasks to evoke brain activities. The most commonly used tasks in BCIs can be roughly classified into motor-related and cognitive tasks. Motor-related tasks include movement execution tasks such as finger tapping, hand squeezing, and knee extension, as well as motor imagery tasks, which involve mental imagination of moving different body parts without actual movements. Motor-related tasks are interesting in BCI applications, as various movement-related (e.g., different directions, different body parts, imagery vs actual movement) commands can be generated. Several studies in fNIRS-based BCIs have employed motor-related tasks for user's intention decoding (Batula et al. 2014, 2017; Erdoğan et al. 2019; Gemignani et al. 2018; Holper and Wolf 2011; Kabir et al. 2018; Nagaoka et al. 2010; Naseer and Hong 2013b; Nguyen et al. 2013; Noori et al. 2017; Peng et al. 2018; Rahman et al. 2019; Robinson et al. 2016; Seo et al. 2012; Shin and Jeong 2014; Stangl et al. 2013; Yin et al. 2015c; Zafar et al. 2019; Zhang et al. 2017). These tasks have also been utilized in BCI-based neurorehabilitation applications (Petracca et al. 2015; Rea et al. 2014a).

Another group of tasks commonly used in BCIs is cognitive tasks. These tasks include mental arithmetic tasks (e.g., mental subtraction, multiplication), (Abibullaev and An 2012; Abibullaev et al. 2011; Hennrich et al. 2015; Holper and Wolf 2011; Naseer et al. 2014, 2016a, b; Power et al. 2010, 2011, 2012; Schudlo et al. 2013; Yoo et al. 2018; Zafar and Hong 2017), mental counting (or backward counting) (Yoo et al. 2018; Zafar and Hong 2017), mental singing (or music imagery) (Chan et al. 2012; Power et al. 2010, 2011), word formation (or verbal fluency) (Abibullaev and An 2012; Abibullaev et al. 2011; Faress and Chau 2013; Hennrich et al. 2015; Schudlo and Chau 2015b), object rotation (Abibullaev and An 2012; Abibullaev et al. 2011; Hennrich et al. 2015), Stroop task (Ho et al. 2019a, b; Schudlo and Chau 2015b; Zafar et al. 2019), picture imagery (Naito et al. 2007), and puzzle solving (Yoo et al. 2018; Zafar and Hong 2017). The cognitive tasks have shown to be effective for some patients in locked-in state who are unable to perform motor-related tasks (Hong et al. 2018a, b).

In some BCI studies, both motor-related and cognitive tasks have been used to increase the number of commands (Hong et al. 2015; Hwang et al. 2014; Stangl et al. 2013).

Once the appropriate tasks are identified, locations for recording the hemodynamic response should be determined, to design the fNIRS probe. For example, for motor-related activities, the fNIRS channels are commonly placed over the motor cortex (Abtahi et al. 2017; Cui et al. 2010; Gemignani et al. 2018; Holper and Wolf 2011; Kabir et al. 2018; Naseer and Hong 2013b; Noori et al. 2017; Robinson et al. 2016; Seo et al. 2012; Shin and Jeong 2014; Yin et al. 2015c; Zafar et al. 2019; Zhang et al. 2017; Zimmermann et al. 2013), while for the cognitive tasks, these channels are generally located over the prefrontal cortex (Abibullaev and An 2012; Abibullaev et al. 2011; Bauernfeind et al. 2011; Chan et al. 2012; Dong and Jeong 2018a, b; Falk et al. 2010; Faress and Chau 2013; Hennrich et al. 2015; Ho et al. 2019a, b, Huang et al. 2018; Naseer et al. 2014, 2016a, b; Noori et al. 2016; Pathan et al. 2019; Power et al. 2010, 2011, 2012; Yoo et al. 2018). In (Schudlo and Chau 2015b), prefrontal and parietal cortices were used for collecting fNIRS data to study cognitive tasks. In studies that considered a combination of motor-related and cognitive tasks as their experimental paradigm, the channles were located at both motor and prefrontal cortices (Hong et al. 2015; Hwang et al. 2014; Stangl et al. 2013).

In some studies, for the classification of motor imagery/execution paradigms, fNIRS data has been recorded from the prefrontal area (Peng et al. 2018; Rahman et al. 2019, 2020). This selection was based on the idea that if in some patients, the motor cortex is damaged; classification of the motor-related tasks might not be possible using the signals recorded from the motor cortex. In this condition, the hemodynamic response from prefrontal cortex was investigated as a possible substitution due to its correlation with voluntary hand movements. Moreover, Wu et al. (2018) reported that the prefrontal cortex plays an important role in motor imagery tasks.

It should be noted that designing a proper channel configuration to cover the regions of interest is very important. Moreover, the source-detector distance is another factor which should be considered in determining the source-detector arrangements (Taga et al. 2007). In this work, we will study the effects of using the hemodynamic response from different brain regions on the classification of fNIRS signals corresponding to motor execution tasks.

1.1.2.2 Data Analysis

After acquiring fNIRS signals, the next step is to design a data processing algorithm to decode different classes of tasks. The data analysis usually starts with removing noise and artifacts from the recordings. Cleaned signals are then converted to $[\Delta HbO_2]$ and $[\Delta HbR]$, using the modified Beer-Lambert law and passed to the next processing step, which is feature extraction, in order to extract informative features which can discriminate various tasks. The final step is the classification algorithm which employs the extracted features to predict the user's intention. In what follows, we will discuss the challenges of each data analysis step in more details.

Pre-processing

The recorded raw signals usually contain noise and artifacts, which are not originated from brain activities and, therefore, need to be removed in order to provide clean and noise-free inputs for the classification problem. Depending on the sources of these unwanted signals, they can be categorized into physiological noise, motion artifacts, and instrumental noise.

In previous studies, various techniques based on adaptive filtering have been proposed for removing motion artifacts (Janani and Sasikala 2017). These techniques include principal component analysis (PCA) (Zhang et al. 2005), Wiener filtering (Izzetoglu et al. 2005), Kalman filtering (Dong and Jeong 2018a, b; Durantin et al. 2016; Izzetoglu et al. 2010), wavelet-based methods (Chiarelli et al. 2015; Molavi and Dumont 2012), and Savitzky-Golay filtering (Nguyen et al. 2013; Shin and Jeong 2014). Dynamic time warping-based averaging has also been proposed to improve the detection power in fNIRS recordings (Zhu and Najafizadeh 2017).

To remove physiological noise such as heartbeat, respiratory rate, and Mayer waves, band-pass filtering has been extensively used in previous studies (Abtahi et al. 2017; Erdoğan et al. 2019; Ho et al. 2019a, b; Hong et al. 2015; Hwang et al. 2014; Noori et al. 2016, 2017; Peng et al. 2018; Schudlo and Chau 2015a, b; Seo et al. 2012; Yoo et al. 2018; Zafar et al. 2019; Zafar and Hong 2017; Zhang et al. 2017). The other methods for removing the physiological noise include adaptive filtering (Kamran and Hong 2013, 2014), PCA (Zhang et al. 2005) and independent component analysis (ICA) (Bauernfeind et al. 2014; Santosa et al. 2013). Some studies employed short-distance fNIRS channels to measure the superficial responses which can be used to remove the scalp-hemodynamics (Gagnon et al. 2011, 2014; Sato et al. 2016; Zhang et al. 2009).

While pre-processing is a very important step in a BCI algorithm and can significantly affect the classification performance, the pre-processing algorithms that are computationally extensive are not generally suitable for real-time BCI applications.

Feature Extraction

Selecting a proper set of features which provide discriminatory information among different tasks is crucial for achieving accurate classification performance. Various time- and frequency-domain features have been employed in fNIRS-based BCIs.

Time-domain features include signal *mean* (Dong and Jeong 2018a, b; Erdoğan et al. 2019; Holper and Wolf 2011; Hong et al. 2015, 2017; Huang et al. 2018; Hwang et al. 2014; Kabir et al. 2018; Khan and Hong 2015; Naseer and Hong 2013b; Naseer et al. 2014, 2016b; Noori et al. 2016, 2017; Peng et al. 2018; Rahman et al. 2019; Robinson et al. 2016; Shin and Jeong 2014; Zafar et al. 2019; Zafar and Hong 2017; Zhang et al. 2017), *max* (*peak*) (Erdoğan et al. 2019; Hong et al. 2017; Huang et al. 2018; Khan and Hong 2015; Naseer et al. 2016b; Noori et al. 2017; Rahman et al. 2019; Zafar et al. 2019), *slope* (Erdoğan et al. 2019; Faress and Chau 2013; Hong et al. 2015; Huang et al. 2018; Kabir et al. 2018; Khan and Hong 2015; Noori et al. 2016, 2017; Naseer et al. 2016a, b; Power et al. 2012; Rahman et al. 2019; Schudlo and Chau 2015a, b; Schudlo et al. 2013; Shin and Jeong 2014; Zafar and Hong 2017; Zhang et al. 2009), *variance* (Holper and Wolf 2011; Huang et al. 2018; Kabir et al. 2018; Noori et al. 2016, 2017; Naseer et al. 2016b; Rahman et al. 2019; Shin and Jeong 2014; Zafar and Hong 2017; Zhang et al. 2017), *skewness* (Erdoğan et al. 2019; Holper and Wolf 2011; Hong et al. 2017; Khan and Hong 2015; Noori et al. 2016, 2017; Naseer et al. 2016b; Zafar and Hong 2017), *kurtosis* (Erdoğan et al. 2019; Holper and Wolf 2011; Khan and Hong 2015; Noori et al. 2016, 2017; Naseer et al. 2016a, b; Zafar and Hong 2017), *min* (Huang et al. 2018; Zafar et al. 2019), and *number of peaks* (Khan and Hong 2015). In Naseer et al. (2016a), all possible two- and three-feature combinations of mean, slope, variance, max, skewness, and kurtosis were evaluated to find the best combination of features for fNIRS classification of mental arithmetic tasks. (Abibullaev and An 2012; Abibullaev et al. 2011; Koo et al. 2016; Pathan et al. 2019; Xu et al. 2011). Features based on fractality of fNRS recordings have also shown to carry discriminatory power (Zhu et al. 2020; Zhu and Najafizadeh 2016). Time-frequency-based features such as wavelet coefficients have also been employed in fNIRS-based BCI algorithms (Abibullaev and An 2012; Abibullaev et al. 2011; Koo et al. 2016; Pathan et al. 2019; Xu et al. 2011). Some studies have extracted the features directly from recorded light intensities rather than using the oxy and deoxy hemoglobin (Luu and Chau 2008; Power et al. 2010, 2011). Signal *mean* and *slope* are the most common features that were used in previous studies. Their results suggest that using a combination of features (e.g., the signal *mean* along with other time-domain features) leads to a better classification performance, compared to the case of using only one type of feature. However, it should be noted that extracting more features requires more computational effort which can negatively affect the speed of the BCI algorithms.

Besides selecting the type(s) of features, the other challenge in feature extraction is to determine the time intervals of the hemodynamic signals that will be used for feature extraction. Due to the natural delay in the hemodynamic response of the brain, time intervals with long durations are usually considered for feature extraction from fNIRS signals. However, while longer intervals may offer a better classification accuracy, it also results in longer required time to generate control commands and, hence, reduce the speed and the practicality of BCIs. Therefore, an algorithm that can decode fNIRS signals with high accuracy using the data acquired over a shorter interval is desirable. Most of the previous studies considered a time interval of 10 s or more for extracting features (Abibullaev and An 2012; Abibullaev et al. 2011; Erdoğan et al. 2019; Falk et al. 2010; Faress and Chau 2013; Gemignani et al. 2018; Hennrich et al. 2015; Hong et al. 2017; Huang et al. 2018; Hwang et al. 2014; Naseer et al. 2014, 2016a, b; Pathan et al. 2019; Peng et al. 2018; Power et al. 2010, 2011; Schudlo et al. 2013; Seo et al. 2012; Yin et al. 2015a, c; Zhang et al. 2017; Zimmermann et al. 2013). Some other studies used shorter intervals of 5–10 s (Cui et al. 2010; Hong et al. 2015; Kabir et al. 2018; Naseer and Hong 2013b; Nguyen et al. 2013; Power et al. 2012; Rahman et al. 2019). However, the duration of 5–10 s is still considered to be long for real-time implementation of a BCI algorithm. Recently, Zafar et al. 2019; Zafar et al. (2017) proposed a method for fNIRS classification of three mental tasks using the initial dip of the hemodynamic response, showing that it significantly improves the speed of the fNIRS-based BCIs. Time domain features of mean, max, slope, skewness, and kurtosis were extracted from time intervals of [0–2.5] and [2–7] s, and the classification accuracy results from these two intervals were compared. The classification accuracy using the [2–7] s interval was about 10% higher than the [0–2.5] s interval. However, considering the [0–2.5] s interval offers the potential of improving the speed of the BCI system for real-time applications.

Classification

In BCI applications, the prediction of user's intentions from their neural signals with high accuracy is very crucial to ensure their safety. Additionally, any differentiable task (e.g., motor-related or cognitive) can be used as a unique command to control the external device. It is known that the discrimination of multiple tasks is more challenging than differentiation among two tasks. However, in BCI applications, differentiation of more tasks results in generating a greater number of commands that can be used to control external devices. To this date, majority of the previous studies have focused on binary classification problems (Bauernfeind et al. 2011; Chan et al. 2012; Cui et al. 2010; Dong and Jeong 2018a, b; Erdoğan et al. 2019; Falk et al. 2010; Faress and Chau 2013; Gemignani et al. 2018; Hennrich et al. 2015; Huang et al. 2018; Hwang et al. 2014; Kabir et al. 2018; Naseer and Hong 2013a; Naseer et al. 2014, 2016a; Noori et al. 2016; Nguyen et al. 2013; Pathan et al. 2019; Power et al. 2010, 2011, 2012; Rahman et al. 2019; Robinson et al. 2016; Schudlo and Chau 2015a; Shin and Jeong 2014; Stangl et al. 2013; Yin et al. 2015c; Zafar et al. 2019; Zhang et al. 2017; Zimmermann et al. 2013). There are a few works which considered multi-class classification of fNIRS signals corresponding to motor-related (Holper and Wolf 2011; Peng et al. 2018; Shin and Jeong 2014; Yin et al. 2015a), cognitive (Abibullaev and An 2012; Abibullaev et al. 2011; Schudlo and Chau 2015b; Yoo et al. 2018; Zafar and Hong 2017), or both tasks (Hong et al. 2015).

Several classifier models have been employed in classification of fNIRS signals. Linear discriminant analysis (LDA) (Abibullaev and An 2012; Bauernfeind et al. 2011; Faress and Chau 2013; Gemignani et al. 2018; Holper and Wolf 2011; Hong et al. 2015; Hwang et al. 2014; Kabir et al. 2018; Naseer and Hong 2013b; Naseer et al. 2014; Noori et al. 2016; Power et al. 2011, 2012; Rahman et al. 2019; Schudlo and Chau 2015a, b; Stangl et al. 2013; Zafar and Hong 2017; Zhang et al. 2017) and support vector machine (SVM) (Abibullaev and An 2012; Cui et al. 2010; Dong and Jeong 2018a, b; Erdoğan et al. 2019; Huang et al. 2018; Naseer et al. 2014; Nguyen et al. 2013; Pathan et al. 2019; Peng et al. 2018; Robinson et al. 2016; Yin et al. 2015c; Zhu et al. 2020) are commonly used classifier models in fNIRS-based BCIs due to their simplicity and good classification performance. Other classifier models that have been used include hidden Markov model (HMM) (Chan et al. 2012; Falk et al. 2010; Power et al. 2010; Zimmermann et al. 2013), artificial neural network (ANN) (Abibullaev and An 2012; Abibullaev et al. 2011; Chan et al. 2012; Erdoğan et al. 2019; Naseer et al. 2016a, b; Nguyen et al. 2013), random forest (RF) (Erdoğan et al. 2019), Naïve Bayes (Shin and Jeong 2014), extreme learning machine (ELM) (Yin et al. 2015a), Deep Neural Network (Hennrich et al. 2015), and long-short-term memory (LSTM) (Yoo et al. 2018; Zafar et al. 2019). Among the abovementioned classification algorithms, LDA, SVM, and ANN are the most commonly used methods that have outperformed other methods in terms of the average classification accuracy.

1.1.3 Objective

In order to implement a BCI system that is practical and efficient, a multi-class classification algorithm which offers a high classification accuracy using features extracted from a short time interval is of great interest. Considering the challenges involved in different steps of data acquisition and analysis in fNIRS-based BCIs and the results of the previous studies, in this work, we aim to study the multi-class classification of motor execution tasks. Moreover, we will explore the effects of various parameter selections on the performance of the BCI algorithm including:

- Location of channels from which the fNIRS signals are recorded
- Duration of the interval used for extracting features as well as its delay from the stimulus onset
- Different types of time-domain features
- Different classification models

1.2 Experiments

1.2.1 Participants

Five healthy and right-handed subjects including three males and two females, aged between 19 and 35 participated in the experiment. All participants had no history of neurologic, psychiatric, and mental disorders. All participants had normal or corrected-to-normal vision. Written informed consents approved by the Rutgers' Institutional Review Board (IRB) were obtained prior to the experiments.

1.2.2 fNIRS Recording

NIRx System (NIRScout, NIRx Medical Technologies, LLC) was used to record hemodynamic responses at a sampling rate of 7.81 Hz and using two wavelengths of near infrared lights (760 and 830 nm). A customized fNIRS cap was designed using 16 sources and 24 detectors, which were placed over the prefrontal, motor, parietal, and occipital cortices (see Fig. 1.1). Considering the source-detector separation of 3 cm, a total of 54 fNIRS measurement channels were formed. It has been shown that a source-detector separation of 3 cm ensures that the photons reach the cortex. Moreover, source-detector separation of higher than 5 cm results in weak signals (Taga et al. 2007). Figure 1.2a–d shows the source-detector arrangements over the prefrontal, motor, parietal, and occipital regions.

1.2.3 Experimental Protocol

Experiments were conducted in the neuroimaging laboratory located in the Department of Electrical and Computer Engineering at Rutgers University. Subjects were asked to sit in a comfortable chair facing a 21.5-inch monitor positioned at a distance of 70 cm. A joystick was placed in front of them so they could move it with their

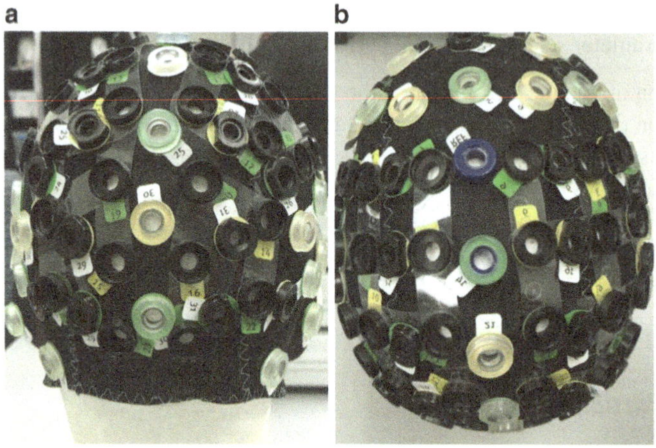

Fig. 1.1 Customized cap designed for fNIRS recordings from (**a**) back and (**b**) top views

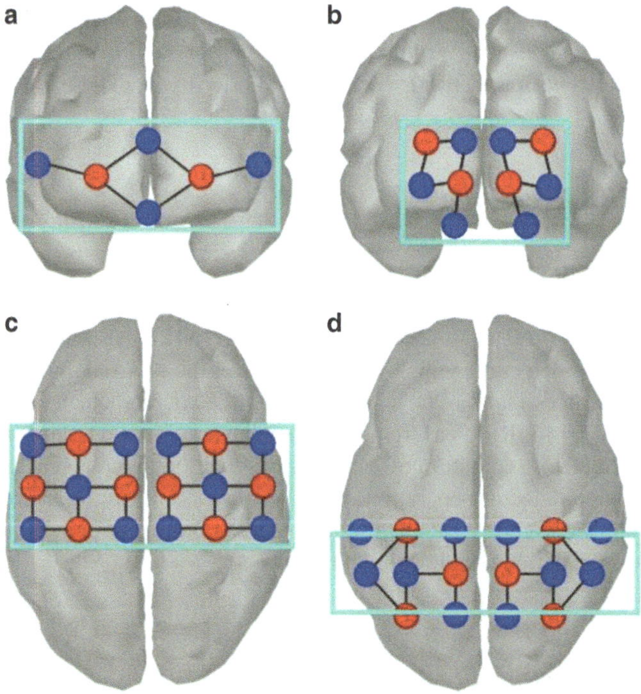

Fig. 1.2 Channel configuration for placement of the probe on (**a**) prefrontal, (**b**) occipital, (**c**) motor, and (**d**) parietal regions

right hand (see Fig. 1.3). The experiment consisted of three blocks. Each block started with 10 s of initial rest. Two types of tasks were considered:

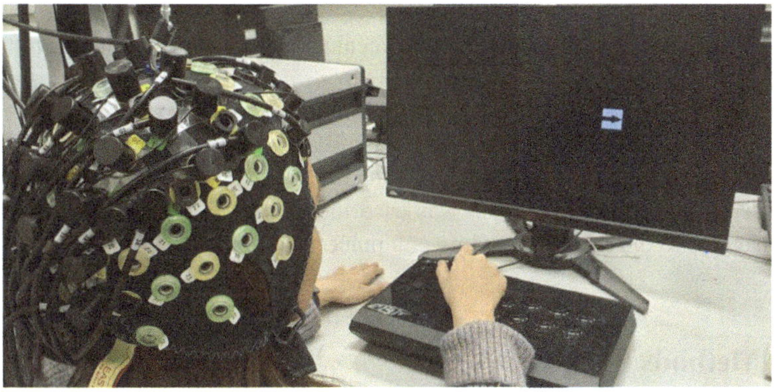

Fig. 1.3 Experimental setup

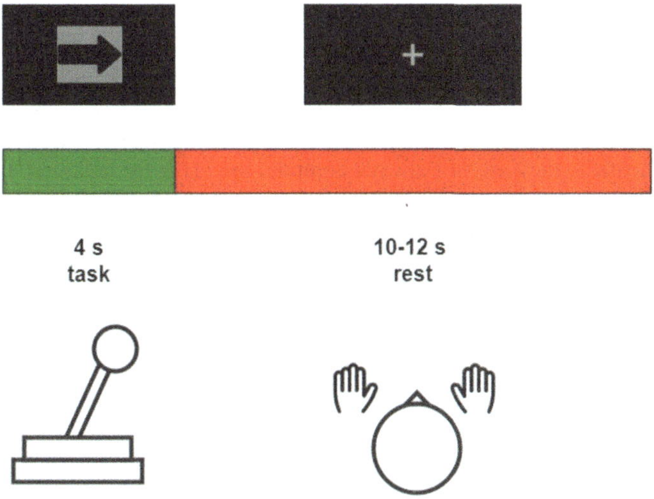

Fig. 1.4 Visual illustration of a single trial

- Dictated motor execution tasks: if a symbol with an arrow inside the square is displayed, subjects had to move the square from the center of the screen towards one of four (up, down, left, and right) directions using the joystick,
- Non-movement task: the subjects were asked do nothing (center) if there was a circle inside the square.

During each block, the subjects performed 75 randomly ordered trials which included 5 classes (4 motor-execution and 1 non-movement) of tasks. Each trial consisted of 4 s post-stimulus motor execution interval followed by a rest interval between 10 and 12 s during which a fixation cross was displayed. The subjects were asked to avoid any body movement during the rest interval. The schematic of the experimental paradigm is shown in Fig. 1.4. The green blocks indicate the motor execution task period, and the red blocks show the inter-trial rest period. In each block, 15 trials of each class (directions/center) were performed by each subject resulting in 45 trials for each class in total.

Prior to the recordings, the participants completed a short training block consisting of five trials of each class to become familiar with the tasks. The total time of the experiment was up to 70 min considering the average rest time of 5 min between the experiment blocks. E-prime 3 was used to display the cues, send the stimulus onset triggers to the fNIRS recording computer, and monitor the joystick responses.

1.3 Methods

1.3.1 *Pre-processing*

fNIRS recordings from the [-1,12] s interval, where 0 is the time of motor execution stimulus onset, were selected from each trial. We tried to minimize the pre-processing steps performed on the raw fNIRS signals. Although noise and artifact removals are important steps in preparing the acquired signals for feature extraction and classification, they are not always computationally affordable in practical and real-time BCI applications. Therefore, in this work, we only performed the basic band-pass filtering with [0.01–0.2] Hz pass band, to remove the cardiac signal and low-frequency oscillations.

After filtering, the modified Beer-Lambert law was utilized to convert the filtered optical intensity data into changes in the concentration of oxy and deoxy hemoglobin ([ΔHbO_2] and [ΔHbR]) (Ardeshirpour et al. 2013; Qureshi et al. 2017; Zhu and Najafizadeh 2017):

$$\begin{bmatrix} \Delta HbO_2 \\ \Delta HbR \end{bmatrix} = \frac{1}{l \times d} \begin{bmatrix} \alpha_{HbO_2}(\lambda_1) & \alpha_{HbR}(\lambda_1) \\ \alpha_{HbO_2}(\lambda_2) & \alpha_{HbR}(\lambda_2) \end{bmatrix}^{-1} \begin{bmatrix} \Delta A(t, \lambda_1) \\ \Delta A(t, \lambda_2) \end{bmatrix}$$

where l is the distance between the source and detector (in mm), d is the differential path length factor, $\Delta A(t, \lambda_i)(i = 1, 2)$ is the optical density variation of the light emitted of wavelength λ_i (in $\mu M^{-1} mm^{-1}$), and $\alpha_{HbO_2}(\lambda_i)$ and $\alpha_{HbR}(\lambda_i)$ are the extinction coefficients of oxy and deoxy hemoglobin, respectively.

Here, we used ([ΔHbO_2] signal for our classification problem, as it generally has a higher SNR as compared to [ΔHbR]. For the baseline correction, the baseline was considered as the mean of the signal from the [−1,0] interval, and it was subtracted from the post-stimulus data ([0–12] s). This baseline-corrected data was then passed to the feature extraction algorithm.

1.3.2 Feature Extraction

Various features were extracted from different time intervals. For each interval, the data was segmented into 1-s windows with 50% overlap. Features extracted from these segments for a specific set of channels formed the feature vectors. For example, if 24 motor channels were considered for classification, the size of feature vectors was 24 × 1.

Time-domain features including "mean," "max," "slope," "variance," "skewness," and "kurtosis" were extracted to evaluate their ability in discriminating motor execution tasks. These features were calculated as follows:

- Mean:

$$\mu\ (X_i) = \frac{1}{N}\sum_{j=1}^{N} X_i(j)$$

- Max (peak):

$$\max\ (X_i) = \max_j \{X_i(j)\}$$

- Slope:

$$\text{slope}\ (X_i) = \frac{X_i(N) - X_i(1)}{W}$$

- Variance:

$$\sigma\,(X_i) = \frac{1}{N-1}\sum_{j=1}^{N} (X_i(j) - \mu)^2$$

- Skewness:

$$\text{sk}\ (X_i) = \frac{1}{N-1}\sum_{j=1}^{N} \left(\frac{X_i(j) - \mu}{\sigma}\right)^3$$

- Kurtosis:

$$\text{kur}\ (X_i) = \frac{1}{N-1}\sum_{j=1}^{N} \left(\frac{X_i(j) - \mu}{\sigma}\right)^4$$

where X_i is the [ΔHbO_2] signal obtained from the ith channel, N is the number of samples in the segment from which the features are being extracted, and W is the duration of the segment. For a selected time interval, these features were calculated for a specific set of channels and put in a vector to form the feature vectors. In the case of using multiple brain regions for feature extraction, the feature vectors from channels over the corresponding regions were concatenated into a vector. Extracted features were passed to the classifier for training and testing steps.

These time-domain features were employed due to their simplicity as well as their effectiveness in fNIRS classification problems in previous studies. Predefined MATLAB functions were used to calculate these features.

1.3.3 Classification

Two well-established classification algorithms, SVM and ANN, were employed for classification, and the accuracy results were compared. Implementation of these algorithms are summarized as follows:

Support vector machine (SVM): SVM is a well-known supervised classifier which has been widely used in classification of fNIRS recordings. The SVM classifier with an appropriate kernel function determines the hyperplanes that maximize the distance between the training data points of classes. In this work, we used an SVM classifier with a second-degree polynomial kernel function, which is also called quadratic SVM (QSVM).

Artificial neural network (ANN): ANN is another commonly used classification algorithm considered in fNIRS classification studies. ANN consists of multiple layers including the input layer, hidden layer (s), and the output layer. To achieve a proper ANN classification algorithm, various parameters should be tuned such as the number of hidden layers, the number of neurons in each layer, the training function, the learning rate, and the number of epochs. To implement the ANN classifier, we employed MATLAB deep learning toolbox. The ANN classifier here consisted of 2 fully connected hidden layers with 20 neurons each and an output layer with 5 neurons (see Fig. 1.5). The Levenberg-Marquardt optimization was used as the network training function.

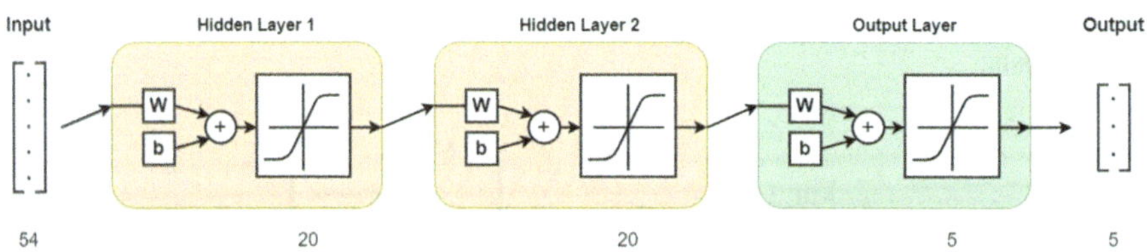

Fig. 1.5 Neural network architecture

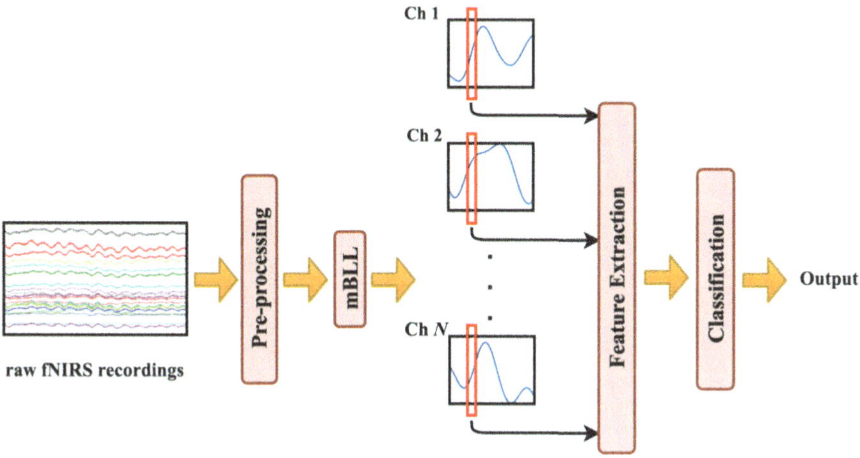

Fig. 1.6 Overview of the data classification steps

For implementing both of the classification algorithms, for each subject, the extracted features from all trials were separated into two randomized groups for training and validation (75%), and testing (25%). A fivefold cross-validation was considered for both classifiers. Note that the classification problem in this study is subject-specific.

An overview of various data analysis steps to predict different tasks from raw fNIRS recordings is illustrated in Fig. 1.6.

1.4 Results and Discussions

Classification was performed under various conditions to investigate the effects of different parameters on the classification accuracy.

To study the effects of the interval duration from which the features were extracted, six intervals with lengths of 2, 4, 6, 8, 10, and 12 s, from the stimulus onset, were considered. We first considered the "mean" of [ΔHbO_2] from these intervals as the feature and considered data from all channels. The classification accuracy results using QSVM for 5 classes (the movement directions of up, down, left, right, and the non-movement) are presented in Table 1.1 for all subjects. The results of the average classification accuracy for 2, 4, 6, 8, 10, and 12 s intervals are 71.49%, 82.06%, 84.48%, 85.48%, 86.41%, and 87.24%, respectively. These results indicate that increasing the length of the interval from which the features are extracted improves the classification accuracy. By comparing the classification accuracy results from consecutive intervals, it can be seen that by increasing the interval length from 2 to 4 s, the accuracy is increased by 10–14% across subjects. However, as the interval duration is increased to 6 s, the accuracy results were

Table 1.1 Classification accuracy results for movement directions of "up," "down," "left," "right," and non-movement, (total of 5 classes), using features extracted from different duration of post-stimulus intervals

	Time window (s)					
	0–2	0–4	0–6	0–8	0–10	0–12
Subject 1	70.22 ± 3.75	80.50 ± 2.21	82.73 ± 1.83	84.14 ± 1.34	85.13 ± 1.18	85.54 ± 1.10
Subject 2	73.69 ± 3.67	83.71 ± 2.07	85.58 ± 1.55	87.30 ± 1.22	88.28 ± 1.06	89.06 ± 1.01
Subject 3	69.47 ± 3.76	79.52 ± 2.12	81.67 ± 1.72	82.53 ± 1.40	82.79 ± 1.21	84.04 ± 1.13
Subject 4	75.73 ± 3.92	84.25 ± 2.11	86.58 ± 1.24	87.25 ± 1.14	88.15 ± 1.15	89.03 ± 0.71
Subject 5	68.34 ± 4.59	82.31 ± 2.37	85.83 ± 1.63	86.17 ± 1.27	87.72 ± 1.29	88.51 ± 1.04
Average	71.49 ± 4.81	82.06 ± 2.83	84.48 ± 2.50	85.48 ± 2.26	86.41 ± 2.44	**87.24 ± 2.29**

For all cases, the features are the "mean" of [ΔHbO_2] from all channels and the classifier is QSVM. The results indicate that by increasing the length of the time window used for feature extraction, the classification accuracy increases. Although the highest average accuracy is achieved from the longest time window ([0–12] s), comparing this accuracy with the average accuracy from [0–6] s window, shows that by doubling the duration of the time window for extracting features, the average accuracy only increases by around 3%. The accuracy improvement is most significant (10% or more) when the duration is increased from [0–2] to [0–4] s

Table 1.2 Classification accuracy results for movement directions of "up," "down," "left," "right," and non-movement, (total of 5 classes), using features extracted from different windows of post-stimulus intervals

	Time window (s)		
	0–2	1–3	2–4
Subject 1	70.22 ± 3.75	76.68 ± 3.40	78.87 ± 3.65
Subject 2	73.69 ± 3.67	80.14 ± 3.48	80.89 ± 3.56
Subject 3	69.47 ± 3.76	72.96 ± 3.91	75.84 ± 4.11
Subject 4	75.73 ± 3.92	81.07 ± 4.51	81.47 ± 3.69
Subject 5	68.34 ± 4.59	74.47 ± 3.69	76.38 ± 4.01
Average	71.49 ± 4.81	77.06 ± 4.92	**78.69 ± 4.42**

For all cases, the features are the "mean" of [ΔHbO_2] from all channels and the classifier is QSVM. The results show that the highest average accuracy is obtained from the [2–4] s interval, which is more delayed from the stimulus onset, compared to the other two intervals. One explanation is that due to the natural delay in the hemodynamic response of the brain, the features extracted from delayed intervals from the stimulus onset provide more discriminatory information for the classification problem

improved only by 2–3%. After 6 s, adding 2 s to the interval length enhanced the accuracy by 1%. These results reveal that although the 12 s interval offers the highest accuracy, the accuracy improvement from 4 to 12 s intervals is only 5% (on average). In other words, by tripling the duration of the interval for feature extraction, the average classification accuracy increases from 82.06% to 87.24%. Therefore, in order to avoid the extra processing effort, it seems more reasonable to use the shorter interval of [0–4] s, which still offers a reasonably high accuracy for the five-class classification problem.

To further investigate the effect of interval selection for feature extraction on the classification results, we divided the [0–4] s interval into three 2-s intervals ([0–2], [1–3], and [2–4] s) to evaluate which part of this interval is more informative in terms of discriminating different classes. For this analysis, the "mean" of the [ΔHbO_2] signal from all channels and the QSVM were considered as features and classifier, respectively. The classification accuracy results are summarized in Table 1.2. The results show that the highest average classification accuracy is achieved form the [2–4] s interval (78.69%), and it is 6–8% higher than the result for the [0–2] s interval (71.49%). This might be due to the natural delay in the hemodynamic response of the brain, which makes the data extracted from later intervals more informative for the classification problem. Given these results, for the rest of the analysis here, we considered the [2–4] s window as the fixed time interval for feature extraction.

After selecting the time window for feature extraction, we investigated the effects of channel locations on the classification results. As discussed earlier, most existing fNIRS studies on classification of movement execution/imagery tasks have used signals recorded over the motor and/or prefrontal cortices. Here, we designed an fNIRS customized cap such that the parts of motor, prefrontal, parietal, and occipital cortices are covered. To evaluate the significance of including fNIRS data from

Table 1.3 Classification accuracy results for movement directions of "up," "down," "left," "right," and non-movement, (total of 5 classes), using features extracted from different channel locations

	Channel locations				
	Prefrontal	Motor	Parietal	Occipital	All channels
Subject 1	35.67 ± 2.96	65.90 ± 3.38	53.90 ± 2.85	44.59 ± 3.49	78.87 ± 3.65
Subject 2	37.32 ± 3.64	68.12 ± 3.47	58.47 ± 3.39	52.21 ± 3.39	80.89 ± 3.56
Subject 3	39.27 ± 3.58	63.47 ± 3.72	56.41 ± 3.94	49.48 ± 4.11	75.84 ± 4.11
Subject 4	35.88 ± 3.77	69.61 ± 3.79	54.81 ± 3.66	47.70 ± 3.76	81.47 ± 3.69
Subject 5	34.77 ± 3.03	64.40 ± 4.30	58.01 ± 3.06	46.88 ± 3.38	76.38 ± 4.01
Average	36.58 ± 3.73	66.30 ± 4.36	56.32 ± 3.81	48.17 ± 4.43	**78.69 ± 4.42**

For all cases, the features are the "mean" of [ΔHbO_2] from [2–4] s post-stimulus interval and the classifier is QSVM. The results indicate that the highest classification accuracy is achieved when features extracted from all the recording channels (placed on prefrontal, motor, parietal, and occipital cortices) are included, which suggests the significance of considering the hemodynamic response from different brain regions rather than just using the data from one specific area (e.g., motor cortex for movement-related tasks)

different locations on the classification accuracy, classification was performed using recordings obtained from different locations and compared to the case were the data from all channels were used. The "mean" of [ΔHbO_2] from the [2–4] s interval was used as the feature. The classification accuracy results are presented in Table 1.3. The highest average classification accuracy when using data from channels placed in one region is achieved from the motor cortex region (66.30%). This is expected, since we are studying the problem of classification of motor-related tasks. For parietal, prefrontal, and occipital cortices, an average accuracy of 56.32%, 36.58%, and 48.17% is obtained, respectively. Interestingly, when the data from all channels were considered, the classification accuracy is significantly increased (78.69%). These observations suggest the data from brain regions other than the motor cortex contain discriminatory information for motor-related tasks. One possible explanation for this finding is that various brain regions are involved in the planning and performing of motor execution tasks (Hanakawa et al. 2008; Kim et al. 2018).

Up to this point, only the "mean" of [ΔHbO_2] was used as feature. We also calculated other time-domain features (max, slope, variance, skewness, and kurtosis) of [ΔHbO_2] from the [2–4] s interval for all channels. The classification performance was evaluated for each choice, and results are given in Table 1.4. As can be seen, the highest classification accuracy is achieved when "mean" (78.69%) and "max" (77.46%) are used as features. Using the "slope" and "variance" of the signal as the feature, the classification accuracy drops to 63.78% and 47.39%, respectively. The classification accuracy results for the "skewness" and "kurtosis" features are 39.44% and 25.61% (the chance level is 20%), respectively. These results for "skewness" and "kurtosis" could have been possibly improved if longer intervals were used for feature extraction. Considering these findings, it can be concluded that for the selected interval, both "mean" and "max" features offer

Table 1.4 Classification accuracy results for movement directions of "up," "down," "left," "right," and non-movement, (a total of 5 classes), using different features

	Time-domain features					
	Mean	Max	Slope	Variance	Skewness	Kurtosis
Subject 1	78.87 $\pm$ 3.65	77.48 $\pm$ 3.86	61.81 $\pm$ 4.25	45.71 $\pm$ 4.06	35.18 $\pm$ 3.26	24.96 $\pm$ 3.17
Subject 2	80.89 $\pm$ 3.56	78.97 $\pm$ 3.59	64.98 $\pm$ 3.60	45.78 $\pm$ 3.21	36.74 $\pm$ 3.57	23.72 $\pm$ 2.71
Subject 3	75.84 $\pm$ 4.11	75.51 $\pm$ 4.01	62.33 $\pm$ 3.66	47.32 $\pm$ 3.63	43.66 $\pm$ 3.28	26.86 $\pm$ 2.58
Subject 4	81.47 $\pm$ 3.69	79.48 $\pm$ 3.19	69.79 $\pm$ 3.31	51.28 $\pm$ 3.65	42.58 $\pm$ 3.80	26.20 $\pm$ 2.67
Subject 5	76.38 $\pm$ 4.01	75.84 $\pm$ 4.00	59.98 $\pm$ 4.07	46.88 $\pm$ 3.81	39.03 $\pm$ 2.91	26.29 $\pm$ 2.84
Average	**78.69** $\pm$ **4.42**	77.46 $\pm$ 4.05	63.78 $\pm$ 5.08	47.39 $\pm$ 4.19	39.44 $\pm$ 4.68	25.61 $\pm$ 3.00

For all cases, the features are extracted from [2–4] s post-stimulus interval, and from all channels, and the classifier is QSVM. Comparing the classification accuracy results using different time-domain features shows that the "mean" and "max" features provide the most discriminatory information across various tasks, whereas the "kurtosis" and "skewness" features result in lowest classification accuracy

Table 1.5 Classification accuracy results for movement directions of "up," "down," "left," "right," and non-movement, (total of 5 classes), using different classifiers

	Classifier type	
	Q-SVM	ANN
Subject 1	78.87 ± 3.65	86.02 ± 4.06
Subject 2	80.89 ± 3.56	86.56 ± 3.28
Subject 3	75.84 ± 4.11	82.36 ± 4.31
Subject 4	81.47 ± 3.69	89.00 ± 3.81
Subject 5	76.38 ± 4.01	82.57 ± 4.56
Average	78.69 ± 4.42	**85.30 ± 4.73**

For all cases, the features are the "mean" of [ΔHbO_2] from the [2–4] s post-stimulus interval from all channels. The classification results show that the ANN algorithm outperforms the QSVM classifier and is a better choice for this classification problem

higher classification accuracies comparing to the other features. For most subjects, the classification accuracy using "mean" is 1–2% higher than using "max" features.

Finally, to study the effects of the classifier model, we compared the classification accuracy results using QSVM with an ANN classifier. The results are presented in Table 1.5. It can be seen that when ANN is used as the classifier, the accuracy is improved by 6–7% across subjects. These results suggest that the ANN offers a higher classification accuracy (85.30%) than QSVM classifier and is a better choice for this multi-class classification problem. The confusion matrices for each subject are depicted in Figs. 1.7 and 1.8 shows the confusion matrix for all subjects.

It is worth mentioning that although in this study the ANN classifier outperformed the QSVM in terms of the classification accuracy, the ANN classification algorithm requires more computational effort compared to QSVM.

The goal of this study was to discriminate multiple movement execution tasks from fNIRS recordings. Using the presented BCI algorithm, we successfully differentiated five classes including four classes of movement execution and one non-movement class. Moreover, we evaluated the effects of changing various parameters related to feature extraction and classification algorithms on the accuracy of decoding the movement execution tasks. The results of our study revealed that by increasing the length of the window from which the features are extracted, the classification accuracy increases. Specifically, by lengthening the time window from [0–2] s to [0–4] s, the classification accuracy increases significantly. However, for time intervals longer than 4 s, the accuracy slightly improves. Interestingly, the classification results revealed that including data from all regions leads to the highest accuracy when classifying motor tasks. Furthermore, the classification accuracy achieved by considering the "mean" of [ΔHbO_2] as the feature was higher compared to the cases where other time domain features were used. These results can be employed for parameter selection in classification of fNIRS recordings.

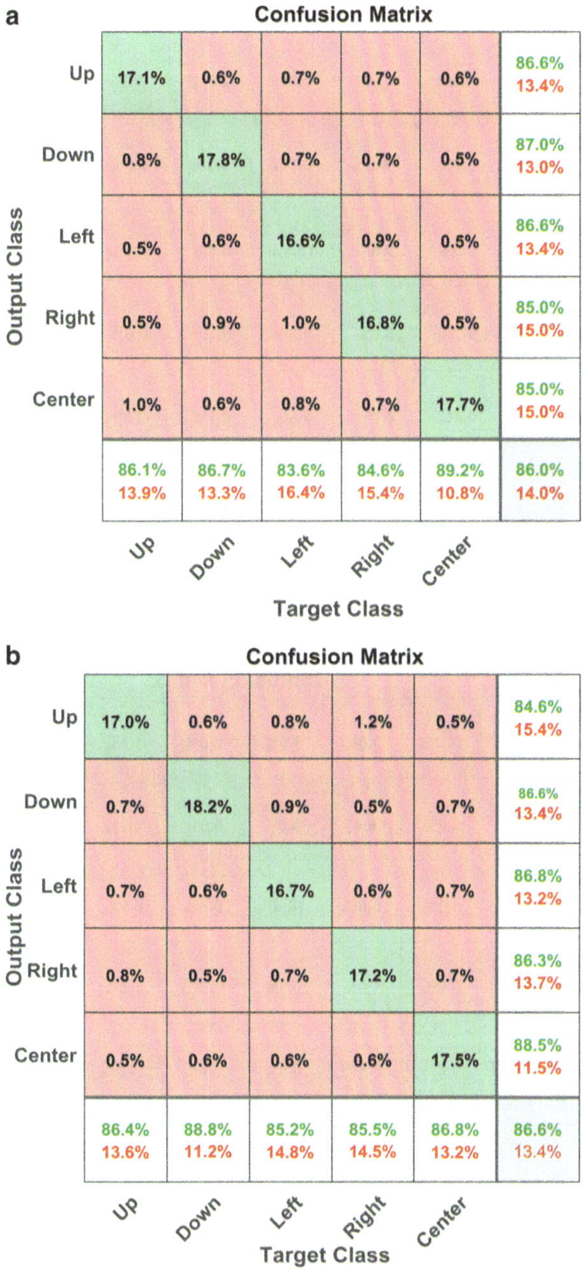

Fig. 1.7 (**a**)–(**e**). Confusion matrix of classification results for subjects 1–5 using the "mean" of the [ΔHbO_2] as feature extracted from the [2–4] s interval and considering all channels. ANN was used as the classifier

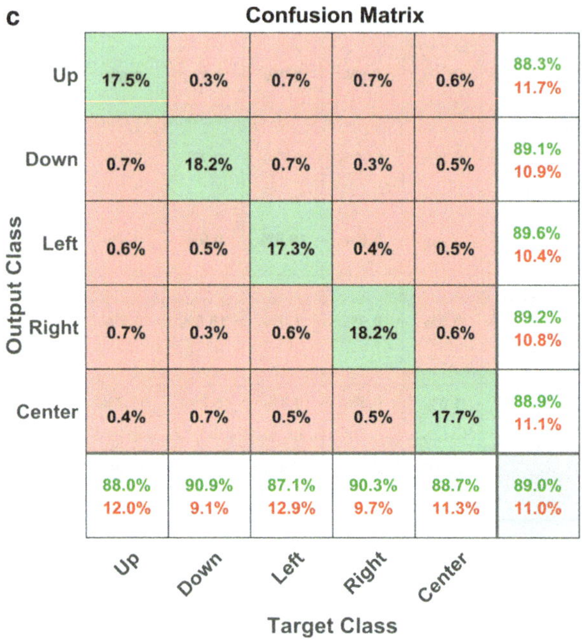

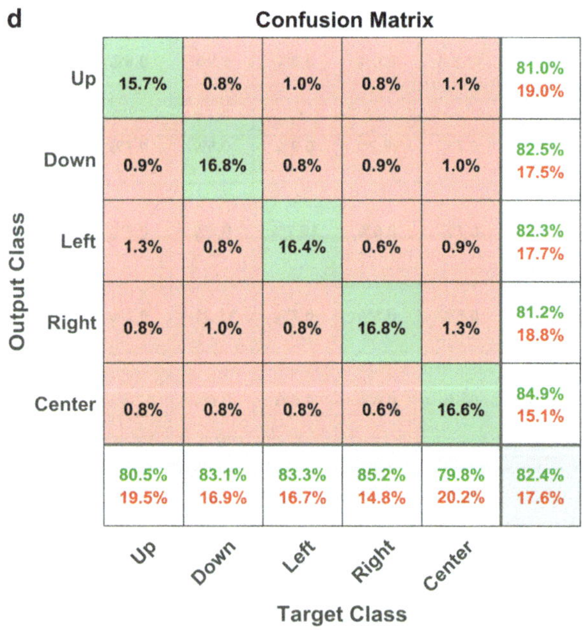

Fig. 1.7 (continued)

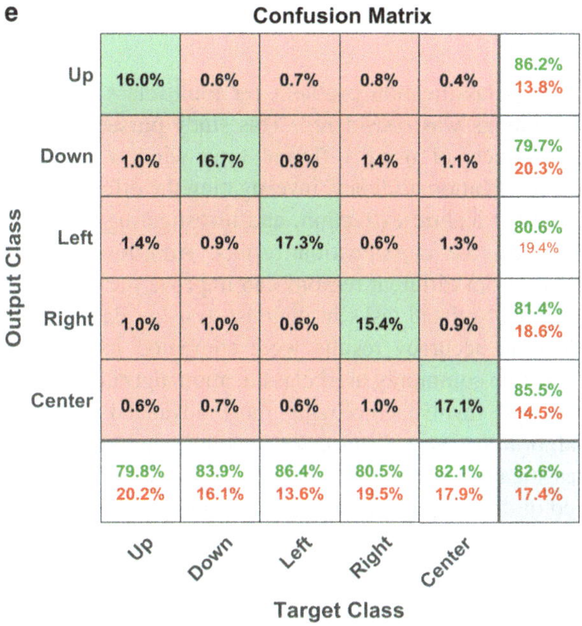

Fig. 1.7 (continued)

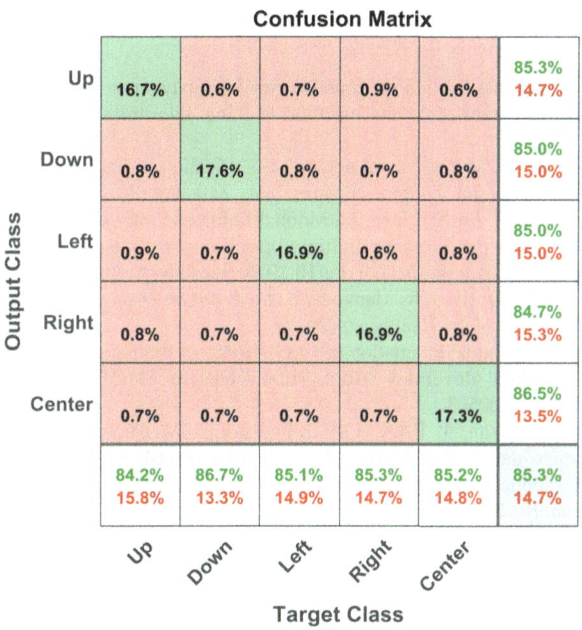

Fig. 1.8 Confusion matrix of classification results for all subjects using the "mean" of the [ΔHbO_2] as feature extracted from the [2–4] s interval and considering all channels. ANN was used as the classifier

1.5 Conclusions

In this chapter, the classification problem for multi-class motor execution tasks using fNIRS recordings was considered. This study pursued the following goals: investigating the effects of using different time window lengths for extracting features on the classification accuracy, investigating the effects of the latency of the time interval used for feature extraction, and investigating the effects of different channel locations on the classification results. Additionally, it was examined whether using data from different regions can improve the results of classification of different movement-related tasks in contrast to using data only from the motor cortex. Classification accuracy results were computed for various time-domain features as well as two commonly used classification algorithms of SVM and ANN.

Future works will involve employing more advanced feature extraction and classification algorithms as well as using feature selection methods in order to improve the classification performance in terms of accuracy, required computational effort, and speed of the BCI algorithm.

Acknowledgments This work is supported by NSF award 1841087. The authors thank Ali Haddad and Jennifer Huang for their help in experimental design and data collection.

References

B. Abibullaev, J. An, Classification of frontal cortex haemodynamic responses during cognitive tasks using wavelet transforms and machine learning algorithms. Med. Eng. Phys. **34**(10), 1394–1410 (2012)

B. Abibullaev, J. An, J.-I. Moon, Neural network classification of brain hemodynamic responses from four mental tasks. Int. J. Optomechatron. **5**(4), 340–359 (2011)

B. Abibullaev, J. An, S.-H. Jin, S.H. Lee, J.I. Moon, Minimizing inter-subject variability in fNIRS-based brain–computer interfaces via multiple-kernel support vector learning. Med. Eng. Phys. **35**(12), 1811–1818 (2013). https://doi.org/10.1016/j.medengphy.2013.08.009

M. Abtahi, A.M. Amiri, D. Byrd, K. Mankodiya, *Hand Motion Detection in fNIRS Neuroimaging Data,* Paper presented at the Healthcare (2017)

S. Ahn, S.C. Jun, Multi-modal integration of EEG-fNIRS for brain-computer interfaces – current limitations and future directions. Front. Hum. Neurosci. **11**(503) (2017). https://doi.org/10.3389/fnhum.2017.00503

F. Amyot, T. Zimmermann, J. Riley, J.M. Kainerstorfer, V. Chernomordik, E. Mooshagian, et al., Normative database of judgment of complexity task with functional near infrared spectroscopy—application for TBI. NeuroImage **60**(2), 879–883 (2012)

K.K. Ang, C. Guan, *Brain-Computer Interface in Stroke Rehabilitation* (2013)

Y. Ardeshirpour, A.H. Gandjbakhche, L. Najafizadeh, Biophotonics techniques for structural and functional imaging, in vivo. Stud. Health Technol. Inform. **185**, 265–297 (2013)

R.N. Aslin, M. Shukla, L.L. Emberson, Hemodynamic correlates of cognition in human infants. Ann. Rev. Psychol. **66**, 349–379 (2015)

S.Y. Baik, J.-Y. Kim, J. Choi, J.Y. Baek, Y. Park, Y. Kim, et al., Prefrontal asymmetry during cognitive tasks and its relationship with suicide ideation in major depressive disorder: An fNIRS study. Diagnostics **9**(4), 193 (2019)

M. Bamdad, H. Zarshenas, M.A. Auais, Application of BCI systems in neurorehabilitation: A scoping review. Disabil. Rehabil. Assist. Technol. **10**(5), 355–364 (2015). https://doi.org/10.3109/17483107.2014.961569

A.M. Batula, H. Ayaz, Y.E. Kim, Evaluating a four-class motor-imagery-based optical brain-computer interface, in *Paper presented at the 2014 36th Annual International Conference of the IEEE Engineering in Medicine and Biology Society* (2014)

A.M. Batula, J.A. Mark, Y.E. Kim, H. Ayaz, Comparison of brain activation during motor imagery and motor movement using fNIRS. Comput. Intell. Neurosci. **2017** (2017)

G. Bauernfeind, R. Scherer, G. Pfurtscheller, C. Neuper, Single-trial classification of antagonistic oxyhemoglobin responses during mental arithmetic. Med. Biol. Eng. Comput. **49**(9), 979 (2011)

G. Bauernfeind, S. Wriessnegger, I. Daly, G. Müller-Putz, Separating heart and brain: On the reduction of physiological noise from multichannel functional near-infrared spectroscopy (fNIRS) signals. J. Neural Eng. **11**(5), 056010 (2014)

A.P. Buccino, H.O. Keles, A. Omurtag, Hybrid EEG-fNIRS asynchronous brain-computer Interface for multiple motor tasks. PLoS One **11**(1), e0146610–e0146610 (2016). https://doi.org/10.1371/journal.pone.0146610

J. Cao, B. Khan, N. Hervey, F. Tian, M.R. Delgado, N.J. Clegg, et al., Evaluation of cortical plasticity in children with cerebral palsy undergoing constraint-induced movement therapy based on functional near-infrared spectroscopy. J. Biomed. Optic **20**(4), 046009 (2015)

J. Chan, S. Power, T. Chau, Investigating the need for modelling temporal dependencies in a brain-computer interface with real-time feedback based on near infrared spectra. J. Near Infrared Spectrosc. **20**(1), 107–116 (2012)

A.M. Chiarelli, E.L. Maclin, M. Fabiani, G. Gratton, A kurtosis-based wavelet algorithm for motion artifact correction of fNIRS data. NeuroImage **112**, 128–137 (2015)

A.M. Chiarelli, P. Croce, A. Merla, F. Zappasodi, Deep learning for hybrid EEG-fNIRS brain–computer interface: Application to motor imagery classification. J. Neural Eng. **15**(3), 036028 (2018)

X. Cui, S. Bray, A.L. Reiss, Speeded near infrared spectroscopy (NIRS) response detection. PLoS One **5**(11) (2010)

S. Dong, J. Jeong, Noise reduction in fNIRS data using extended Kalman filter combined with short separation measurement, in *Paper presented at the 2018 6th international conference on brain-computer Interface (BCI)* (2018a, January 15–17)

S. Dong, J. Jeong, Onset classification in hemodynamic signals measured during three working memory tasks using wireless functional near-infrared spectroscopy. IEEE J. Select. Topic. Quant. Electron. **25**(1), 1–11 (2018b)

G. Durantin, S. Scannella, T. Gateau, A. Delorme, F. Dehais, Processing functional near infrared spectroscopy signal with a Kalman filter to assess working memory during simulated flight. Front. Hum. Neurosci. **9**, 707 (2016)

A.C. Ehlis, B. Barth, J. Hudak, H. Storchak, L. Weber, A.C.S. Kimmig, et al., Near-infrared spectroscopy as a new tool for neurofeedback training. Appl. Psychiatr. Methodolog. Consider. **60**(4), 225–241 (2018)

S.B. Erdoğan, E. Özsarfati, B. Dilek, K.S. Kadak, L. Hanoğlu, A. Akin, Classification of motor imagery and execution signals with population-level feature sets: Implications for probe design in fNIRS based BCI. J. Neural Eng (2019)

T.H. Falk, M. Guirgis, S. Power, T.T. Chau, Taking NIRS-BCIs outside the lab: Towards achieving robustness against environment noise. IEEE Trans. Neural Syst. Rehabil. Eng. **19**(2), 136–146 (2010)

A. Faress, T. Chau, Towards a multimodal brain–computer interface: Combining fNIRS and fTCD measurements to enable higher classification accuracy. NeuroImage **77**, 186–194 (2013)

M. Ferrari, V. Quaresima, A brief review on the history of human functional near-infrared spectroscopy (fNIRS) development and fields of application. NeuroImage **63**(2), 921–935 (2012)

L. Gagnon, K. Perdue, D.N. Greve, D. Goldenholz, G. Kaskhedikar, D.A. Boas, Improved recovery of the hemodynamic response in diffuse optical imaging using short optode separations and state-space modeling. NeuroImage **56**(3), 1362–1371 (2011)

L. Gagnon, M.A. Yücel, D.A. Boas, R.J. Cooper, Further improvement in reducing superficial contamination in NIRS using double short separation measurements. NeuroImage **85**, 127–135 (2014)

P. Gajbhiye, R.K. Tripathy, A. Bhattacharyya, R.B. Pachori, Novel approaches for the removal of motion Artifact from EEG recordings. IEEE Sensors J. **19**(22), 10600–10608 (2019). https://doi.org/10.1109/JSEN.2019.2931727

S. Ge, Q. Yang, R. Wang, P. Lin, J. Gao, Y. Leng, et al., A brain-computer interface based on a few-channel EEG-fNIRS bimodal system. IEEE Access **5**, 208–218 (2017). https://doi.org/10.1109/ACCESS.2016.2637409

J. Gemignani, E. Middell, R.L. Barbour, H.L. Graber, B. Blankertz, Improving the analysis of near-infrared spectroscopy data with multivariate classification of hemodynamic patterns: A theoretical formulation and validation. J. Neural Eng. **15**(4), 045001 (2018)

M.A. Gramlich, S.M. Neer, D.C. Beidel, C.J. Bohil, C.A. Bowers, A functional near-infrared spectroscopy study of trauma-related auditory and olfactory cues: Posttraumatic stress disorder or combat experience? *Dissertation***30**(6), 656–665 (2017)

Y. Gu, S. Miao, J. Han, K. Zeng, G. Ouyang, J. Yang, X.J. Li, Complexity analysis of fNIRS signals in ADHD children during working memory task. Sci. Rep. **7**(1), 1–10 (2017)

Y. Gu, S. Miao, J. Han, Z. Liang, G. Ouyang, J. Yang, X.J. Li, Identifying ADHD children using hemodynamic responses during a working memory task measured by functional near-infrared spectroscopy. J. Neur. Eng. **15**(3), 035005 (2018)

T. Hanakawa, M.A. Dimyan, M. Hallett, Motor planning, imagery, and execution in the distributed motor network: A time-course study with functional MRI. Cereb. Cortex **18**(12), 2775–2788 (2008)

M. Hatakenaka, I. Miyai, M. Mihara, S. Sakoda, K.J.N. Kubota, Frontal regions involved in learning of motor skill—A functional NIRS study. **34**(1), 109–116 (2007)

M. Hatakenaka, I. Miyai, M. Mihara, H. Yagura, N.J.N. Hattori, Impaired motor learning by a pursuit rotor test reduces functional outcomes during rehabilitation of poststroke ataxia. Neurorehabilit. Neu. Repair **26**(3), 293–300 (2012)

J. Hennrich, C. Herff, D. Heger, T. Schultz, Investigating deep learning for fNIRS based BCI, in *Paper Presented at the 2015 37th Annual International Conference of the IEEE Engineering in Medicine and Biology Society (EMBC)* (2015)

C. Herff, D. Heger, F. Putze, J. Hennrich, O. Fortmann, T. Schultz, Classification of mental tasks in the prefrontal cortex using fNIRS, in *Paper Presented at the 2013 35th Annual International Conference of the IEEE Engineering in Medicine and Biology Society (EMBC)* (2013, July 3–7)

T.K.K. Ho, J. Gwak, C.M. Park, A. Khare, J.-I. Song, Deep leaning-based approach for mental workload discrimination from multi-channel fNIRS, in *Recent Trends in Communication, Computing, and Electronics*, (Springer, 2019a), pp. 431–440

T.K.K. Ho, J. Gwak, C.M. Park, J.-I. Song, Discrimination of mental workload levels from multi-channel fNIRS using deep leaning-based approaches. IEEE Access **7**, 24392–24403 (2019b)

L. Holper, M. Wolf, Single-trial classification of motor imagery differing in task complexity: A functional near-infrared spectroscopy study. J. Neuroeng. Rehabil. **8**(1), 34 (2011)

K.-S. Hong, N. Naseer, Y.-H. Kim, Classification of prefrontal and motor cortex signals for three-class fNIRS–BCI. Neurosci. Lett. **587**, 87–92 (2015)

K.-S. Hong, M.R. Bhutta, X. Liu, Y.-I. Shin, Classification of somatosensory cortex activities using fNIRS. Behav. Brain Res. **333**, 225–234 (2017)

K.-S. Hong, M.J. Khan, M.J. Hong, Feature extraction and classification methods for hybrid fNIRS-EEG brain-computer interfaces. Front. Hum. Neurosci. **12**(246) (2018a). https://doi.org/10.3389/fnhum.2018.00246

K.-S. Hong, M.J. Khan, M.J. Hong, Feature extraction and classification methods for hybrid fNIRS-EEG brain-computer interfaces. Front. Hum. Neurosci. **12**, 246 (2018b)

F. Hosomi, M. Yanagi, Y. Kawakubo, N. Tsujii, S. Ozaki, O. Shirakawa, Capturing spontaneous activity in the medial prefrontal cortex using near-infrared spectroscopy and its application to schizophrenia. Sci. Rep. **9**(1), 5283 (2019). https://doi.org/10.1038/s41598-019-41739-4

R. Huang, E. Kavichai, K.-S. Hong, Comparison of Kernels in online SVM classification of fNIRS data, in *Paper Presented at the 2018 18th International Conference on Control, Automation and Systems (ICCAS)* (2018)

H.-J. Hwang, J.-H. Lim, D.-W. Kim, C.-H. Im, Evaluation of various mental task combinations for near-infrared spectroscopy-based brain-computer interfaces. J. Biomed. Opt. **19**(7), 077005 (2014)

M. Izzetoglu, A. Devaraj, S. Bunce, B. Onaral, Motion artifact cancellation in NIR spectroscopy using wiener filtering. IEEE Trans. Biomed. Eng. **52**(5), 934–938 (2005)

M. Izzetoglu, P. Chitrapu, S. Bunce, B. Onaral, Motion artifact cancellation in NIR spectroscopy using discrete Kalman filtering. Biomed. Eng. Online **9**(1), 16 (2010)

A. Janani, M. Sasikala, Investigation of different approaches for noise reduction in functional near-infrared spectroscopy signals for brain–computer interface applications. Neural Comput. Applic. **28**(10), 2889–2903 (2017)

A. Janani, M. Sasikala, Classification of fNIRS signals for decoding right- and left-arm movement execution using SVM for BCI applications, in *Paper Presented at the Computational Signal Processing and Analysis, Singapore* (2018)

M.F. Kabir, S.M.R. Islam, M.A. Rahman, Accuracy improvement of fNIRS based motor imagery movement classification by standardized common spatial pattern, in *Paper Presented at the 2018 4th International Conference on Electrical Engineering and Information & Communication Technology (iCEEiCT)* (2018)

M.A. Kamran, K.-S. Hong, Linear parameter-varying model and adaptive filtering technique for detecting neuronal activities: An fNIRS study. J. Neural Eng. **10**(5), 056002 (2013)

M.A. Kamran, K.-S. Hong, Reduction of physiological effects in fNIRS waveforms for efficient brain-state decoding. Neurosci. Lett. **580**, 130–136 (2014)

H. Kato, M. Izumiyama, H. Koizumi, A. Takahashi, Y.J.S. Itoyama, Near-infrared spectroscopic topography as a tool to monitor motor reorganization after hemiparetic stroke: A comparison with functional MRI. Stroke J. Am. Heart Assoc **33**(8), 2032–2036 (2002)

M.J. Khan, K.-S. Hong, Passive BCI based on drowsiness detection: An fNIRS study. Biomed. Opt. Express **6**(10), 4063–4078 (2015)

Y.K. Kim, E. Park, A. Lee, C.-H. Im, Y.-H. Kim, Changes in network connectivity during motor imagery and execution. PLoS One **13**(1) (2018)

K.L.M. Koenraadt, E.G.J. Roelofsen, J. Duysens, N.L.W. Keijsers, Cortical control of normal gait and precision stepping: An fNIRS study. NeuroImage **85**, 415–422 (2014). https://doi.org/10.1016/j.neuroimage.2013.04.070

B. Koo, H.-G. Lee, Y. Nam, H. Kang, C.S. Koh, H.-C. Shin, S. Choi, A hybrid NIRS-EEG system for self-paced brain computer interface with online motor imagery. J. Neurosci. Method **244**, 26–32 (2015). https://doi.org/10.1016/j.jneumeth.2014.04.016

B. Koo, H. Vu, H. Lee, H. Shin, S. Choi, Motor imagery detection with wavelet analysis for NIRS-based BCI, in *Paper Presented at the 2016 4th International Winter Conference on Brain-Computer Interface (BCI)* (2016, February 22–24)

C.Q. Lai, H. Ibrahim, M.Z. Abdullah, J.M. Abdullah, S.A. Suandi, A. Azman, Artifacts and noise removal for electroencephalogram (EEG): A literature review, in *Paper Presented at the 2018 IEEE Symposium on Computer Applications & Industrial Electronics (ISCAIE)* (2018, April 28–29)

P. Lapborisuth, X. Zhang, A. Noah, J.J.N. Hirsch, Neurofeedback-based functional near-infrared spectroscopy upregulates motor cortex activity in imagined motor tasks. Neurophotonics **4**(2), 021107 (2017)

R. Li, T. Potter, W. Huang, Y. Zhang, Enhancing performance of a hybrid EEG-fNIRS system using channel selection and early temporal features. Front. Hum. Neurosci. **11**(462) (2017). https://doi.org/10.3389/fnhum.2017.00462

T. Liu, X. Liu, L. Yi, C. Zhu, P.S. Markey, M. Pelowski, Assessing autism at its social and developmental roots: A review of autism spectrum disorder studies using functional near-infrared spectroscopy. NeuroImage **185**, 955–967 (2019)

F. Lotte, L. Bougrain, A. Cichocki, M. Clerc, M. Congedo, A. Rakotomamonjy, F. Yger, A review of classification algorithms for EEG-based brain–computer interfaces: A 10 year update. J. Neural Eng. **15**(3), 031005 (2018)

S. Luu, T. Chau, Decoding subjective preference from single-trial near-infrared spectroscopy signals. J. Neural Eng. **6**(1), 016003 (2008)

J.R. Mahoney, R. Holtzer, M. Izzetoglu, V. Zemon, J. Verghese, G.J. Allali, The role of prefrontal cortex during postural control in Parkinsonian syndromes a functional near-infrared spectroscopy study. Brain Res **1633**, 126–138 (2016)

I. Maidan, H. Bernad-Elazari, E. Gazit, N. Giladi, J.M. Hausdorff, A.J. Mirelman, Changes in oxygenated hemoglobin link freezing of gait to frontal activation in patients with Parkinson disease: an fNIRS study of transient motor-cognitive failures. J. Neurol **262**(4), 899–908 (2015)

A.-M. Marx, A.-C. Ehlis, A. Furdea, M. Holtmann, T. Banaschewski, D. Brandeis, et al., Near-infrared spectroscopy (NIRS) neurofeedback as a treatment for children with attention deficit hyperactivity disorder (ADHD)—A pilot study. Front. Human Neurosci **8**, 1038 (2015)

A. Mazzoni, R. Grove, V. Eapen, R.K. Lenroot, J.J. Bruggemann, The promise of functional near-infrared spectroscopy in autism research: What do we know and where do we go? Soc. Neurosci **14**(5), 505–518 (2019)

D. McFarland, J. Wolpaw, EEG-based brain–computer interfaces. Curr. Opinion Biomed. Eng **4**, 194–200 (2017)

M. Mihara, I.J.N. Miyai, Review of functional near-infrared spectroscopy in neurorehabilitation. Neurophotonics **3**(3), 031414 (2016)

M. Mihara, N. Hattori, M. Hatakenaka, H. Yagura, T. Kawano, T. Hino, I.J.S. Miyai, Near-infrared spectroscopy–mediated neurofeedback enhances efficacy of motor imagery–based training in poststroke victims: A pilot study. Stroke **44**(4), 1091–1098 (2013)

J. Minguillon, M.A. Lopez-Gordo, F. Pelayo, Trends in EEG-BCI for daily-life: Requirements for artifact removal. Biomed. Signal Process. Control **31**, 407–418 (2017). https://doi.org/10.1016/j.bspc.2016.09.005

B. Molavi, G.A. Dumont, Wavelet-based motion artifact removal for functional near-infrared spectroscopy. Physiol. Meas. **33**(2), 259 (2012)

T. Nagaoka, K. Sakatani, T. Awano, N. Yokose, T. Hoshino, Y. Murata, et al., Development of a new rehabilitation system based on a brain-computer interface using near-infrared spectroscopy, in *Oxygen Transport to Tissue XXXI* (Springer, 2010), pp. 497–503

M. Naito, Y. Michioka, K. Ozawa, Y. Ito, M. Kiguchi, T. Kanazawa, A communication means for totally locked-in ALS patients based on changes in cerebral blood volume measured with near-infrared light. IEICE Trans. Inf. Syst. **90**(7), 1028–1037 (2007)

N. Naseer, K.-S. Hong, Classification of functional near-infrared spectroscopy signals corresponding to the right- and left-wrist motor imagery for development of a brain–computer interface. Neurosci. Lett **553**, 84–89 (2013a). https://doi.org/10.1016/j.neulet.2013.08.021

N. Naseer, K.-S. Hong, Classification of functional near-infrared spectroscopy signals corresponding to the right-and left-wrist motor imagery for development of a brain–computer interface. Neurosci. Lett. **553**, 84–89 (2013b)

N. Naseer, K.-S. Hong, Functional near-infrared spectroscopy based discrimination of mental counting and no-control state for development of a brain-computer interface, in *Paper Presented at the 2013 35th Annual International Conference of the IEEE Engineering in Medicine and Biology Society (EMBC)* (2013c, July 3–7)

N. Naseer, K.-S. Hong, fNIRS-based brain-computer interfaces: A review. Front. Hum. Neurosci. **9**(3) (2015a). https://doi.org/10.3389/fnhum.2015.00003

N. Naseer, K.-S. Hong, fNIRS-based brain-computer interfaces: A review. Front. Hum. Neurosci **9**, 3 (2015b)

N. Naseer, M.J. Hong, K.-S. Hong, Online binary decision decoding using functional near-infrared spectroscopy for the development of brain–computer interface. Exp. Brain Res. **232**(2), 555–564 (2014)

N. Naseer, F.M. Noori, N.K. Qureshi, K.-S. Hong, Determining optimal feature-combination for LDA classification of functional near-infrared spectroscopy signals in brain-computer interface application. Front. Hum. Neurosci. **10**, 237 (2016a)

N. Naseer, N.K. Qureshi, F.M. Noori, K.-S. Hong, Analysis of different classification techniques for two-class functional near-infrared spectroscopy-based brain-computer interface. Comput. Intell. Neurosci, 2016 (2016b)

H.T. Nguyen, C.Q. Ngo, K. Truong Quang Dang, V.T. Vo, Temporal hemodynamic classification of two hands tapping using functional near—infrared spectroscopy. Front. Hum. Neurosci. **7**, 516 (2013)

L.F. Nicolas-Alonso, J. Gomez-Gil, Brain computer interfaces, a review. Sensors **12**(2), 1211–1279 (2012)

Y. Nishizawa, T. Kanazawa, Y. Kawabata, T. Matsubara, S. Maruyama, M. Kawano, et al., fNIRS assessment during an emotional stroop task among patients with depression: Replication and extension. Psychiatr. Invest. **16**(1), 80–86 (2019). https://doi.org/10.30773/pi.2018.11.12.2

F.M. Noori, N.K. Qureshi, R.A. Khan, N. Naseer, Feature selection based on modified genetic algorithm for optimization of functional near-infrared spectroscopy (fNIRS) signals for BCI, in *Paper Presented at the 2016 2nd International Conference on Robotics and Artificial Intelligence (ICRAI)* (2016, November 1–2)

F.M. Noori, N. Naseer, N.K. Qureshi, H. Nazeer, R.A. Khan, Optimal feature selection from fNIRS signals using genetic algorithms for BCI. Neurosci. Lett. **647**, 61–66 (2017)

N.S. Pathan, M. Foysal, M.M. Alam, Efficient mental arithmetic task classification using wavelet domain statistical features and SVM classifier, in *Paper Presented at the 2019 International Conference on Electrical, Computer and Communication Engineering (ECCE)* (2019)

M. Peifer, L. Zhu, L. Najafizadeh, Real-time classification of actual vs imagery finger tapping using fNIRS, in *Paper Presented at the Biomedical Optics* (2014)

H. Peng, J. Chao, S. Wang, J. Dang, F. Jiang, B. Hu, D. Majoe, Single-trial classification of fNIRS signals in four directions motor imagery tasks measured from prefrontal cortex. IEEE Trans. Nanobioscience **17**(3), 181–190 (2018)

D. Perpetuini, R. Bucco, M. Zito, A. Merla, Study of memory deficit in Alzheimer's disease by means of complexity analysis of fNIRS signal. Neurophotonics **5**(1), 011010 (2017)

A. Petracca, M. Carrieri, D. Avola, S.B. Moro, S. Brigadoi, S. Lancia, et al, A virtual ball task driven by forearm movements for neuro-rehabilitation, in *Paper Presented at the 2015 International Conference on Virtual Rehabilitation (ICVR)* (2015, June 9–12)

S.D. Power, T.H. Falk, T. Chau, Classification of prefrontal activity due to mental arithmetic and music imagery using hidden Markov models and frequency domain near-infrared spectroscopy. J. Neural Eng. **7**(2), 026002 (2010)

S.D. Power, A. Kushki, T. Chau, Towards a system-paced near-infrared spectroscopy brain–computer interface: Differentiating prefrontal activity due to mental arithmetic and mental singing from the no-control state. J. Neural Eng. **8**(6), 066004 (2011)

S.D. Power, A. Kushki, T. Chau, Intersession consistency of single-trial classification of the prefrontal response to mental arithmetic and the no-control state by NIRS. PLoS One **7**(7) (2012)

N.K. Qureshi, N. Naseer, F.M. Noori, H. Nazeer, R.A. Khan, S. Saleem, Enhancing classification performance of functional near-infrared spectroscopy-brain–computer Interface using adaptive estimation of general linear model coefficients. Front. Neurorobot. **11**, 33 (2017)

M.A. Rahman, F. Khanam, M. Ahmad, Detection of effective temporal window for classification of motor imagery events from prefrontal hemodynamics, in *Paper Presented at the 2019 International Conference on Electrical, Computer and Communication Engineering (ECCE)* (2019)

M.A. Rahman, M.M. Haque, A. Anjum, M.N. Mollah, M. Ahmad, Classification of motor imagery events from prefrontal hemodynamics for BCI application, in *Paper Presented at the Proceedings of International Joint Conference on Computational Intelligence* (2020)
M. Rea, M. Rana, N. Lugato, P. Terekhin, L. Gizzi, D. Brötz, et al., Lower limb movement preparation in chronic stroke: A pilot study toward an fNIRS-BCI for gait rehabilitation. Neurorehabil. Neural Repair **28**(6), 564–575 (2014a)
M. Rea, M. Rana, N. Lugato, P. Terekhin, L. Gizzi, D. Brötz, et al., Lower limb movement preparation in chronic stroke: a pilot study toward an fNIRS-BCI for gait rehabilitation. Neurorehabilit. Neur. Repair **28**(6), 564–575 (2014b)
N. Robinson, A.D. Zaidi, M. Rana, V.A. Prasad, C. Guan, N. Birbaumer, R. Sitaram, Real-time subject-independent pattern classification of overt and covert movements from fNIRS signals. PLoS One **11**(7) (2016)
D. Rosenbaum, A. Haipt, K. Fuhr, F.B. Haeussinger, F.G. Metzger, H.-C. Nuerk, et al., Aberrant functional connectivity in depression as an index of state and trait rumination. Sci. Rep. **7**(1), 2174–2174 (2017). https://doi.org/10.1038/s41598-017-02277-z
H. Santosa, M. Jiyoun Hong, S.-P. Kim, K.-S. Hong, Noise reduction in functional near-infrared spectroscopy signals by independent component analysis. Rev. Sci. Instrum. **84**(7), 073106 (2013)
T. Sato, I. Nambu, K. Takeda, T. Aihara, O. Yamashita, Y. Isogaya, et al., Reduction of global interference of scalp-hemodynamics in functional near-infrared spectroscopy using short distance probes. NeuroImage **141**, 120–132 (2016). https://doi.org/10.1016/j.neuroimage.2016.06.054
G. Schalk, E.C. Leuthardt, Brain-computer interfaces using electrocorticographic signals. IEEE Rev. Biomed. Eng. **4**, 140–154 (2011)
L.C. Schudlo, T. Chau, Single-trial classification of near-infrared spectroscopy signals arising from multiple cortical regions. Behav. Brain Res. **290**, 131–142 (2015a)
L.C. Schudlo, T. Chau, Towards a ternary NIRS-BCI: Single-trial classification of verbal fluency task, Stroop task and unconstrained rest. J. Neural Eng. **12**(6), 066008 (2015b)
L.C. Schudlo, S.D. Power, T. Chau, Dynamic topographical pattern classification of multichannel prefrontal NIRS signals. J. Neural Eng. **10**(4), 046018 (2013)
Y.-W. Seo, S.-D. Lee, D.-K. Koh, B.-M. Kim, Partial least squares-discriminant analysis for the prediction of hemodynamic changes using near infrared spectroscopy. J. Opt. Soc. Kor **16**(1), 57–62 (2012)
F. Shamsi, L. Najafizadeh, *Multi-class classification of motor execution tasks using fNIRS*, in *Paper presented at the 2019 IEEE Signal Processing in Medicine and Biology Symposium (SPMB)* (2019)
F. Shamsi, L. Najafizadeh, On the effects of pain on fNIRS classification, in *Paper presented at the Optics and the Brain* (2020)
J. Shin, C.-H. Im, Performance improvement of near-infrared spectroscopy-based brain-computer interface using regularized linear discriminant analysis ensemble classifier based on bootstrap aggregating. Front. Neurosci. **14**, 168 (2020)
J. Shin, J. Jeong, Multiclass classification of hemodynamic responses for performance improvement of functional near-infrared spectroscopy-based brain–computer interface. J. Biomed. Opt. **19**(6), 067009 (2014)
J. Shin, J. Kwon, C.-H. Im, A ternary hybrid EEG-NIRS brain-computer Interface for the classification of brain activation patterns during mental arithmetic, motor imagery, and idle state. Front. Neuroinform. **12**(5) (2018). https://doi.org/10.3389/fninf.2018.00005
B. Singh, H. Wagatsuma, A removal of eye movement and blink artifacts from EEG data using morphological component analysis. Comput. Math. Methods Med. **2017** (2017)
M. Soltanlou, M.A. Sitnikova, H.-C. Nuerk, T.J. Dresler, Applications of functional near-infrared spectroscopy (fNIRS) in studying cognitive development: The case of mathematics and language. Front. Psychol **9**, 277 (2018)
H. Song, L. Chen, R. Gao, I.I.M. Bogdan, J. Yang, S. Wang, Automatic schizophrenic discrimination on fNIRS by using complex brain network analysis and SVM. BMC Med. Inform. Dec. Making **17**(3), 166 (2017)

M. Stangl, G. Bauernfeind, J. Kurzmann, R. Scherer, C. Neuper, A haemodynamic brain–computer interface based on real-time classification of near infrared spectroscopy signals during motor imagery and mental arithmetic. J. Near Infrared Spectrosc. **21**(3), 157–171 (2013)

D. Steyrl, R.J. Kobler, G.R. Müller-Putz, On similarities and differences of invasive and non-invasive electrical brain signals in brain-computer interfacing. J. Biomed. Sci. Eng. **9**(08), 393 (2016)

G. Taga, F. Homae, H. Watanabe, Effects of source-detector distance of near infrared spectroscopy on the measurement of the cortical hemodynamic response in infants. NeuroImage **38**(3), 452–460 (2007)

H. Takakura, H. Nishijo, A. Ishikawa, H.J. Shojaku, Cerebral hemodynamic responses during dynamic posturography: Analysis with a multichannel near-infrared spectroscopy system. Front. Hum.Neurosci. **9**, 620 (2015)

K. Takeda, Y. Gomi, I. Imai, N. Shimoda, M. Hiwatari, H.J.N.R. Kato, Shift of motor activation areas during recovery from hemiparesis after cerebral infarction: A longitudinal study with near-infrared spectroscopy. Neurosci. Res. **59**(2), 136–144 (2007)

F. Tian, A. Yennu, A. Smith-Osborne, F. Gonzalez-Lima, C.S. North, H. Liu, Prefrontal responses to digit span memory phases in patients with post-traumatic stress disorder (PTSD): A functional near infrared spectroscopy study. NeuroImage. Clin. **4**, 808–819 (2014). https://doi.org/10.1016/j.nicl.2014.05.005

S. Waldert, Invasive vs. non-invasive neuronal signals for brain-machine interfaces: Will one prevail? Front. Neurosci. **10**, 295 (2016)

S. Wu, J. Li, L. Gao, C. Chen, S. He, Suppressing systemic interference in fNIRS monitoring of the hemodynamic cortical response to motor execution and imagery. Front. Hum. Neurosci. **12**, 85 (2018)

B. Xu, Y. Fu, L. Miao, Z. Wang, H. Li, Classification of fNIRS data using wavelets and support vector machine during speed and force imagination, in *Paper Presented at the 2011 IEEE International Conference on Robotics and Biomimetics* (2011, December 7–11

A. Yennu, F. Tian, A. Smith-Osborne, R.J. Gatchel, F.L. Woon, H. Liu, Prefrontal responses to Stroop tasks in subjects with post-traumatic stress disorder assessed by functional near infrared spectroscopy. Sci. Rep. **6**(1), 30157 (2016). https://doi.org/10.1038/srep30157

X. Yin, B. Xu, C. Jiang, Y. Fu, Z. Wang, H. Li, G. Shi, Classification of hemodynamic responses associated with force and speed imagery for a brain-computer Interface. J. Med. Syst. **39**(5), 53 (2015a). https://doi.org/10.1007/s10916-015-0236-0

X. Yin, B. Xu, C. Jiang, Y. Fu, Z. Wang, H. Li, G. Shi, A hybrid BCI based on EEG and fNIRS signals improves the performance of decoding motor imagery of both force and speed of hand clenching. J. Neural Eng. **12**(3), 036004 (2015b)

X. Yin, B. Xu, C. Jiang, Y. Fu, Z. Wang, H. Li, G. Shi, NIRS-based classification of clench force and speed motor imagery with the use of empirical mode decomposition for BCI. Med. Eng. Phys. **37**(3), 280–286 (2015c). https://doi.org/10.1016/j.medengphy.2015.01.005

S.-H. Yoo, S.-W. Woo, Z. Amad, Classification of three categories from prefrontal cortex using LSTM networks: fNIRS study, in *Paper Presented at the 2018 18th International Conference on Control, Automation and Systems (ICCAS)* (2018)

A. Zafar, K.-S. Hong, Detection and classification of three-class initial dips from prefrontal cortex. Biomed. Opt. Express **8**(1), 367–383 (2017)

A. Zafar, U. Ghafoor, M. Yaqub, K.-S. Hong, Initial-dip-based classification for fNIRS-BCI. in *Paper Presented at the Neural Imaging and Sensing 2019* (2019)

P.V. Zephaniah, J.G. Kim, Recent functional near infrared spectroscopy based brain computer interface systems: Developments, applications and challenges. Biomed. Eng. Lett. **4**(3), 223–230 (2014). https://doi.org/10.1007/s13534-014-0156-9

F. Zhang, H.J. Roeyers, Exploring brain functions in autism spectrum disorder: A systematic review on functional near-infrared spectroscopy (fNIRS) studies. Int. J. Psychophysiol **137**, 41–53 (2019)

Y. Zhang, D.H. Brooks, M.A. Franceschini, D.A. Boas, Eigenvector-based spatial filtering for reduction of physiological interference in diffuse optical imaging. J. Biomed. Opt. **10**(1), 011014 (2005)

Q. Zhang, G.E. Strangman, G. Ganis, Adaptive filtering to reduce global interference in non-invasive NIRS measures of brain activation: How well and when does it work? NeuroImage **45**(3), 788–794 (2009)

S. Zhang, Y. Zheng, D. Wang, L. Wang, J. Ma, J. Zhang, et al., Application of a common spatial pattern-based algorithm for an fNIRS-based motor imagery brain-computer interface. Neurosci. Lett. **655**, 35–40 (2017)

L. Zhu, L. Najafizadeh, Temporal dynamics of fNIRS-recorded signals revealed via visibility graph, in *Paper Presented at the Cancer Imaging and Therapy* (2016)

L. Zhu, L. Najafizadeh, Dynamic time warping-based averaging framework for functional near-infrared spectroscopy brain imaging studies. J. Biomed. Opt. **22**(6), 066011 (2017)

L. Zhu, S. Haghani, L. Najafizadeh, On fractality of functional near-infrared spectroscopy signals: Analysis and applications. Neurophotonics **7**(2), 025001 (2020)

R. Zimmermann, L. Marchal-Crespo, J. Edelmann, O. Lambercy, M.-C. Fluet, R. Riener, et al., Detection of motor execution using a hybrid fNIRS-biosignal BCI: A feasibility study. J. Neuroeng. Rehabil. **10**(1), 4 (2013)

Chapter 2
A Comparative Study of End-To-End Discriminative Deep Learning Models for Knee Joint Kinematic Time Series Classification

M. Abid, Y. Ouakrim, A. Mitiche, P. A. Vendittoli, N. Hagemeister, and N. Mezghani

2.1 Introduction

The knee is a complex joint that requires perfectly coupled three-dimensional (3D) motions for proper function. As a result, reliable diagnosis of knee-joint pathologies is a difficult task, requiring in many cases a combination of clinical examinations and imaging, such as magnetic resonance imaging and computed tomography. Such methods provide little direct objective information on the functional aspects of the knee-joint and are not typically performed during knee movement. For this reason, biomechanical gait analysis has become essential in knee-joint pathology diagnosis: it provides quantitative information about the structure and motion of the knee-joint to complement the usual evaluation methods for more accurate diagnosis (Medved 2000). 3D knee kinematic signals, measuring knee flexion/extension, abduction/adduction, and internal/external rotation during locomotion, are now commonly used in gait analysis to assist knee-joint pathology diagnosis. Knee kinematic gait signals can be acquired in a normal clinical setting, using a commercially available treadmill and a motion capture system. Motion

M. Abid (✉) · Y. Ouakrim · N. Mezghani
Laboratoire LIO, Centre de Recherche du CHUM, Montreal, QC, Canada

Centre de Recherche LICEF, TELUQ University, Montreal, QC, Canada
e-mail: Mariem.Abid@etsmtl.ca

A. Mitiche
Institut National de la Recherche Scientifique (INRS), Centre Énergie, Matériaux et Télécommunications, Montreal, QC, Canada

P. A. Vendittoli
Centre de recherche Hôpital Maisonneuve-Rosemont, Montreal, QC, Canada

N. Hagemeister
Laboratoire LIO, Centre de Recherche du CHUM, Montreal, QC, Canada

I. Obeid et al. (eds.), *Biomedical Signal Processing*,
https://doi.org/10.1007/978-3-030-67494-6_2

capture systems are generally composed of optoelectronic cameras which track 3D coordinates from active or passive markers 1 fixed onto the knee segments (e.g., femur and tibia). These marker data are transformed into knee-joint angles, which describe the relative motion between knee segments over time, such as the angular displacement of the tibia with respect to the femur (de Guise et al. 2011; Phinyomark et al. 2016). As functions of time, the data can be viewed as time series. Their analysis has concentrated on classification to distinguish asymptomatic and pathological knee function. The overall classification system flow consists generally of three steps: pre-processing to put the measurements in easily usable form, feature extraction and selection to describe the data by characteristics, and classification into different categories. Classification faces the challenge of data high-dimensionality, and variability, which several studies have addressed explicitly (Chau 2001a; Mezghani et al. 2018). High dimensionality has been addressed by dimensionality reduction using feature extraction and selection (Abid et al. 2019a). Local features, most often considered, are characteristic points on the kinematic signals, such as flexion angle peak values from the kinematic data of locomotion. Global features consider the shape of the whole kinematic signal, rather a few characteristic points on it. Classification is then performed based on the elected features using machine learning methods (Abid et al. 2019a). Measured patterns of locomotion are characterized by high within-subject and stride-to-stride variability. For each subject, several measurements are repeated a number of times, giving a family of curves that can differ from each other, some possibly affected by outliers. Variability analysis is generally done as a pre-processing task. Standard deviation band (Labbe et al. 2008) and functional boxplot (Mechmeche et al. 2016), for instance, have been used for estimating this variability. An outlier is any curve that is more than two standard deviations away from the mean or that is outside the maximum non-outlying envelope. However, the mean itself of the data can be significantly affected by outliers, and the band-depth computation is very complex.

In general, current studies include manual feature extraction as an essential step. Feature design is often time-consuming, can be unreliable when there are few training data, and generally does not exploit temporal information. Recent investigations have obtained good results but have been tested on small datasets, which limits the generality of their conclusions. For instance, 40 knee osteoarthritis (OA) subjects and 40 healthy subjects participated in a study in which 3D knee kinematics data (flexion/extension, abduction/adduction, and internal/external rotation) were recorded (Mezghani et al. 2018). The authors examined a set of 70 specific kinematic features to determine the most discriminant to be used. Regression tree representation gave 85% accuracy in discriminating knee OA subjects from healthy subjects.

The aim of this study is to investigate deep neural networks (LeCun et al. 2015) for automatic classification of asymptomatic (AS) and knee OA kinematic data using the entire pre-processed signal and a relatively large dataset compared to previous studies of biomechanical data classification (Abid et al. 2019a). Pre-processing is to determine representative patterns of a subject's kinematic signals by averaging these after addressing variability so as to improve data objectivity. Deep

Table of abbreviations

Abbreviation	Meaning
ICC	Intraclass correlation
OA	Osteoarthrosis
3D	Three-dimensional
MTS	Multivariate time series
GRF	Ground reaction force
IQR	Inter-quartile range
CMC	Coefficient of multiple correlation
ANOVA	Analysis of variance
KS	Knee straining
RTs	Regression trees
KL	Kellgren and lawrence
CART	Classification and regression tree
SVD	Singular value decomposition
PCA	Principal component analysis
WT	Wavelets transform
AS	ASymptomatic
ACL	Anterior cruciate ligament
ACL-R	Anterior cruciate ligament reconstructed
PCs	Principal components
LR	Logistic regression
FR	Femero-Rotulian
FT	Femero-tibial
DBSCAN	Density-based spatial clustering of applications with noise
SVM	Support vector machine
SSA	Singular spectrum analysis
HS	Heel strike
TO	Toe-off
MS	Mid-swing
RMSE	Root mean square error
CNN	Convolutional neural network
time-CNN	Time convolutional neural network
t-LeNet	Time le-net
FCN	Fully convolutional neural network
ResNet	Residual network
ReLU	Rectified linear unit
PReLU	Parametric ReLU
TP	True positives
FP	False positives
FN	False negatives
TN	True negatives
ROM	Range of motion
CAM	Class activation map
MLP	Multilayer perceptron

Nomenclature

Symbol	Meaning
X	Knee kinematic time series
y	Labels
T	Time steps
D	Knee kinematic time series dataset
N	Number of samples in the dataset
j	Time instance
m	Number of features

learning obviates the need for feature engineering. The motivation for investigating deep neural networks in knee kinematic data classification is their success in classification of time series at large on UCR (Dau et al. 2018) and/or MTS (Baydogan 2015) time series archive datasets (Wang et al. 2017; Fawaz et al. 2019) from different domains such as human activity recognition and sleep stage identification. The advantage of deep neural networks is their ability for automatic feature extraction from raw, complex, and high-dimensional data. In this work, pre-processed knee kinematic data signals are the inputs to deep neural networks to learn kinematic features capable of discriminating knee OA patients from AS participants. The proposed methodology is depicted schematically in Fig. 2.1. Data collection is followed by pre-processing steps of gait events detection, normalization, outlier detection, and cycle selection. This allows us to determine the most representative shape by considering the within-subject variability, defined as the fluctuation in gait parameters from one stride to the next. Afterward, pre-processed knee kinematic data signals (entire gait cycle) are input to deep neural networks. Our investigation provides a comparison of the effectiveness of various deep neural networks in knee kinematic time series classification problem. To the best of our knowledge, this is the first study on classifying raw knee kinematic time series data using end-to-end discriminative deep learning classifiers.

2.2 Related Work

In this section, we first present related work at each step of the pre-processing flowchart depicted in Fig. 2.1. Then, we provide a review on knee-joint kinematic data analysis for knee pathology classification.

2.2.1 Kinematic Data Pre-processing

The choice of an appropriate method in each step of kinematic data pre-processing, while significantly affecting performance, is not always obvious and requires a combination of experience and trial-and-error (Chau 2001b). Any gait events,

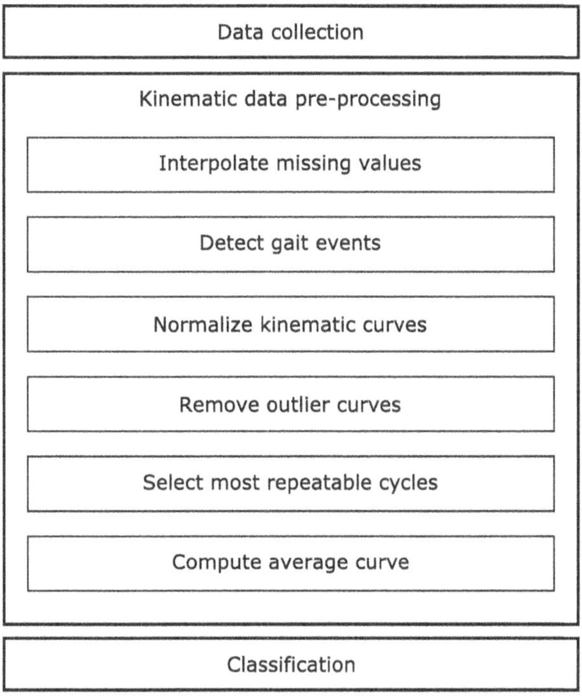

Fig. 2.1 The flowchart describes the knee kinematic data classification process. Data collection is followed by pre-processing steps of gait events detection, normalization, outlier detection, and cycle selection. Afterward, pre-processed knee kinematic data signals (entire gait cycle) are input to deep neural networks, to distinguish between asymptomatic (AS) subjects and knee osteoarthritis (OA) patients

outliers detection, and cycle selection methods developed must therefore be both accurate and reliable.

- Gait Events Detection. Several methods of determining gait events from knee kinematic curves have been shown in the literature. Kinetics-based gait event detection methods have been widely used. That is, a force plate is conventionally used to identify gait events instants, whereby a vertical ground reaction force (GRF) threshold of 2% of the patients' body weight is defined (Labbe et al. 2008; Boivin 2010; Gaudreault et al. 2013). Velocity-based algorithms was also used to determine when gait events occur with relatively successful results. For example, using the foot velocity algorithm proposed by O'Connor et al. (2007), the beginning and the final of each cycle are determined using the vertical velocity signals, derived from heel markers placed on each foot (Leporace et al. 2012). When instrumentation is not available to determine gait events timing, some studies rely on kinematics-based gait event detection methods (Zeni et al. 2008; Hreljac and Marshall 2000).

- Outlier Removal. Within a sample of single-cycle gait curves, there is both phase and amplitude variation. The literature refers to lateral displacements in curve features as phase variation, as opposed to amplitude variation in curve height. Typically, when we describe variability in gait curves, we refer to amplitude variability. Mechmeche et al. (2016) proposed to deal with phase variability in knee kinematic curves using curve registration. A popular approach to estimating curve variability is to peg prediction bands around a group of curves. However, the presence of a small fraction of outliers can unduly inflate our estimates of gait variability and subsequent analysis. Johnson (1998) defines an outlier to be "an observation in a data set which appears to be inconsistent with the remainder of that set of data." One common way of estimating curve variability in knee kinematics is the calculation of the standard deviation band and then to mark as a potential outlier any curve that is more than two standard deviations away from the mean (Labbe et al. 2008). The problem with this method is that the mean of the data can be greatly affected by outliers. Other related work for detecting outlying observations consists of the construction of a functional boxplot based on the concept of band-depth and then to mark as a potential outlier any curve that is outside the maximum non-outlying envelope obtained by inflating the inter-quartile range (IQR) 1.5 times (Mechmeche et al. 2016). One of the main limitations of the band-depth computation is its computational complexity.
- Most Repeatable Cycles Selection. Two similarity indices that attempt to assess the within-subject repeatability of knee kinematic data were considered in the literature: the coefficient of multiple correlation (CMC) and the intraclass correlation coefficient (ICC). The CMC represents the root square of the adjusted coefficient of multiple determination (Kadaba et al. 1989). It was used to identify the most repeatable 15 curves (Fuentes-Dupré 2010; Mezghani et al. 2015). The limitations of the use of CMC to assess within-subject repeatability in kinematic gait data have been discussed (Røislien et al. 2012), notably the influence of the range of motion of the joint. The intraclass correlation coefficient (ICC) has also been used to determine which representative curves to select (Duhamel et al. 2004). For each participant, a minimum of four and a maximum of 10 gait cycles were obtained for each knee angle. In his work the computation of the ICC is based on a one-way, random, linear model and doesn't take into account the correlation between the repeated measurements.
- Averaging. Once the outliers removed, traditionally, the average curve of all observations was used as a representative gait cycle (Mezghani et al. 2012). Two gait cycles were included to represent the variability of the individual gait instead of using the average of some gait cycles (Leporace et al. 2012). A representative data curve was also determined by a variational method to characterize a subject (Ben Nouma et al. 2018). Other related works average over the most repeatable 15 cycles among all observations (Gaudreault et al. 2013; Mezghani et al. 2016a).

2.2.2 *Classification*

Knee kinematic data classification is aimed at distinguishing automatically between the normal subjects and pathological knee patients. Two broad types of approaches can be distinguished: statistical methods and machine learning methods. Both local and global features can serve dimensionality reduction. A comparison table (Table 2.1) is given that inform on data acquisition techniques and accuracies.

Table 2.1 Knee kinematic data classification-related studies

Study	Pathology	Population	Data acquisition	Feature ext/select	Classification	Accuracy
Li et al. (2005)	OA	35 OA 107 AS	3D Knee Analyzer	Local rep.	ANOVA	–
Ouakrim (2011)	OA	30 OA 14 AS	KneeKG	Local rep global rep	SVD	77.27% 93.18%
Mezghani et al. (2012)	OA	30 OA 14 AS	KneeKG	Global rep	SVD	93.1%
Leporace et al. (2012)	ACL-R	6 ACL-R 10 AS	Four cameras motion analysis system (INNOVI-SION)	Global rep **PCA**	LR	93.75%
Gaudreault et al. (2013)	OA	18 KS 20 non-KS	KneeKG	Local rep	Student t test	–
Mezghani et al. (2013)	AS	111 AS	KneeKG	Global rep **PCA**	Discriminant model based on PCs' sign	–
Mezghani et al. (2015)	OA	25 KS 25 non-KS 29 OA	KneeKG	–	Bayes classifier	–
Mezghani et al. (2016a)	OA	44 S 40 non-S	KneeKG	Local rep	CART	84.7%
Mezghani et al. (2016b)	OA	100 OA	KneeKG	Local repn	RTs	88%
Christian et al. (2016)	ACL	7 ACL 7 AS	Vicon motion analysis system	PCA	SVM	100%
Mezghani et al. (2018)	OA	100 OA 40 AS	KneeKG	Local rep	RTs	85
Zgolli et al. (2018)	AS	165 AS	KneeKG	Isometric mapping	DBSCA	–
Ben Nouma et al. (2019)	OA	63 OA	KneeKG	WT	Kohnen neural network	90.47%

Several biomechanical studies on discriminating patients with knee-joint OA from normal subjects using local approaches are available in the literature. The maximum knee flexion, abduction angles during three daily activities were analyzed, using ANOVA, to know whether there were statistically significant differences between normal and OA groups at different disease severity levels (Li et al. 2005). In Gaudreault et al. (2013), specific kinematic parameters, such as knee angle at initial foot contact, peak angles, minimal angles and angle range, were extracted, which concord with those identified in the knee-joint gait literature (Astephen et al. 2008; Teixeira and Olney 1996). A student t-test has been performed to investigate the differences between workers exposed to Knee Straining (KS) postures and non-KS for gait kinematic variables (peak, ranges, and minimum values). In recent studies, a set of 70 features were extracted from 3D kinematic patterns based on variables routinely assessed in clinical biomechanical studies of knee OA populations, such as maximums, minimums, varus and valgus thrust, angles at initial contact, mean values, and range of motion throughout gait cycles or gait cycle sub-phases (Mezghani et al. 2016a,b, 2018). Within these features, a set of 14 features have been identified as diagnostic and burden of disease biomarkers for knee OA characterization. Regression Trees (RTs) have then been applied to feature-based OA vs non-OA discrimination and to grade OA severity (according to the Kellgren and Lawrence (KL) grades from 1 to 4) (Mezghani et al. 2016b, 2018). The success rate of the RTs classifier was 86% to distinguish KL1-2 from KL3-4 grades, 88.2% for KL1 from KL2 grades, and 88% for KL3 from KL4 grades. Using features extracted from the waveforms, another study investigated the Classification and Regression Tree (CART) to classify surgical versus non-surgical patients with a primary diagnosis of moderate to severe knee OA and scheduled for arthroplasty consult (Mezghani et al. 2016a). In contrast to local approaches, waveform methods for global feature extraction such as Singular Value Decomposition (SVD), Principal Component Analysis (PCA), and Wavelets Transform (WT) are outlined.

SVD was used to characterize the kinematic waveform while also identifying gait sub-cycles for a better discrimination between AS and OA groups and for assessing the severity of the disease of OA patients into KL1-2 and KL3-4 categories according to the Kellgren and Lawrence (KL) scale (Mezghani et al. 2012; Ouakrim 2011). The kinematic waveforms were characterized using 14 points of interest (Ouakrim 2011). For AS/OA classification, the analysis showed that the most discriminant sub-cycle was during the stance phase. Concerning the knee-joint OA severity assessment, the most discriminant sub-cycle was during the swing phase of the frontal kinematic waveform, and the success rate was 93.2%. For the discrimination of Anterior Cruciate Ligament Reconstructed (ACL-R) subjects and healthy subjects, PCA was applied on kinematic waveforms (Leporace et al. 2012). The ACL-R subjects had a mean of 12 ± 2 months time from surgery and had incurred a complete ACL tear. All ACL-R subjects had a unilateral tear of their ligament, with no previous ligament injury of either knee, and no history of knee surgery. Differences were found between groups in the frontal and transverse planes. Then, the principal components (PCs) of the three planes were retained for classifying the status of normality using Logistic Regression (LR). Only the frontal plane kinematics had high importance for classifying the status of normality. PCA was also used to extract meaningful patterns representative of the AS gait to separate the entire kinematic waveforms in the sagittal, transverse and frontal planes into homogenous groups (Mezghani et al. 2013). A wavelet representation of kinematic data extracted in each plane separately (sagittal, frontal, and transverse planes) has been used to train a sample-encoding Kohonen network to distinguish between two types of knee OA pathologies, namely, femero-rotulian (FR) and femero-tibial (FT) (Ben Nouma et al. 2019).

Few studies have investigated clustering techniques for knee biomechanical patterns. The PCs clustering model was applied to the frontal, sagittal, and transverse plane kinematic data (Mezghani et al. 2013), which led to the identification of four distinct patterns in normal gait. The clustering quality has been verified based on the analysis of the silhouette width and with statistical evaluation by hypothesis testing. The density-based spatial clustering of applications with noise (DBSCAN) algorithm has been applied to the frontal, sagittal, and transverse plane kinematic data, which led to the identification of two representation patterns for each plane. Cluster divisions are evaluated using the silhouette index, the Dunn index, and connectivity (Zgolli et al. 2018).

A Bayes classifier has been applied to determine if workers exposed to KS have knee kinematic data that resemble those of knee OA patients rather than of non-KS workers on the first 20-gait cycle percentages of the kinematic waveforms (Mezghani et al. 2015). A Support Vector Machine (SVM) was also trained to distinguish kinematics of patients with an ACL injured knee from healthy subjects (Christian et al. 2016). ACL patients had either a knee extension or flexion deficit or a combination of both in the affected limb, but were able to walk without a walking aid for a minimum of 10 m, and sustained a complete unilateral ACL rupture within a period of 21 days (13 (SD 5) days) prior to the experiment.

2.3 Methods and Materials

2.3.1 Data Collection

This study has been approved by ethics committee of the Centre de Recherche du Centre Hospitalier de l'Université de Montréal (CRCHUM) and the École de Technologie Supérieure (ÉTS), Hôpital Maisonneuve-Rosemont (HMR). All subjects provided an informed consent before participation.

We used 3D knee kinematics of 239 subjects collected in different centers. The first group included 49 asymptomatic (AS) subjects. The second group included 190 knee osteoarthritis (OA) patients. The demographic characteristics of the data in the two classes are shown in Table 2.2. Statistical analyses were performed using the two-sample t-test. A p value below 0.05 was considered statistically significant.

Table 2.2 Demographic characteristics of AS and OA groups

Characteristics	AS group	OA group	P value
Age (years) (Mean ± SD)	60.4 ± 4.2	63 ± 9	0.05
Height (cm) (Mean ± SD)	167.4 ± 11.2	167.3 ± 9.6	0.944
Weight (kg) (Mean ± SD)	86.1 ± 19.1	82.7 ± 14.8	0.182
BMI (kg/m^2) (Mean ± SD)	30.5 ± 5.4	29.5±4.5	0.181
Sex ratio (Male:Female)	16:33	78:112	0.285

SD Standard Deviation, *BMI* body mass index

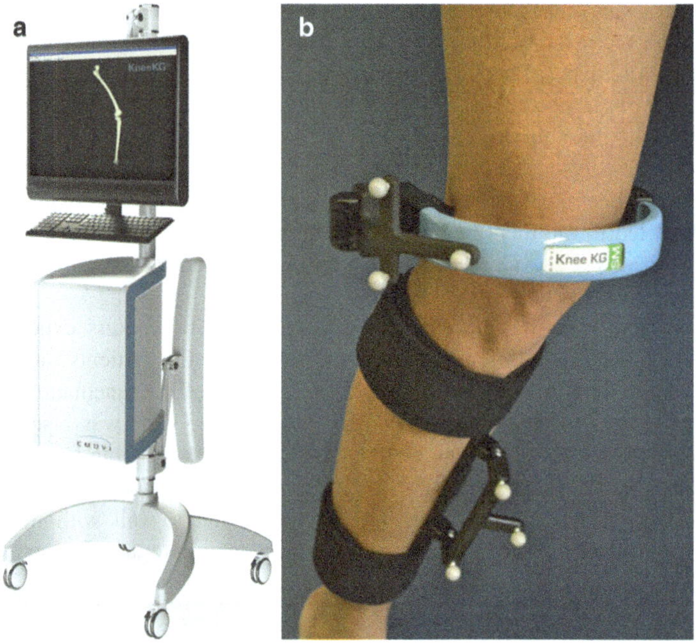

Fig. 2.2 Knee motion analysis recording equipment setup using the$KneeKG^{TM}$: (**a**) The $KneeKG^{TM}$ is composed of an infrared motion capture system (Polaris Spectra camera, Northern Digital Inc.) and a computer equipped with the Knee3D software suite (Emovi, Inc.). The camera and computer can both be mounted on a cart making the entire system mobile. (**b**) Exoskeleton of the $KneeKG^{TM}$ system fixed on the participant's lower limb. The harness lies on the femoral condyles, and the plate is fixed on the tibial crest

3D knee kinematics are acquired with the $KneeKG^{TM}$ system (Emovi Inc. Canada) during gait on a treadmill (45 s duration). KneeKG is a non-invasive knee-marker attachment system consisting of an exoskeleton, an infrared camera, and a computer equipped with the $KneeKG^{TM}$ software (Lustig et al. 2012) (Fig. 2.2). The exoskeleton is composed of a femoral arch with lateral markers and a tibial marker attachment. The exoskeleton, designed to reduce skin-motion artifacts (Labbe et al. 2008), is placed on the participant's lower limb. The 3D positions and movements of the markers are captured at a frequency rate of 60 Hz by the

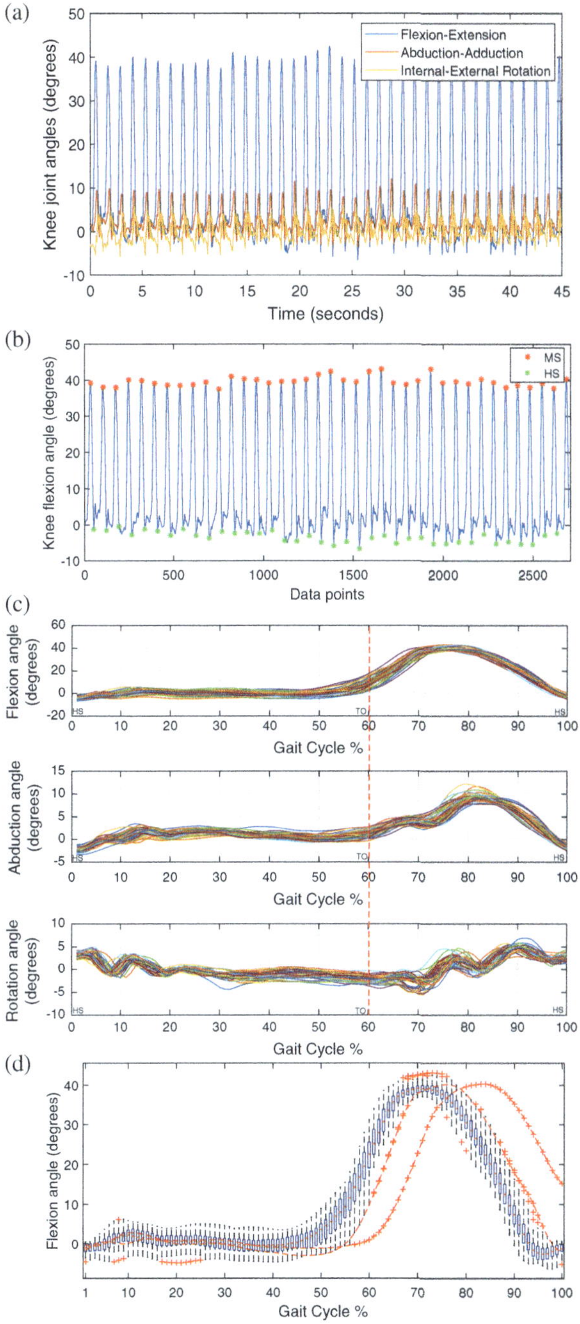

Fig. 2.3 (**a**) Plot of measured knee-joint angles (flexion-extension, abduction-adduction, and internal-external rotations) during a 45 s walking trial on the treadmill for one AS subject. (**b**) The detection of the HS and MS instants based on the knee flexion extrema of one AS subject. (**c**) Depicted are gait cycles for one AS subject, beginning at HS and ending at the next HS, for knee joint angles in all three planes. (**d**) Boxplot (in blue) of knee flexion angles, for one AS subject, highlighting outliers (in red)

infrared camera (Lustig et al. 2012). Kinematic data were used to generate knee-joint angles with the $KneeKG^{TM}$ software (Emovi Inc.): knee flexion-extension, abduction-adduction, and internal-external rotation, representing the motion of the tibia relative to the femur, according to the knee-joint coordinate system as defined by Grood and Suntay (Grood and Suntay 1983). The accuracy (Sati et al. 1996), reproducibility (Hagemeister et al. 1999), repeatability (Hagemeister et al. 2005), and reliability (Labbe et al. 2008) of the system have been studied. Each participant undergoes a series of successive gait trials during a given session. In each trial, the motion trajectories in the sagittal, frontal, and transverse planes of the knee reference system are recorded. These data are filtered using a non-parametric time series analysis called Singular Spectrum Analysis (SSA) (Aissaoui et al. 2006) and transformed into 3D knee-joint angles (Hagemeister et al. 2005). The $KneeKG^{TM}$ software produces a dataset for each subject represented by a standardized KKG file format stored in an SQLite database format. The dataset contains the 3D knee-joint angles, namely, flexion-extension, abduction-adduction, and internal-external rotation, in the form of time series, i.e., the time-varying angle values (Fig. 2.3a). In the knee-joint coordinate system, flexion-extension occurs about the femoral axis in the sagittal plane, internal-external rotation occurs about the tibial axis in the transverse plane, and abduction-adduction occurs about an axis that is perpendicular to the femoral and tibial axes in the frontal plane.

2.3.2 Kinematic Data Pre-processing

Once data collection is complete, the raw kinematic data (Fig. 2.3a) are pre-processed in order to find robust representative patterns for each participant, via steps of missing data interpolation, gait events detection, normalization, outlier detection, cycles' selection, and averaging (Abid et al. 2020). The time series is interpolated by cubic spline interpolation to fill gaps that may be present between data point measurements.

- Gait events detection. The raw kinematic curves of each participant are then divided into distinct gait cycles. The gait cycle is the time between two successive heel contacts of the same foot and consists of a stance and swing phase (Fig. 2.4). Analysis of knee kinematics relies on the accurate determination of the timing of key gait events such as heel strike (HS), the time at which the heel first hits the walking surface, toe-off (TO), the time at which the foot leaves the walking surface, and mid-swing (MS), the maximum knee flexion. In the context of kinematics-based gait event detection methods, our approach center around the location of local maxima values in the sagittal plane curve, since the data from the sagittal plane are more reproducible than those from the other two planes (Yu et al. 1997). MS points correspond to local maxima. HS points are the first local minima after the local maxima and are specified as the start of each gait cycle

(Fig. 2.3b). By convention, HS initiates the cycle, TO initiates the swing phase, and stance is followed by swing phases (Fig. 2.3c).

- Normalization. Knowing gait events allows for normalization of the resulting knee kinematic curves over percentages of the gait cycle rather than absolute time. A typical gait cycle normalized in time is represented on a linear 1–100% scale, therefore giving 100 sample points. That is, HS is generally taken as the starting point of a complete gait cycle (0%); TO occurs at about 60–62%, denoting the initiation of the swing phase; and the end of the cycle (100%) occurs with the next HS which will be the HS of the next cycle. Thus, for each knee angle, the superposed normalized cycles (about 30 to 40 cycles depending on the person's stride) constitute the observations to describe with representative patterns characterizing the given participant (Fig. 2.3c).
- Outlier removal. These observations correspond to a family of curves each one slightly different from the other, due to within-subject variability from stride-to-stride. In this work, we first propose to use cross-validation to quantify the true achieved coverage probability for a robust estimate of the spread of the sample of gait curves (Lenhoff et al. 1999). We argued that bootstrap prediction bands provide inadequate coverage probability toward boxplot, when applied to the knee angle curves of AS and knee OA subjects employed in this study. A boxplot is a schematic plot, a box, and whiskers plot, made up of five components, that give a robust summary of the distribution of a dataset: the minimum, the maximum, the median, and the first and third quartiles. Afterward, the variability among the group of curves, as estimated by boxplot, is minimized

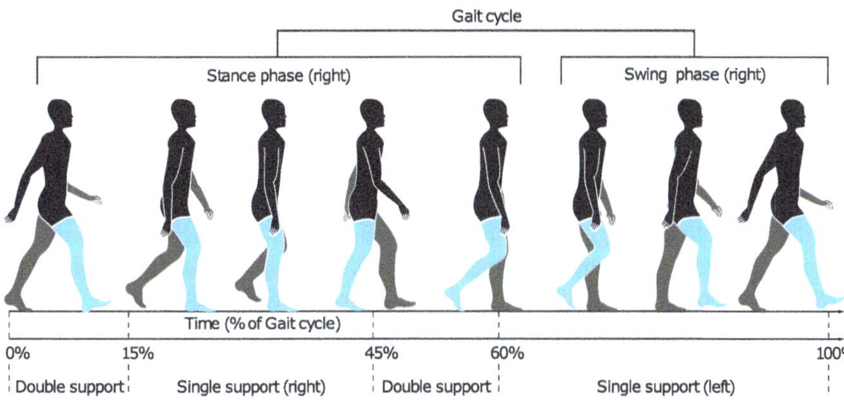

Fig. 2.4 An illustration of gait phases. The gait cycle involves two main phases, the stance phase when the foot is in contact with the ground and the swing phase when the foot is not in contact with the ground. The stance phase generally corresponds to the first 60% of the gait cycle, and the swing phase to the remaining last 40%. The stance phase is further composed of a period of double stance during the first and last 10% of the stance phase, when both feet contact the ground, and a period of single stance during the remainder of the stance phase when only one foot is in contact with the ground. The swing phase also has three parts: the initial swing, the mid swing, and the terminal swing

by the subsequent removal of outlying curves in all three planes of motion. In case of gait curves, the outlier is not a single point, but an entire curve (Fig. 2.3d). In order to affirm that a curve is an outlier, we apply the Chebyshev's theorem stating the percentage of data points falling outside the sample values that are a factor k of the IQR below the 25th percentile or above the 75th percentile, i.e., the first and third quartiles.

- Most repeatable cycles selection. After estimating within-subject variability, we evaluate the similarity of curves to decide which curves can be selected as characterizing the subject. In other words, we intend to determine whether these curves are repeatable, i.e., sufficiently similar to consider that their mean estimates the true, unknown curve (Duhamel et al. 2004). In this study, a cross-validation methodology was applied to the set of observations. The idea is to remove one curve from the original dataset, then calculate the Root Mean Square Error (RMSE) on the remaining curves. The number of RMSE calculated is equal to the number of curves in the dataset. The curve resulting in the highest RMSE is removed. A set of 15 curves for each knee angle is selected that demonstrate the best repeatability (Boivin 2010).
- Averaging. In this study, each subject is represented by a single gait curve, which is the mean of the 15 most repeatable cycles, as proposed in Gaudreault et al. (2013) and Mezghani et al. (2016a).

The proposed pre-processing steps have been performed on each subject of the two population databases (OA and AS), for ease of analysis and visualization. Figure 2.5 shows the knee kinematic signals in the sagittal plane, frontal plane, and transverse plane, for each population separately.

2.3.3 *Classification*

The purpose is to classify knee kinematic signals using deep neural networks in order to discriminate between AS and OA subjects. We tested various end-to-end discriminative deep learning models of time series classification, in order to find which model works best for knee kinematic signals classification (Abid et al. 2019b). In contrast to feature engineering, discriminative deep learning directly learns a mapping between the raw input and outputs a class probability distribution. This is important in our study because it avoids the bias due to handcrafted features.

More formally, let (X, y) be an instance with $T = 100$ observations (time steps) $X = (X^1, \ldots, X^T)$ (the knee kinematic time series) and a discrete class variable y which takes 2 possible values (the labels, i.e., AS or OA). Target values are 0 for the AS class and 1 for the OA class. A dataset D is a set of N (samples) such instances: $D = \{(X_1, y_1), (X_2, y_2), \ldots, (X_N, y_N)\}$. The task of classifying knee kinematic time series data consists of learning a classifier on D in order to map from the space of possible inputs $\{X\}$ to a probability distribution over the classes y. Each data observation X^j, $(j = 1, \ldots, T)$ of a time series X can be a list of one or more data

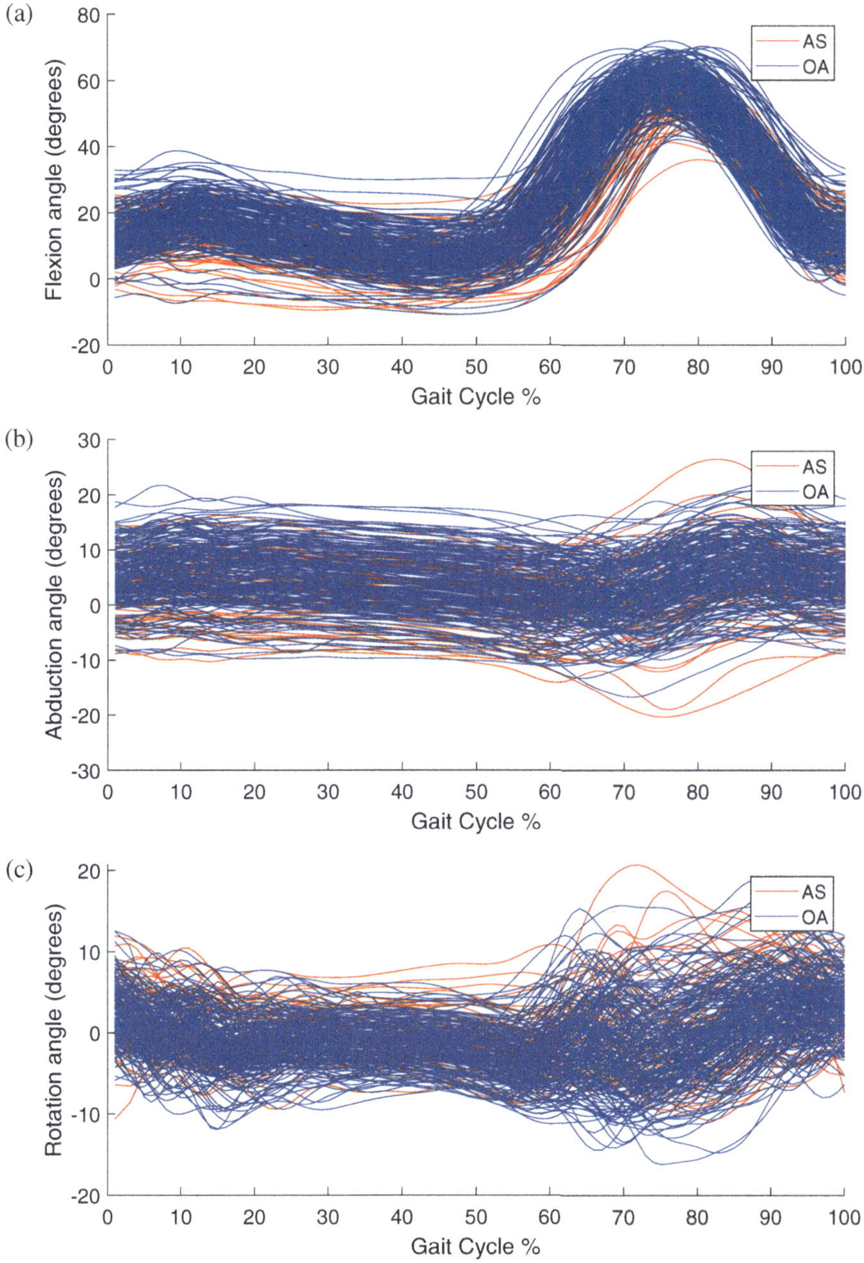

Fig. 2.5 Plots of pre-processed knee kinematic signals for AS population (in red) and OA population (in blue), in all three planes flexion-extension, abduction-adduction, and internal-external rotation

measurements (features), i.e., $X^j = (X_{1j}, \ldots, X_{mj})$ for m data measurements, all taken at the jth time instance. Elements X_{mj} are real numbers corresponding to the knee kinematic angles. An m-dimensional multivariate (m-variate) time series (MTS) $X = (X^1, \ldots, X^T)$ consists of T ordered elements $X^j \in \mathbb{R}^m$. A univariate time series X of length T is simply an MTS with $m = 1$, i.e. $X^j \rightarrow X^j \in \mathbb{R}$ and $X = (X^1, \ldots, X^T)$.

A deep neural network has an input layer, an output layer, and more than two hidden layers. A layer is a collection of neurons. A neuron takes a group of weighted inputs, applies an activation function, and returns an output.

The input layer has Txm neurons. Like in image classification problems, we consider multidimensional time series, $y \in \mathbb{R}^{N \times T \times m}$. A tensor is a multidimensional array. Vectors and matrices are first-order and second-order tensors, respectively, where order is the number of ways or modes of the tensor. When m equals 1, we train one feature at a time (flexion/extension, abduction/adduction, or internal/external rotation), at each time step for each sample. When m equals 3, the 3-variate time series is jointly trained (flexion/extension, abduction/adduction, and internal/external rotation, together).

Hidden layers of a deep network are designed to learn hierarchical feature representations of the data. During training, a set of hyper-parameters is optimized, and the weights are initialized randomly (LeCun et al. 2012). By gradient descent, the weights are updated using the back propagation algorithm, in a way that minimizes the cost function on the training set. The choice of the model, the architecture, and the cost function are crucial for obtaining a network that generalizes well and are generally problem and data dependent. We trained five deep learning models, which have convolutional neural network (CNN)-based architecture (LeCun and Bengio 1998), and designed specifically for time series classification.

CNN combines three architectural ideas: local receptive fields, shared weights, and pooling. Convolutional neural networks (CNNs) consist of alternating convolutional layers and pooling layers. The convolutional layer implements the receptive field and shared weights concepts. Neurons in the convolutional layers are locally connected to neurons inside its receptive field in the previous layer. Neurons in a layer are organized in planes within which all the neurons share the same set of weights (also called filters or kernels). The set of outputs of the neurons in such a plane is called a feature map. The number of feature maps is the same as the number of filters. A pooling layer performs either average sub-sampling (mean-pooling) or maximum sub-sampling (max-pooling). For a time series, the pooling layers simply reduce the length and thus the resolution, of the feature maps.

The different hyper-parameters of CNN are the optimization algorithm (momentum), the number of epochs, the number of layers, the number of filters, the filter size, the activation function, the cost function, the batch size, and the weight initialization. Here the following are the deep learning models (Fig. 2.6) that we investigated to determine their ability to discriminate between knee kinematic signals of patients with OA and AS participants.

- Time convolutional neural network (time-CNN) (Zhao et al. 2017): Convolution and pooling operations are alternately used to generate deep features of the raw data. Then the features are connected to a multilayer perceptron (MLP) to perform classification. Figure 2.6a summarizes the architecture of the time-CNN model. There are three layers in this network including two convolutional blocks and one fully connected layer, with a Sigmoid activation function. The convolutional block consists of a convolution layer, a Sigmoid layer, and an average pooling layer with pooling size 3. The number of filters {6, 12} and the filter size {7, 7} in each block. The following parameters were tuned: convolutional filter size in set {5, 7, 9}, the pooling size in {2, 3, 4, 5}, the pooling method in {mean-pooling, max-pooling}, and the number of convolution filters in {2, 3, 4, 6, 9, 12, 15}.
- Time Le-Net (t-LeNet) (Le Guennec et al. 2016): is a time series-specific version of leNet model (Lecun et al. 1998). Figure 2.6b summarizes the architecture of the t-LeNet model. There are 4 layers in this network including 2 convolution blocks, 1 fully connected layer with 500 neurons and a rectified linear unit (ReLU)activation function, and finally a Softmax layer. The convolutional block

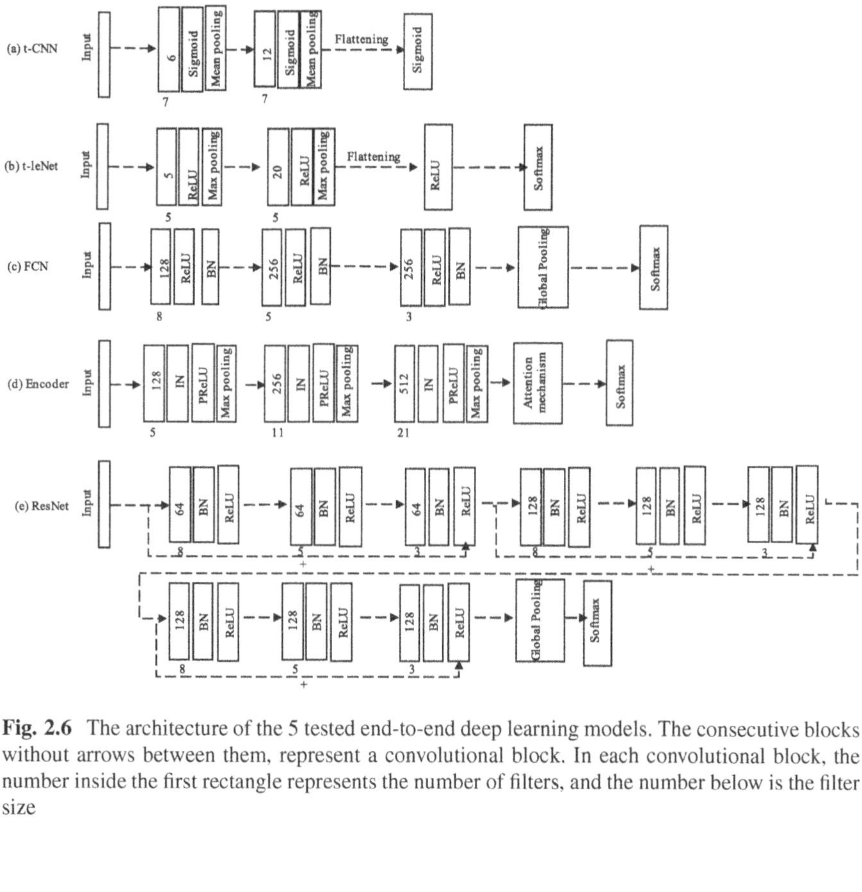

Fig. 2.6 The architecture of the 5 tested end-to-end deep learning models. The consecutive blocks without arrows between them, represent a convolutional block. In each convolutional block, the number inside the first rectangle represents the number of filters, and the number below is the filter size

consists of a convolution layer, a ReLU layer, and a max pooling layer with pooling size 2 and 4 on the first and second block, respectively. The number of filters {5, 20} and the filter size {5, 5} in each block. Two data augmentation techniques have been proposed namely window slicing and window warping.

- Fully Convolutional Neural Network (FCN) (Wang et al. 2017): Fig. 2.6c summarizes the architecture of the FCN model. There are 5 layers in this network including 3 convolution blocks, 1 global average pooling layer, and finally a Softmax layer. The convolutional block consists of a convolution layer, a batch normalization layer, and a ReLU activation layer. The number of filters {128, 256, 128} and the filter size {8, 5, 3} in each block.
- Encoder (Serrà et al. 2018): is a standard convolutional network, with a convolutional attention mechanism to summarize the time-axis and a final fully connected layer to set the desired representation dimensionality. Figure 2.6d summarizes the architecture of the encoder model. There are five layers in this network including three convolution blocks, one attention mechanism, and finally a Softmax layer. The convolutional block consists of a convolution layer, an instance normalization layer, a Parametric ReLU (PReLU) activation layer, a max pooling layer with pooling size 2, and a dropout of 0.2. The number of filters {128, 256, 512} and the filter size {5, 11, 21}.
- Residual Network (ResNet) (Wang et al. 2017): extends the neural networks towards deeper architectures by adding the shortcut connection to enable the gradient flow directly through the bottom layers. Figure 2.6e summarizes the architecture of the ResNet model. There are 11 layers in this network including 9 convolution blocks, 1 global average polling layer, and finally a Softmax layer. The convolutional block consists of a convolution layer, a batch normalization layer, and a ReLU activation layer. The number of filters {64, 64, 64, 128, 128, 128, 128, 128, 128} and the filter size {8, 5, 3, 8, 5, 3, 8, 5, 3}.

All deep learning models have an output layer with two neurons, corresponding to the binary classification in this application.

2.3.4 *Weighting Imbalanced Classes*

We can notice the imbalance of the dataset (49 asymptomatic (AS) subjects vs. 190 knee osteoarthritis (OA) patients). We do not include any oversampling to handle the class imbalance problem, but an algorithm-level method. That is, a class weighting is added to automatically assign higher weights to the minority classes in the learning process, in order to reduce bias toward the majority group (Krawczyk 2016; Johnson and Khoshgoftaar 2019).

2.3.5 Cross-Validation

To find the best hyper-parameters, we performed hyperband searches (Li et al. 2016) with the Keras Tuner Python package,[1] using double cross-validation (Bengio 2012). Keras Tuner is a library to easily perform hyper-parameter tuning with Tensorflow 2.0. Hyperband uses early-stopping to speed up the hyper-parameter tuning process. The main idea is to fit a large number of models for a small number of epochs and to only continue training for the models achieving the highest accuracy on the validation set. Double cross-validation applies recursively the idea of cross-validation, using an outer loop cross-validation to evaluate generalization error and then applying an inner loop cross-validation inside each outer loop split's training subset (i.e., splitting it again into training and validation folds) in order to select hyper-parameters for that split. Table 2.3 summarizes the optimized hyper-parameters configuration for each model. We trained the deep learning models presented above with 10 different runs each. The validation is performed using a stratified ten-fold cross-validation of the knee kinematic dataset D, to preserve the class distribution in the train and test sets for each evaluation of a given model. The model is fit on nine fold as the training dataset and evaluated on the holdout fold as the testing dataset. Instead of averaging the performance measure computed on each holdout fold, predictions are made and stored in a list. Then, at the end of the run, the predictions are compared to the expected values for each holdout test set and a single performance measure is reported (Fig. 2.6).

All models were initialized randomly using the Glorot's uniform initialization method (Glorot and Bengio 2010). The number of epochs (training iterations) is optimized using the principle of early stopping (Bengio 2012). Early stopping allows to specify an arbitrary large number of training epochs and stop training once the model performance stops improving on a holdout validation dataset. The batch size is set equal to the training set size (batch gradient descent).

Table 2.3 Hyper-parameters' optimization for knee kinematic signals dataset

Model	Cost function	Learning rate	Optimizer	Activation function
Time-CNN	MSE	0.001	Adam	Sigmoid
t-leNet	Entropy	0.01	Adam	ReLU
FCN	Entropy	0.001	Adam	ReLU
Encoder	Entropy	0.00001	Adam	PReLU
ResNet	Entropy	0.001	Adam	ReLU

[1]http://keras-team.github.io/keras-tuner/

2.3.6 Performance Measures

Metrics of accuracy, precision, recall, and $F1$ score were used for model selection, i.e., the ability of the model to discriminate between AS and OA participants. These metrics are defined in Equation 2.1–2.4. In these equations, TP stands for true positives, i.e., the number of OA participants correctly classified as OA participants. TN stands for true negatives, i.e., the number of AS participants correctly classified as AS participants. FP stands for false positives, i.e., the number of AS participants misclassified as OA participants, and FN stands for false negatives, i.e., the number of OA participants misclassified as AS participants.

$$Accuracy = \frac{TP + TN}{TP + TN + FP + FN} \tag{2.1}$$

$$Precision = \frac{TP}{TP + FP} \tag{2.2}$$

$$Recall = \frac{TP}{TP + FN} \tag{2.3}$$

$$F1 = 2 * \frac{precision * recall}{precision + recall} \tag{2.4}$$

In all reported experiments, the prediction metrics of the models are calculated as the average of the repeated stratified ten-fold cross-validation.

In order to compare the five end-to-end deep learning models over the four datasets, following Fawaz et al. (2019), we conduct statistical analysis by using the Friedman test to reject the null hypothesis. The test addresses the hypothesis that all methods perform equally well. For the post hoc analysis, following the recent recommendations in Benavoli et al. (2016), we perform the pairwise comparisons of the post-hoc analysis using the Wilcoxon signed rank test instead of the average rank comparison. In order to visualize the comparison, we used a critical difference diagram (Demšar 2006) to visualize the results of these statistical tests projected onto the average rank axis, with a thick horizontal line showing a clique of classifiers that are not significantly different (Fawaz et al. 2019). Following Fawaz et al. (2019), we perform the pairwise comparisons of the post hoc analysis using the Wilcoxon signed rank test (Benavoli et al. 2016). We used the Python code provided in Fawaz et al. (2019).

2.4 Results

In the following, we present the experimental results obtained using the methodology detailed above. We first present the results of the proposed pre-processing steps, by measuring the reliability of the subjects' curves before and after pre-processing. In the second subsection, we present the performance of the described end-to-end deep learning models to determine their ability to discriminate between knee kinematic signals of patients with OA and AS participants.

2.4.1 *Kinematic Data Pre-processing*

For each subject, the gait curve reliability was gauged by fulfilling the following steps: (1) summarize the variability within the time-normalized curves of the subject, which is further reduced by the subsequent removal of outlying curves; (2) identify a subset of representative curves for the subject; (3) compute the intraclass correlation (ICC) (Mcgraw and Wong 1996) estimates and their 95% confidence intervals for knee kinematics of a multicenter dataset of 239 knee OA and AS subjects (presented in Sect. 2.3.1), in order to measure the reliability of the subjects' curves before and after pre-processing. These pre-processing steps are implemented in Matlab. To summarize the variability, we have adopted a displaying of the distribution via boxplot. Based on the true achieved coverage estimation, boxplot is a robust measurement of variability in knee angle curves of AS and knee OA subjects employed in this study. In Fig. 2.3d, the curves of this subject are graphically superimposed in order to visually assess reliability. We observe that two curves seem to be different from the others. Using interquartile range, we detect with no doubt that these curves can be considered as outliers. Figure 2.7 shows, for each plane, the frequency distribution of the ICC computed on the dataset before and after processing, for all the subjects. The graph shows that the subset of the 15 curves selected to represent the gait of the subject are perfectly reliable ($ICC \geq 0.7$) (Koo and Li 2016).

2.4.2 *Classification*

Tables 2.4, 2.5, 2.6, and 2.7 summarize the accuracy, precision, recall, and F1 score of the compared deep learning models: time-CNN, t-leNet, FCN, encoder, and ResNet, applied for each plane separately, namely, the sagittal (flexion/extension), frontal (Abduction/adduction), and transverse (Internal/external rotation) planes, and trained jointly as well. The compared deep learning models are available in an open-source deep learning framework which is implemented using the open-source deep learning library Keras with the Tensorflow back-end. The corresponding critical difference diagram is depicted in Fig. 2.8, where the statistical test failed to find any significant difference between the five end-to-end deep learning models.

In a nutshell, we presented deep learning models that take univariate and multivariate time series. That is, in univariate time series classification, the model is trained for each knee kinematic data plane separately, i.e., m=1. In multivariate time

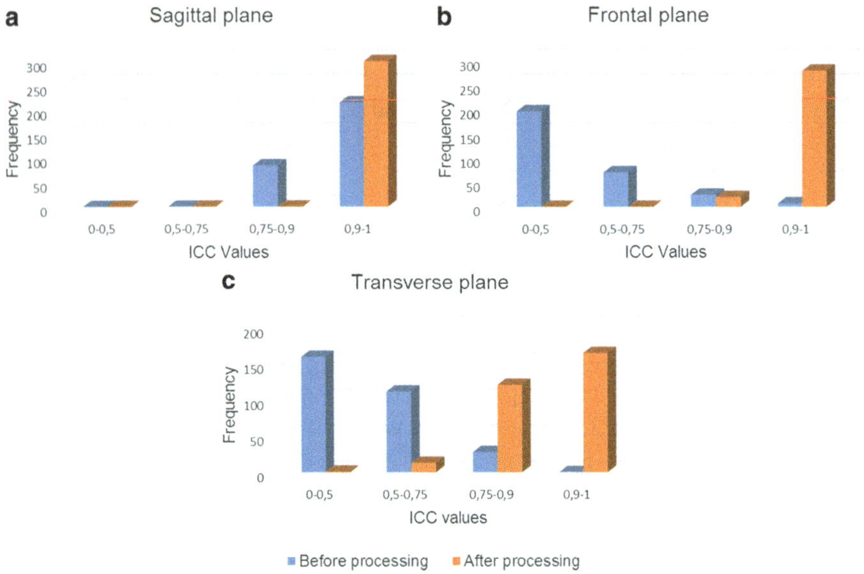

Fig. 2.7 ICC Values and their 95% confident intervals based on a single measurement, absolute agreement, 2-way mixed-effects model, of knee kinematics for all subjects in all three planes, before processing (in blue), and after processing (in orange). ICC values less than 0.5 are indicative of poor repeatability, values between 0.5 and 0.75 indicate moderate repeatability, values between 0.75 and 0.9 indicate good repeatability, and values greater than 0.90 indicate excellent repeatability

Table 2.4 The results of applying five end-to-end deep learning models on the sagittal plane (flexion/extension), in terms of mean and standard deviation of Precision, Accuracy, Recall, and F1 score, for classifying OA (190 subjects) and AS (49 subjects). The out-of-fold prediction metrics of the models are calculated as the average of the repeated (10 runs) stratified ten-fold cross-validation

Model	Precision	Accuracy	Recall	F1
Time-CNN	92.11 ± 0.11	93.77 ± 0.09	98.15 ± 0.008	94.66 ± 0.07
t-leNet	49.99 ± 0.0	50 ± 0.0	1.0 ± 0.0	66.66 ± 1.11
FCN	60.27 ± 0.17	57.36 ± 0.15	74.31 ± 0.20	62.92 ± 0.12
Encoder	74.46 ± 0.09	73.76 ± 0.06	74.47 ± 0.04	74.16 ± 0.05
ResNet	72.97 ± 0.15	76.69 ± 0.16	92.36 ± 0.11	80.70 ± 0.12

series classification, the model is jointly trained for all three planes (sagittal, frontal, and transverse), i.e., m=3. We observed an average improvement on multivariate time series classification in comparison with univariate time series classification, which proves advantageous for knee kinematic data classification, and specifically for small datasets, and necessitates further investigation.

Table 2.5 The results of applying 5 end-to-end deep learning models on the plane frontal plane (abduction/adduction), in terms of mean and standard deviation of Precision, Accuracy, Recall, and F1 score, for classifying OA (190 subjects) and AS (49 subjects). The out-of-fold prediction metrics of the models are calculated as the average of the repeated (10 runs) stratified ten-fold cross-validation

Model	Precision	Accuracy	Recall	F1
Time-CNN	93.31 ± 0.12	94.84 ± 0.11	99.68 ± 0.003	95.90 ± 0.07
t-leNet	95.49 ± 0.13	95.89 ± 0.12	99.94 ± 0.001	97.07 ± 0.08
FCN	65.02 ± 0.09	67.80 ± 0.11	80.10 ± 0.13	71.18 ± 0.10
Encoder	64.52 ± 0.05	67.51 ± 0.05	79.52 ± 0.05	71.04 ± 0.04
ResNet	62.40 ± 0.09	68.02 ± 0.11	92.57 ± 0.13	74.29 ± 0.09

Table 2.6 The results of applying five end-to-end deep learning models on the transverse plane (internal/external rotation), in terms of mean and standard deviation of Precision, Accuracy, Recall, and F1 score, for classifying OA (190 subjects) and AS (49 subjects). The out-of-fold prediction metrics of the models are calculated as the average of the repeated (10 runs) stratified ten-fold cross-validation

Model	Precision	Accuracy	Recall	F1
Time-CNN	91.94 ± 0.12	93.78 ± 0.11	99.21 ± 0.007	94.96 ± 0.08
t-leNet	95.53 ± 0.13	95.93 ± 0.12	99.63 ± 0.011	97.03 ± 0.08
FCN	66.33 ± 0.21	66.68 ± 0.22	83.57 ± 0.12	73.10 ± 0.17
Encoder	88.96 ± 0.12	89.09 ± 0.11	90.63 ± 0.12	89.24 ± 0.11
ResNet	93.91 ± 0.14	94.25 ± 0.15	97.68 ± 0.06	95.44 ± 0.11

Table 2.7 The results of applying five end-to-end deep learning models on the three-variate knee kinematic time series jointly, in terms of mean and standard deviation of Precision, Accuracy, Recall, and F1 score, for classifying OA (190 subjects) and AS (49 subjects). The out-of-fold prediction metrics of the models are calculated as the average of the repeated (10 runs) stratified ten-fold cross-validation

Model	Precision	Accuracy	Recall	F1
Time-CNN	88.36 ± 0.11	91.81 ± 0.09	98.73 ± 0.009	92.29 ± 0.07
t-leNet	95.65 ± 0.13	96.14 ± 0.11	99.84 ± 0.004	97.18 ± 0.08
FCN	86.57 ± 0.14	89.76 ± 0.11	97.89 ± 0.03	91.35 ± 0.09
Encoder	83.17 ± 0.16	86.25 ± 0.15	95.15 ± 0.08	88.33 ± 0.12
ResNet	90.95 ± 0.12	93.11 ± 0.11	98.68± 0.01	94.24 ± 0.08

2.5 Discussion and Conclusion

In this study we investigated the application of machine learning techniques to differentiate between gait patterns of OA patients and AS participants using raw knee kinematic data. To the best of our knowledge, the present study is the first to explore the application of deep learning approaches, which obviates the need for feature engineering. The developed techniques have been tested on a database collected from different sites to have a larger number of OA patients and

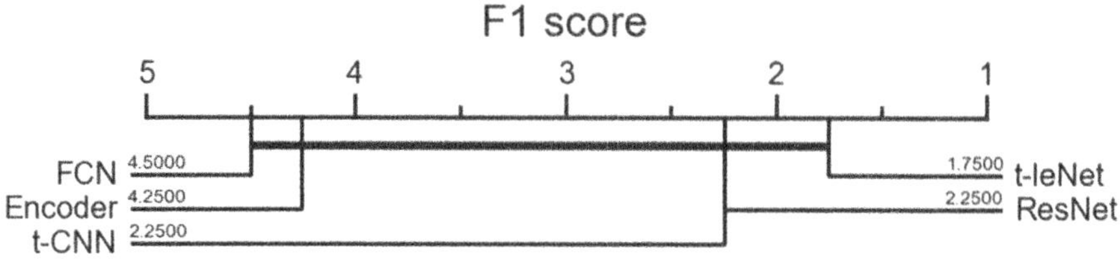

Fig. 2.8 Statistical comparison of classifiers over multiple datasets: a critical difference diagram showing pairwise statistical difference comparison of 5 end-to-end deep learning models on the sagittal, frontal, and transverse knee kinematic datasets, and the three-variate time series as well. Average ranks of examined models are presented. A thick horizontal line shows a group of classifiers that are not-significantly different in terms of accuracy

AS participants compared to previous studies, which gives better generalization capabilities (Mezghani et al. 2018).

We believe that gait curves classification relies heavily on the output of the pre-processing step. That is why, we performed pre-processing steps for summarizing the knee kinematic signals of asymptomatic and osteoarthritis subjects. Our analysis takes into consideration the within-subject variability. The proposed methods make it possible to solve two main problems encountered in clinical practice: the removal of outliers and the selection of reliable curves to represent the gait of a given subject. The robust estimation of variability in a family of gait curves is itself a non-trivial challenge. For this issue, we supported the use of boxplot which provide adequate coverage to the kinematic curves employed in this study. We demonstrated that the variability among a subject's family of curves, as estimated by boxplot, can be minimized by the removal of outlying curves and further reduced by the subsequent selection of the most repeatable cycles as representative of a subject's gait. We point out that reducing variability has been used to obtain representative patterns. However, it is worth mentioning that the within-subject variability from stride-to-stride carries important information and is an important predictor for various neurological (such as cerebral palsy) and age-related diseases, which lead to inflated stride-to-stride variability during gait. In these contexts, pre-processing techniques should be performed prudently for addressing variability issues.

Descriptive statistics such as peak angles are commonly extracted from the gait signal. In this study, the entire signal is employed as the initial features. End-to-end deep learning approaches come to remove the bias due to handcrafted features, thus enabling the network to learn the most discriminative useful features for the classification problem. We started from the most successful existing deep learning models applied in various time series domains in order to answer the question of selecting the most appropriate and best-performing model for the knee kinematic time series classification problem to distinguish knee OA and AS participants. We discovered how to fit five end-to-end deep learning models to a univariate (one plane of motion at a time) and multivariate knee kinematic time series (multiple planes of motion at a time) classification problem. An average improvement on multivariate time series classification has been observed in comparison with univariate time series classification. In the literature, the focused analysis using each plane data separately corroborates that the abduction/adduction patterns are the most discriminative patterns that are able to distinguish OA and AS participants (Cooke et al. 2007; Cerejo et al. 2002; Sharma et al. 2001; Mezghani et al. 2015). Additionally, we used a 3-D $N \times T \times m$ tensor to represent the time series data, in which N is the number of samples or depth, T is the time step, and m is the number of features. Besides, we dealt with imbalance problem in the classification stage. Even though we found promising results for knee kinematics time series classification using end-to-end deep learning models, the problem remains challenging. Further studies, using different datasets, will be needed before confident general conclusions about the relative suitability of different deep learning models can be given. A first perspective is to fine-tune the deep learning models with much larger datasets and conduct more extensive experiments on knee kinematic time series.

In a future work, we intend to consider each participant in the dataset to be represented by a vector of 15 cycles and not their mean, as a data augmentation solution. Moreover, features could be learned independently on each plane, then the learned features would be concatenated and fed into the classifier. We could also look in more details at multivariate time series classification, where models are jointly trained for all three planes (sagittal, frontal, and transverse). We intend also to compare the deep learning models toward traditional machine learning algorithms applied to a set 70 handcrafted features from the knee kinematic data curves (Mezghani et al. 2018; Cherif et al. 2018). The feature extraction methods is based on variables routinely assessed in clinical biomechanical studies of knee OA populations, such as maximums, minimums, varus and valgus thrust, angles at initial contact, mean values, and range of motion (ROM) throughout gait cycles (Mezghani et al. 2018). It is common practice to extract subsequences from time series to do classification. However, in our case, we should take into consideration the gait cycle events and phases, to segment appropriately. In our problem settings, the gait cycle event-based segmentation techniques would be more adequate than the sliding window segmentation technique. The former would split the knee kinematic signal based on the gait cycle events (Heel Strike, toe-off, etc.), whereas the latter split the signal into windows of a fixed size. A suggested hypothesis is to find a sub-cycle or phase of the overall gait signal which contains the relevant information for the correct discrimination of subjects from different groups.

We intend also to understand the learned features by the deep learning models by applying Class Activation Map (CAM) (Zhou et al. 2016), after improving accuracy, and compare them to the previously cited handcrafted features.

Acknowledgments This research was supported by the Canada Research Chair on Biomedical Data Mining (950-231214).
The authors would like to thank Gerald Parent for his technical assistance regarding the automated internal tool developed in the Imaging and Orthopaedics Research Laboratory (LIO), which provides a framework for biomechanical data analysis. The authors would also to thank Julien Clément for making the data collected from Hôpital Maisonneuve-Rosemont (HMR) available.

Conflict of Interest The authors declare no conflict of interest.

References

M. Abid, N. Mezghani, A. Mitiche, Knee joint biomechanical gait data classification for knee pathology assessment: a literature review. Appl. Bionics Biomech. **2019**, 14 (2019a)

M. Abid, A. Mitiche, Y. Ouakrim, P.A. Vendittoli, A. Fuentes, N. Hagemeister, N. Mezghani, A comparative study of end-to-end discriminative deep learning models for knee joint kinematic time series classification. In: 2019 IEEE signal processing in medicine and biology symposium (spmb) (2019b), pp. 1–6

M. Abid, Y. Ouakrim, P.-A. Vendittoli, N. Hagemeister, N. Mezghani, Representative knee kinematic patterns identification using within-subject variability analysis, in *Computer Methods, Imaging and Visualization in Biomechanics and Biomedical Engineering*, ed. by G.A. Ateshian, K.M. Myers, J.M.R.S. Tavares (Springer International Publishing, Cham, 2020), pp. 483–494

R. Aissaoui, S. Husse, H. Mecheri, G. Parent, J.A. de Guise, Automatic filtering techniques for three-dimensional kinematics data using 3D motion capture system, in *2006 IEEE International Symposium on Industrial Electronics* (Vol. 1, pp. 614–619). (2006)

J.L. Astephen, K.J. Deluzio, G.E. Caldwell, M.J. Dunbar, Biomechanical changes at the hip, knee, and ankle joints during gait are associated with knee osteoarthritis severity. J. Orthop. Res. **26**(3), 332–341 (2008)

M.G. Baydogan, Multivariate time series classification datasets (2015). http://www.mustafabaydogan.com

A. Benavoli, G. Corani, F. Mangili, Should we really use post-hoc tests based on mean-ranks? J. Mach. Learn. Res. **17**(5), 1–10 (2016)

Y. Bengio, Practical recommendations for gradient-based training of deep architectures, in *Neural networks: Tricks of the trade: Second edition*, ed. by G. Montavon, G.B. Orr, K.-R. Müller(Springer, Berlin/Heidelberg, 2012), pp. 437–478

B. Ben Nouma, N. Mezghani, A. Mitiche, Y. Ouakrim, A variational method to determine the most representative shape of a set of curves and its application to knee kinematic data for pathology classification, in *Proceedings of the 2nd Mediterranean Conference on Pattern Recognition and Artificial Intelligence*, New York, 2018, pp. 22–26

B. Ben Nouma, A. Mitiche, N. Mezghani, A sample-encoding generalization of the kohonen associative memory and application to knee kinematic data representation and pathology classification. Appl. Sci. **9**(9), 1741 (2019)

K. Boivin, Développement d'une approche d'évaluation clinique de la cinématique tridimensionnelle du genou durant la marche pour des patients gonarthrosiques (Doctoral dissertation, École Polytechnique de Montréal) (2010). Retrieved from https://publications.polymtl.ca/317/

R. Cerejo, D.D. Dunlop, S. Cahue, D. Channin, J. Song, L. Sharma, The influence of alignment on risk of knee osteoarthritis progression according to baseline stage of disease. Arthritis Rheum. **46**(10), 2632–2636 (2002)

T. Chau, A review of analytical techniques for gait data. part 1: Fuzzy, statistical and fractal methods. Gait Posture **13**, 49–66 (2001a)

T. Chau, A review of analytical techniques for gait data. part 2: Neural network and wavelet methods. Gait Posture **13**, 102–120 (2001b)

N. Cherif, Y. Ouakrim, A. Benazza-Benyahia, N. Mezghani, Physical activity classification using a smart textile, in *2018 IEEE life sciences conference (lsc)* (2018), pp. 175–178

J. Christian, J. Kroll, G. Strutzenberger, N. Alexander, M. Ofner, H. Schwameder, Computer aided analysis of gait patterns in patients with acute anterior cruciate ligament injury. Clin. Biomech. **33**, 55–60 (2016)

T.D.V. Cooke, E.A. Sled, R.A. Scudamore, Frontal plane knee alignment: a call for standardized measurement. J. Rheumatol. **34**(9), 1796–1801 (2007)

H.A. Dau, E. Keogh, K. Kamgar, C.-C.M. Yeh, Y. Zhu, S. Gharghabi, G. Batista, The ucr time series classification archive (2018). https://www.cs.ucr.edu/~eamonn/time_series_data_2018/

J. de Guise, N. Mezghani, R. Aissaoui, N. Hagemeister, New comprehensive methods for the biomechanical analysis of knee osteoarthritis. In Understanding osteoarthritis from 610 bench to bedside (2011), pp. 85–102
J. Demšar, Statistical comparisons of classifiers over multiple data sets. J. Mach. Learn. Res. **7**, 1–30 (2006)
A. Duhamel, J. Bourriez, P. Devos, P. Krystkowiak, A. Destée, P. Derambure, L. Defebvre, Statistical tools for clinical gait analysis. Gait Posture **20**(2), 204–212 (2004)
I.H. Fawaz, G. Forestier, J. Weber, L. Idoumghar, P.A. Muller, Deep learning for time series classification: a review. Data Min. Knowl. Disc. **33**, 917–963 (2019)
A. Fuentes-Dupré, Apport d'une évaluation biomécanique 3D du genou dans la prise en charge orthopédique de patients ayant une rupture du ligament croisé antérieur. (Unpublished doctoral dissertation). Université de Montréal(Faculté de médecine) (2010)
N. Gaudreault, N. Hagemeister, S. Poitras, J.A. de Guise, Comparison of knee gait kinematics of workers exposed to knee straining posture to those of non-knee straining workers. Gait Posture **38**(2), 187–191 (2013)
X. Glorot, Y. Bengio, Understanding the difficulty of training deep feedforward neural networks, in *Proceedings of the International Conference on Artificial Intelligence and Statistics (aistats'10). Society for Artificial Intelligence and Statistics* (2010)
E. Grood, W. Suntay, A joint coordinate system for the clinical description of three-dimensional motions: application to the knee. J. Biomech. Eng. **105**, 136–144 (1983)
N. Hagemeister, G. Parent, M.V. de Putte, N. St-Onge, N. Duval, J. de Guise, A reproducible method for studying three-dimensional knee kinematics. J. Biomech. **38**(9), 1926–1931 (2005)
N. Hagemeister, L. Yahia, N. Duval, J. de Guise, In vivo reproducibility of a new non-invasive diagnostic tool for three-dimensional knee evaluation. The Knee **6**(3), 175–181 (1999)
A. Hreljac, R.N. Marshall, Algorithms to determine event timing during normal walking using kinematic data. J. Biomech. **33**(6), 783–786 (2000)
J. Johnson, T. Khoshgoftaar, Survey on deep learning with class imbalance. J. Big Data **6**, 27 (2019)
R.A. Johnson, *Applied Multivariate Statistical Analysis* (Prentice Hall, Upper Saddle River, 1998)
M.P. Kadaba, H.K. Ramakrishnan, M.E. Wootten, J. Gainey, G. Gorton, G.V.B. Cochran, Repeatability of kinematic, kinetic, and electromyographic data in normal adult gait. J. Orthop. Res. **7**(6), 849–860 (1989)
T.K. Koo, M.Y. Li, A guideline of selecting and reporting intraclass correlation coefficients for reliability research. J. Chiropr. Med. **15**(2), 155–163 (2016)
B. Krawczyk, Learning from imbalanced data: open challenges and future directions. Prog. Artif. Intell. **5**, 221–232 (2016)
D.R. Labbe, N. Hagemeister, M. Tremblay, J. de Guise, Reliability of a method for analyzing three-dimensional knee kinematics during gait. Gait & Posture **28**(1), 170–174 (2008)
Y. LeCun, Y. Bengio, *The Handbook of Brain Theory and Neural Networks*, M.A. Arbib ed. by (MIT Press, Cambridge, 1998), pp. 255–258
Y. LeCun, Y. Bengio, G. Hinton, Deep learning. Nature **512**, 436–444 (2015)
Y. Lecun, L. Bottou, Y. Bengio, P. Haffner, Gradient-based learning applied to document recognition, in *Proceedings of the IEEE* (1998), pp. 2278–2324
Y.A. LeCun, L. Bottou, G.B. Orr, K.-R. Müller, Efficient backprop, in *Neural Networks: Tricks of the Trade: Second edition*, ed. by G. Montavon, G.B. Orr, K.-R. Müller (Springer, Berlin/Heidelberg, 2012), pp. 9–48
A. Le Guennec, S. Malinowski, R. Tavenard, Data augmentation for time series classification using convolutional neural networks, in *ECML/PKDD Workshop on Advanced Analytics and Learning on Temporal Data*, Riva Del Garda (2016)
M.W. Lenhoff, T.J. Santner, J.C. Otis, M.G. Peterson, Bootstrap prediction and confidence bands: a superior statistical method for analysis of gait data. Gait Posture **9**, 10–7 (1999)
G. Leporace, L.A. Batista, A.M. Muniz, G. Zeitoune, T. Luciano, L. Metsavaht, J. Nadal, Classification of gait kinematics of anterior cruciate ligament reconstructed subjects using principal

component analysis and regressions modelling, in *2012 Annual International Conference of the IEEE Engineering in Medicine and Biology Society* (2012), pp. 6514–6517
Y. Li, R. Aissaoui, K. Boivin, K. Turcot, N. Duval, A. Roy, R. Pontbriand, N. Hagemeister, J.A. de Guise, Development of a tool for analyzing 3d knee kinematic characteristics of different daily activities, in *2005 IEEE Engineering in Medicine and Biology 27th Annual Conference*, Shanghai, 2005, pp. 7451–7454
L. Li, K. Jamieson, G. DeSalvo, A. Rostamizadeh, A. Talwalkar, Hyperband: A novel bandit-based approach to hyperparameter optimization (2016)
S. Lustig, R.A. Magnussen, L. Cheze, P. Neyret, The kneekg system: a review of the literature. Knee Surg. Sports Traumatol. Arthrosc. **20**(4), 633–638 (2012)
K. Mcgraw, S. Wong, Forming inferences about some intraclass correlation coefficients. Psychol. Methods **1**, 30–46 (1996)
I. Mechmeche, A. Mitiche, Y. Ouakrim, J.A.D. Guise, N. Mezghani, Data correction to determine a representative pattern of a set of 3D knee kinematic measurements, in *2016 38th Annual International Conference of the IEEE Engineering in Medicine and Biology Society (EMBC)* (2016), pp. 884–887
V. Medved, *Measurement of Human Locomotion* (CRC Press, Hoboken, 2000)
N. Mezghani, A. Fuentes, N. Gaudrealt, A. Mitiche, R. Aissaoui, N. Hagmeister, J.A. De Guise, Identification of knee frontal plane kinematic patterns in normal gait by pricipal component analysis. J. Mech. Med. Biol. **13**(03), 1350026 (2013)
N. Mezghani, N. Gaudreault, L. Mitiche, A. Ayoubian, Y. Ouakrim, N. Hagemeister, J.A. De Guise, Kinematic gait analysis of workers exposed to knee straining postures by bayes decision rule. Artif. Intell. **4**(2), 106–111 (2015)
N. Mezghani, M. Dunbar, Y. Ouakrim, A. Fuentes, A. Mitiche, S. Whynot, G. Richardson, Biomechanical signal classification of surgical and non-surgical candidates for knee arthroplasty, in *2016 International Symposium on Signal, Image, Video and Communications (ISIVC)* (2016a), pp. 287–290
N. Mezghani, Y. Ouakrim, A. Fuentes, A. Mitiche, N. Hagmeister, P. Venditolli, J. Guise, Severity grading mechanical biomarkers of knee osteoarthritis. Osteoarthr. Cartil. **24**, S125–S126 (2016b)
N. Mezghani, I. Mechmeche, A. Mitiche, Y. Ouakrim, J. de Guise, An analysis of 3D knee kinematic data complexity in knee osteoarthritis and asymptomatic controls. PLoS ONE **13**, e0202348 (2018)
N. Mezghani, Y. Ouakrim, A. Fuentes, N. Hagemeister, R. Aissaoui, M. Pelletier, J. de Guise, Knee osteoarthritis severity assessment using knee kinematic data classification. Osteoarthr. Cartil. **20**, S97 (2012)
N. Mezghani, Y. Ouakrim, A. Fuentes, A. Mitiche, N. Hagemeister, P.-A. Vendittoli, J. de Guise, Mechanical biomarkers of medial compartment knee osteoarthritis diagnosis and severity grading: discovery phase. J. Biomech. **52**, 106–112 (2018)
C.M. O'Connor, S.K. Thorpe, M.J. O'Malley, C.L. Vaughan, Automatic detection of gait events using kinematic data. Gait Posture **25**(3), 469–474 (2007)
Y. Ouakrim, Classification de sujets asymptomatiques et gonarthrosiques en fonction des données cinématiques: comparaison de l'approche globale et de l'approche locale (Mémoire de maîtrise électronique). École de technologie supérieure, Montréal (2011)
A. Phinyomark, S. Osis, R. Ferber, Analysis of big data in running biomechanics: application of multivariate analysis and machine learning methods. CMBES in Proc. of the 39th Canadian Medical and Biological Engineering Conf., Calgary, Canada, pp. 1–4 (2016)
J. Røislien, O. Skare, A. Opheim, L. Rennie, Evaluating the properties of the coefficient of multiple correlation (cmc) for kinematic gait data. J. Biomech. **45**(11), 2014–2018 (2012)
M. Sati, J. de Guise, S. Larouche, G. Drouin, Improving in vivo knee kinematic measurements: application to prosthetic ligament analysis. The Knee **3**(4), 179–190 (1996)
J. Serrà, S. Pascual, A. Karatzoglou, Towards a universal neural network encoder for time series. In Ccia (2018)

L. Sharma, J. Song, D.T. Felson, S. Cahue, E. Shamiyeh, D.D. Dunlop, The role of knee alignment in disease progression and functional decline in knee osteoarthritis. JAMA **286**(2), 188–195 (2001)

L.F. Teixeira, S.J. Olney, Relationship between alignment and kinematic and kinetic measures of the knee of osteoarthritic elderly subjects in level walking. Clin. Biomech. **11**(3), 126–134 (1996)

Z. Wang, W. Yan, T. Oates, Time series classification from scratch with deep neural networks: a strong baseline, in *2017 International Joint Conference on Neural Networks (IJCNN)* (2017), pp. 1578–1585

B. Yu, T. Kienbacher, E.S. Growney, M.E. Johnson, K.-N. An, Reproducibility of the kinematics and kinetics of the lower extremity during normal stair-climbing. J. Orthop. Res. **15**(3), 348–352 (1997)

J.A. Zeni, J.G. Richards, J.S. Higginson, Two simple methods for determining gait events during treadmill and overground walking using kinematic data. Gait Posture **27**(4), 710–4 (2008)

F. Zgolli, K. Henni, R. Haddad, A. Mitiche, Y. Ouakrim, N. Hagemeister, P-A. Venditolli, A. Fuentes, N. Mezghani, Kinematic data clustering for healthy knee gait characterization, in *2018 IEEE Life Sciences Conference* (LSC) (2018), pp. 239–242

B. Zhao, H. Lu, S. Chen, J. Liu, D. Wu, Convolutional neural networks for time series classification. J. Syst. Eng. Electron. **28**(1), 162–169 (2017)

B. Zhou, A. Khosla, A. Lapedriza, A. Oliva, A. Torralba, Learning deep features for discriminative localization, in *2016 IEEE Conference on Computer Vision and Pattern Recognition (CVPR)* (2016), pp. 2921–2929

Chapter 3
Nonlinear Smoothing of Core Body Temperature Data with Random Gaps and Outliers (DRAGO)

A. Parekh, I. W. Selesnick, A. Baroni, O. M. Bubu, A. W. Varga, D. M. Rapoport, I. Ayappa, E. M. Blessing, and R. S. Osorio

3.1 Introduction

Circadian rhythms are physiologic and behavioral cycles with a period of approximately 24 h in healthy individuals (Zee et al. 2013). These physiologic and behavioral cycles are generated by the endogenous biological pacemacker, the suprachiasmatic nucleus (SCN), located in the anterior hypothalamus (Golombek and Rosenstein 2010). The biological processes of sleep-wake cycle and body temperature follow in sync by the circadian rhythms, and alterations in these rhythms can lead to circadian rhythm disorders such as an irregular sleep-wake rhythm disorder, which is prevalent in subjects with traumatic brain injury (Zee and Vitiello 2009). Moreover, circadian rhythm alterations may also be observed in neurodegenerative diseases such as Alzheimer's disease (Zee and Vitiello 2009; Skene and Swaab 2003; Dowling et al. 2008; Monk et al. 1995).

A. Parekh (✉) · A. W. Varga · D. M. Rapoport · I. Ayappa
Division of Pulmonary, Critical Care and Sleep Medicine, Department of Medicine, Icahn School of Medicine at Mount Sinai, New York, NY, USA
e-mail: ankit.parekh@mssm.edu

I. W. Selesnick
Department of Electrical and Computer Engineering, NYU Tandon School of Engineering, Brooklyn, NY, USA

A. Baroni
Child and Adolescent Psychiatry, NYU Langone Health, New York, NY, USA

O. M. Bubu · E. M. Blessing · R. S. Osorio
Department of Psychiatry, NYU Langone Health, New York, NY, USA

I. Obeid et al. (eds.), *Biomedical Signal Processing*,
https://doi.org/10.1007/978-3-030-67494-6_3

3.1.1 Measuring Core Body Temperature

Core body temperature (CBT) is considered an objective measure of the human circadian rhythm and is known to characterize their circadian phase (Wever 1975). The CBT is typically measured from either the esophagus, nasopharynx, rectum, or tympanum/auditory meatus (Fulbrook 1993). While rectal measurements of the CBT are considered to be the gold standard, compliance and duration of recording are the common challenges complicating reliable measurements. In recent years, there is a growing interest in utilizing ingestible capsules such as the CorTemp ingestible pill (CorTemp® HQ Inc., Palmetto, FL, USA.) for measuring CBT (Monnard et al. 2017). The CorTemp® ingestible pill sensor wirelessly transmits temperature measurements to a recorder worn on the waist as it travels through the digestive tract. The CBT measured using the ingestible pill has a good agreement with the rectal core body temperature, which is a gold standard method of circadian rhythm measurement (Byrne and Lim 2007; Duffy et al. 1999). Moreover, the circadian profile classically exhibited in free-living humans was also seen using CBT measured with the CorTemp pill (Monnard et al. 2017). The CBT recordings using the CorTemp pill can be extended over several days with the usage of multiple pills taken successively.

The measurement of CBT using CorTemp pill, while feasible and accurate, suffers from numerous challenges. Most noteworthy is the issue of fast "turbo" gut transit (Monnard et al. 2017): one in every five subjects discharge the pill in < 15 h after ingestion. As a result, any measurement of a roughly 24-h circadian rhythm is challenging. During sleep it has been known that homeotherms conserve energy by lowering body temperature. However, when recording CBT using the CorTemp pill during sleep, it was also reported that body movements may count for individual variations in the expected nocturnal decline of CBT (Monnard et al. 2017).

As noted before, the CorTemp pill wirelessly transmits CBT data to a waist-worn recorder. This waist-worn recorder must be in close proximity to the pill at all times. It has been reported that due to this limitation of the CorTemp pill, large temperature swings outside of normal ranges can be observed (Monnard et al. 2017). Notably, these swings were increasingly observed in subjects with abdominal adiposity (waist circumference > 100 cm). Previous studies have discarded values >2 standard deviations (SD) from the mean in a moving window to correct for these temperature swings. However, this resulted in many data points being unusable for analyses (Monnard et al. 2017). Moreover, ingestion of hot liquids also results in these temperature swings.

In addition to the noise in CBT due to physiologic changes, the CorTemp pill data also consists of noise because of the way the data is collected. The CorTemp pill data contains missing values whenever the waist-worn receiver is out of range (e.g., during showers). Furthermore, electromagnetic interference from the surroundings also impacts the CorTemp pill data resulting in outliers (spikes). The presence of random gaps and outliers in the raw CBT signal can lead to inaccurate measurements of several features of an individual's circadian rhythm, (e.g., period, mean temperature, timing of peak and nadir temperatures, etc.) (Refinetti et al.

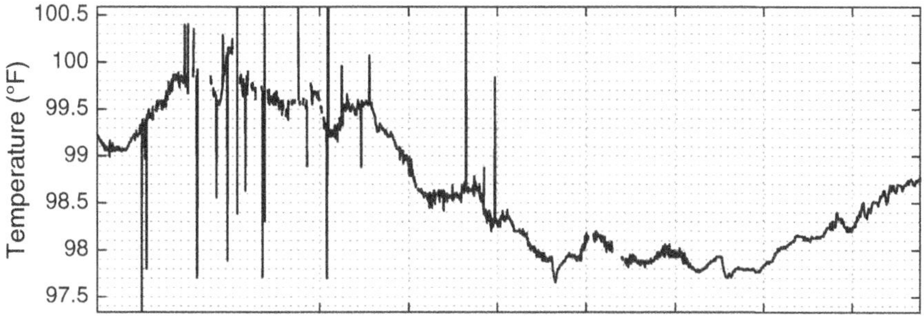

Fig. 3.1 An 18-hour segment of core body temperature (CBT) measured using the CorTemp ingestible pill. The data consists of random gaps (missing data) and outliers (spikes)

2007). As a result, it is not uncommon to either discard the entire CBT data or in some cases repeat the CBT measurements. Figure 3.1 shows an 18-hour segment of CBT data collected using CorTemp pill. Random gaps and outliers (spikes) can be seen throughout the recording. In addition, variations of < 0.05°F are constantly seen throughout the CBT data segment.

The CorTemp pill receiver allows the user to specify a sampling rate that can range from 1 sample every 10 s (0.1 Hz) to an hourly sampling rate. The higher sampling rates allow for a better temporal resolution but the resulting measurements are highly sensitive to the various forms of noise described previously. On the other hand, an hourly sampling rate does not allow for studying the micro-oscillations in the CBT. The CBT data is uniformly sampled with the prespecified sampling rate; however, the data obtained can be non-uniformly sampled as well. Notably, any interaction with the receiver to check for the temperature measurements results in the measurements being non-uniformly sampled. As an example, if the sampling rate is set to 1 sample every 10 s and if the receiver sends a signal requesting the temperature at 25 s, then the data collection resets and starts collecting 1 sample every 10 s starting at 25 s, i.e., the next 3 samples would be at 35, 45, and 55, instead of 30, 40, and 50, which would have been the case if the receiver didn't send a signal requesting the current temperature.

3.1.2 Analysis of Core Body Temperature Measurements

The CBT data is always pre-processed. The pre-processing of CBT data ensures signal integrity. Briefly, the steps involved in pre-processing are:

1. Re-gridding: As described previously, often the CBT data collected using the CorTemp pill is non-uniformly sampled. As a first step, it is often beneficial to re-grid the data to a uniformly sampled grid. Common interpolating techniques such as linear or spline interpolation can be used for re-gridding (Akima 1970).

2. Missing Data: Missing data up to a few samples, generally less than 20% of the entire duration of the signal, can be imputed based on traditional methods such as averaging, similar response pattern imputation, and maximum likelihood estimation (Enders 2010). However, most of these methods assume that the underlying data is stationary, which is not met in the case of CBT signals. Newer methods such as wavelet-lifting (Knight et al. 2012) can be used to handle missing or non-uniformly sampled data as well.
3. Outlier removal: Traditional methods for outlier removal consist of either replacing them with more moderate values (e.g., mean of few preceding samples) or treating them as missing values and imputing as above. However, if the data are not missing completely at random, which is the case for CBT data, such outliers removal techniques bias the underlying signal model.

Pre-processing of the CBT data as described above is imperative to analyze its periodicity. In addition to Fourier and Wavelet-based methods, other periodogram-based approaches involve the Lomb-Scargle periodogram (Leise 2013; Scargle 1982; Lomb 1976). The Lomb-Scargle periodogram can handle missing data as well as non-uniformly sampled data. However, in the event of outliers (spikes) which result in a sub-optimal signal-to-noise ratio, the estimates obtained by the Lomb-Scargle periodogram may not be reliable (VanderPlas 2017).

3.1.3 Contribution

In this chapter, we propose a pre-processing method for the CBT data collected using CorTemp pill. We propose a principled convex optimization based framework. The proposed framework nonlinearly smoothes the CBT data while correcting for missing data and random gaps in the data. To our knowledge, this is the first such unified framework proposed for pre-processing the CBT signal that is capable of tackling both random gaps and outliers in a single pass. We hypothesize that the proposed framework improves SNR of the CBT signal thereby leading to a better estimate of the period using the Lomb-Scargle Periodogram. It is worth noting that the proposed framework can be applied to other time-series signal that exhibit similar behavior: smooth signal with random gaps and outliers.

The rest of the chapter is organized as follows. In Sect. 3.2, we describe the preliminaries for encoding random gaps in the input signal. In Sect. 3.3, we define the signal model and an objective function for estimating the underlying smooth signal. Here we also propose an iterative algorithm using the majorization-minimization procedure and demonstrate its performance on simulated data. In Sect. 3.4, we show the utility of the proposed framework in estimating circadian rhythm using CBT data from the CorTemp ingestible pill from fully entrained cognitively normal elderly subjects.

3.2 Preliminaries

3.2.1 Notation

We denote vectors and matrices by lower and upper case letters, respectively. The N-point signal y is represented by the vector

$$y = \left[y_0, \ldots, y_{N-1}\right]^T, \qquad y \in \mathbb{R}^N, \tag{3.1}$$

where $[\cdot]^T$ represents the transpose. The ℓ_1 and ℓ_2 norm of the vector y are defined as

$$\|y\|_1 := \sum_n |y_n|, \qquad \|y\|_2 := \left(\sum_n |y_n|^2\right)^{1/2} \tag{3.2}$$

We define the second-order difference matrix D as

$$D = \begin{bmatrix} 1 & -2 & 1 & & & \\ & 1 & -2 & 1 & & \\ & & \ddots & & \ddots & \\ & & & 1 & -2 & 1 \end{bmatrix}. \tag{3.3}$$

Using the matrix D of size $(N-1) \times N$, the second-order difference of an N-point discrete signal x is given by Dx.

3.2.2 Encoding Random Gaps in the Input Signal

Suppose only K samples of an N-point input signal q are observed, where $K < N$. This is particularly true when a given signal q contains gaps that are randomly distributed or when non-uniformly sampled data is re-gridded to a uniform grid. We express the observed values $\hat{q}$ as

$$\hat{q} = Sq, \qquad \hat{q} \in \mathbb{R}^K, q \in \mathbb{R}^N, \tag{3.4}$$

where $S \in \mathbb{R}^{K \times N}$ is a sampling matrix. As an example, if only the first, second, and last elements of a 5-point signal q are observed, then the matrix S is given by

$$S = \begin{bmatrix} 1 & 0 & 0 & 0 & 0 \\ 0 & 1 & 0 & 0 & 0 \\ 0 & 0 & 0 & 0 & 1 \end{bmatrix}. \tag{3.5}$$

Note that the matrix S is deduced from the input data by simply deleting the relevant rows from an N- by-N identity matrix. For the example shown above, the third and fourth rows of a 5-by-5 identity matrix are deleted to derive the matrix S. The matrix S satisfies the properties listed below. We will use these properties throughout the paper.

1. The matrix S satisfies the following identities:

$$SS^T = I, \tag{3.6}$$

   where I is the $K \times K$ identity matrix.
2. The matrix S satisfies

$$S^T S = \text{diag}(s), \qquad s \in \mathbb{R}^N, \tag{3.7}$$

   where diag(s) denotes a diagonal matrix with s as its diagonal. For example, with S in (3.5), we have

$$S^T S = \begin{bmatrix} 1\,0\,0\,0\,0 \\ 0\,1\,0\,0\,0 \\ 0\,0\,0\,0\,0 \\ 0\,0\,0\,0\,0 \\ 0\,0\,0\,0\,1 \end{bmatrix}, \tag{3.8}$$

   which can be expressed as $S^T S = \text{diag}\,([1, 1, 0, 0, 1])$.
3. The matrix S^T represents zero-filling. As an example, for the matrix S in (3.5), we have

$$S^T y = \begin{bmatrix} 1\,0\,0 \\ 0\,1\,0 \\ 0\,0\,0 \\ 0\,0\,0 \\ 0\,0\,1 \end{bmatrix} \cdot \begin{bmatrix} y_0 \\ y_1 \\ y_2 \end{bmatrix} = \begin{bmatrix} y_0 \\ y_1 \\ 0 \\ 0 \\ y_2 \end{bmatrix}. \tag{3.9}$$

3.2.3 *Majorization-Minimization*

Majorization-minimization (MM) is an approach that is widely used to solve optimization problems which cannot be solved directly (Figueiredo et al. 2007). Here instead of minimizing the objective function, the MM approach solves a sequence of optimization problems. With $F(x)$ as the objective function, the MM approach solves $G_k(x)$, $k = 0, 1, 2, \ldots$ with the rationale that solving G is easier to solve than F. As a result, the MM approach produces a sequence x_k that is obtained by minimizing $G_{k-1}(x)$. In order to use the MM approach, at every iteration, a suitable function G_k must be specified which satisfies the following properties:

1. G_k must be convex for all k.
2. Each G_k must be a majorizer of F,

$$G_k(x) \geqslant F(x), \qquad \forall x, \tag{3.10}$$

3. G_k agrees with F at x_k

$$G_k(x_k) = F(x_k) \tag{3.11}$$

An example majorizer $G(x) = ax^2 + b$ of a convex function $F(x) = |x|$ is shown in Fig. 3.2.

The MM approach to minimize the function F can then be summarized as follows:

(a) Set $k = 0$. Initialize x_0.
(b) Choose $G_k(x)$ such that it satisfies the properties above.
(c) Set x_{k+1} as the minimizer of $G_k(x)$, i.e.,

$$x_{k+1} = \arg\min_x G_k(x) \tag{3.12}$$

(d) Set $k = k + 1$ and go to step (b)

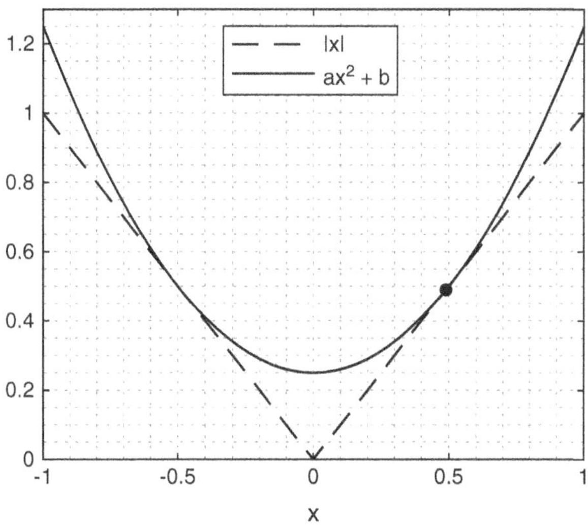

Fig. 3.2 Majorization of $f(x) = |x|$ by a quadratic function $g(x) = ax^2 + b$. Note that $g(x) \geqslant f(x)$ for all x values and $g(x) = f(x)$ for $x = 0.49$ in this example

When F is a convex function, then under mild conditions, the sequence x_k generated as result of the MM iterations convergers to the minimizer of F (see Figueiredo et al. 2007 and the references therein). Note that if the initial value of x_0 is zero, the subsequent MM iterations converge to zero. This is commonly referred to as the "zero-locking" issue. In order to prevent zero-locking, the initial value of x_0 should be set appropriately.

3.3 Nonlinear Smoothing of Data with Random Gaps and Outliers (DRAGO)

In this section, we derive the objective function for nonlinear smoothing of data with random gaps and outliers. We then proceed to derive an algorithm using the MM approach and evaluate its performance on a simulated example.

3.3.1 Problem Formulation

We assume that the underlying true CBT data is smooth, i.e., with finite energy, and that the observed smooth signal contains random gaps and outliers (spikes). To this end, let y be the N-point observed signal with random gaps and outliers in presence of additive white Gaussian noise. The signal model can then be written as

$$Sy = Sf + x + w, \tag{3.13}$$

where f is the smooth signal, x is the sparse signal representing outliers, S is the given sampling matrix, and w represents additive white Gaussian noise (AWGN) with a standard deviation of σ. The matrix S encodes the position of the gaps, and we assume it to be known. In order to estimate the underlying smooth signal f, we consider the following sparse-regularized optimization problem

$$\{\hat{f}, \hat{x}\} = \arg\min_{f,x} \left\{ F(f, x) := \frac{1}{2}\|Sy - Sf - x\|_2^2 + \frac{\lambda_1}{2}\|x\|_1 + \frac{\lambda_2}{2}\|Df\|_2^2 \right\}, \tag{3.14}$$

where λ_1 and λ_2 are the regularization parameters. The objective function in (3.14) promotes the sparsity of the signal x using the ℓ_1 norm while preserving the smoothness of f using the energy of its second-order derivative. If $x = 0$, i.e., the observed signal does not contain outliers, then the resulting optimization problem $F(f)$ reduces to a smoothing operation using least squares weighted regularization. On the other hand, if $f = 0$, i.e., the observed signal is not smooth, but is sparse and contains outliers, then the optimization problem reduces to an instance of the ℓ_1 norm regularized least squares. It is worth noting that the proposed objective function does not require the input signal to be stationary.

3.3.2 Algorithm

We derive an algorithm for the proposed objective function in (3.14) using the majorization-minimization (MM) procedure (Figueiredo et al. 2007). Note that the proposed objective function (3.14) is convex, and hence global minimum of (3.14) can be reliably obtained. As described in Sect. 3.2.3, the MM principle consists of the iteration

$$\{f^{(i+1)}, x^{(i+1)}\} = \arg\min_{f,x} F^{\mathrm{M}}(f, x; x^{(i)}), \tag{3.15}$$

where i is the iteration index and F^{M} denotes a majorizer of the objective function F. In particular, we have

$$F^{\mathrm{M}}(f, x; v) \geqslant F(f, x), \qquad \text{for all} \quad f, x, v, \tag{3.16}$$

$$F^{\mathrm{M}}(f, v; v) = F(f, v), \qquad \text{for all} \quad v. \tag{3.17}$$

We define the majorizer F^{M} as

$$\begin{aligned} F^{\mathrm{M}}(f, x; v) :=& \frac{1}{2}\|S(y-f) - x\|_2^2 + \frac{\lambda_2}{2}\|Df\|_2^2 \\ &+ \frac{\lambda_1}{2} x^T \big[W(v)\big] x, \end{aligned} \tag{3.18}$$

where $W(v)$ is a diagonal matrix defined as

$$\big[W(v)\big]_{n,n} = \frac{1}{|v_n|}. \tag{3.19}$$

To obtain the solution to (3.15), we minimize (3.15) with respect to f and x alternatively. Minimizing F^{M} with respect to x gives

$$x = \big(I + \lambda_1 [W(v)]\big)^{-1} S(y-f). \tag{3.20}$$

Equivalently,

$$x_n = \frac{1}{1 + \lambda_1 [W(v)_{n,n}]} [S(y-f)]_{n,n} \tag{3.21}$$

$$= \frac{1}{1 + \lambda_1 / |v_n|} [S(y-f)]_{n,n} \tag{3.22}$$

$$= \frac{|v_n|}{|v_n| + \lambda_1} [S(y-f)]_{n,n} \,. \tag{3.23}$$

Using (3.20) in (3.18) gives

$$F^{\mathrm{M}}(f;v) = \frac{1}{2}\|S(y-f) - \big(I + \lambda_1[W(v)]\big)^{-1}S(y-f)\|_2^2$$
$$+ \frac{\lambda_2}{2}\|Df\|_2^2 + \bigg(\frac{\lambda_1}{2}(y-f)^T S^T \big(I + \lambda_1[W(v)]\big)^{-1}$$
$$\times [W(v)]\big(I + \lambda_1[W(v)]\big)^{-1}S(y-f)\bigg), \tag{3.24}$$

which can be re-written as

$$F^{\mathrm{M}}(f;v) = \frac{1}{2}\|A_1(v)S(y-f)\|_2^2 + \frac{\lambda_2}{2}\|Df\|_2^2$$
$$+ \frac{1}{2}(y-f)^T S^T [A_2(v)]S(y-f), \tag{3.25}$$

where A_1 and A_2 are diagonal matrices defined as

$$[A_1(v)] := I - \Big(I + \lambda_1[W(v)]\Big)^{-1} \tag{3.26}$$

$$[A_2(v)] := \lambda_1\Big(I + \lambda_1[W(v)]\Big)^{-1} \times$$
$$[W(v)]\Big(I + \lambda_1[W(v)]\Big)^{-1} \tag{3.27}$$

The matrices A_1 and A_2 can be written alternatively using (3.23) as

$$[A_1(v)]_{n,n} = \frac{\lambda_1}{|v_n| + \lambda_1}, \tag{3.28}$$

$$[A_2(v)]_{n,n} = \frac{\lambda_1|v_n|}{(|v_n| + \lambda_1)^2}. \tag{3.29}$$

On the other hand, minimizing F^{M} with respect to f gives

$$f = \big[S^T([A_1(v)]^2 + [A_2(v)])S + \lambda_2 D^T D\big]^{-1}$$
$$\times S^T([A_1(v)]^2 + [A_2(v)])Sy. \tag{3.30}$$

Note that

$$[A_1(v)]_{n,n}^2 + [A_2(v)]_{n,n} = \left(\frac{\lambda_1}{|v_n| + \lambda_1}\right)^2 + \frac{\lambda_1|v_n|}{(|v_n| + \lambda_1)^2} \tag{3.31}$$

Algorithm 1 DRAGO iterative algorithm for smoothing of data with random gaps and outliers. The objective function is given in (3.14)

input: $y \in \mathbb{R}^N, \lambda_1, \lambda_2$
initialize: $x = Sy$
repeat
    $A_{n,n} = \lambda_1 / (|x_n| + \lambda_1)$
    $B = S^T A S + \lambda_2 D^T D$
    $f = B^{-1} S^T A S y$
    $x_n = |x_n| \, [S(y - f)]_n \, / \, (|x_n| + \lambda_1)$
until convergence

$$= \frac{\lambda_1}{|v_n| + \lambda_1}. \tag{3.32}$$

As a result, we have

$$f = \left(S^T [A(v)] S + \lambda_2 D^T D\right)^{-1} S^T [A(v)] S y, \tag{3.33}$$

where $[A(v)]$ is a diagonal matrix with entries

$$[A(v)]_{n,n} = \frac{\lambda_1}{|v(n) + \lambda_1|}. \tag{3.34}$$

Note that the matrix to be inverted in (3.33) is banded.[1] As a result, the equation (3.33) can be implemented efficiently.

The MM procedure (3.15) gives rise to the following iterative algorithm for smoothing of data with random gaps and outliers (DRAGO), which is also summarized in Table 1.

$$[A^{(i)}]_{n,n} = \frac{\lambda_1}{|x_n^{(i)}| + \lambda_1}, \tag{3.35a}$$

$$f^{(i+1)} = \left(S^T A^{(i)} S + \lambda_2 D^T D\right)^{-1} S^T A^{(i)} S y, \tag{3.35b}$$

$$x_n^{(i+1)} = \frac{|x_n^{(i)}|}{|x_n^{(i)}| + \lambda_1} \left[S(y - f^{(i+1)})\right]_{n,n}. \tag{3.35c}$$

[1] A banded matrix is a sparse matrix whose non-zero entries are confined to a diagonal band and zero or more diagonals on either side.

In order to avoid the zero-locking issue, wherein a chosen value for $x^{(0)}$ results in all subsequent iterations to be zero, i.e., $x_n^{i+1} = 0, i > 0$, for all$n$, we set the initial value for the iterative algorithm as $x^{(0)} = Sy$.

3.3.3 Simulated Example

We illustrate the performance of the proposed DRAGO method for smoothing data with random gaps and outliers using the following simulated example. Shown in Fig. 3.3a is the simulated data which consists of two low-frequency sinusoids that are uniformly sampled. Figure 3.3b shows the observed data y with missing data (random gaps; 45% missing) and outliers(spikes). Running the DRAGO iterative algorithm in Table 1 with y as the input results in the estimated signal f shown in Fig. 3.3c, with the input signal y shown in the background (light gray) and the error in estimation is given by root mean square error (RMSE), defined as follows:

$$\mathrm{RMSE}(x_{\mathrm{org}}, x_{\mathrm{est}}) := \frac{\|x_{\mathrm{org}} - x_{\mathrm{est}}\|_2^2}{\|x_{\mathrm{org}}\|_2^2}. \tag{3.36}$$

The estimated outliers x are shown in Fig. 3.3d and the residual $y - (x + f)$ is shown in Fig. 3.3e. It can be seen that residual does not contain any outliers or components (peaks) of the smooth signal. Further, the estimated smooth signal f is free of any random gaps or outliers.

The Lomb-Scargle power spectral density (PSD) estimate of the simulated data s is shown in Fig. 3.4a. The Lomb-Scargle PSD estimate shows prominent peaks (red circles in Fig. 3.4a) at the two fundamental frequencies of x. As noted previously, the Lomb-Scargle PSD estimate can be calculated in the presence of outliers (spikes) and random gaps (missing data). The Lomb-Scargle PSD estimate of the observed signal y without any pre-processing is shown in Fig. 3.4b. It can be seen that a false peak appears at 0.018 Hz. While it may be possible to still detect the two peaks corresponding to the fundamental frequencies of x, this example highlights the issues with using the Lomb-Scargle PSD estimate without any pre-processing. On the other hand, the DRAGO pre-processed estimate f retains the two prominent peaks at the fundamental frequencies of x while at the same time showing the attenuation at higher frequencies as observed in the Lomb-Scargle PSD estimate of the simulated data s (see Fig. 3.4c). The progression of the DRAGO iterative algorithm using the MM procedure for the input data y in Fig. 3.3a is shown in Fig. 3.5. It can be seen that the algorithm converges in about five iterations.

In order to further evaluate the robustness of the proposed DRAGO iterative algorithm, we assess its performance across various levels of (a) missing data and (b) additive white Gaussian noise (AWGN). Figure 3.6 shows the RMSE as a function of % missing data for the simulated data s in Fig. 3.3a. The error stays relatively low when up to 50% of the data is missing, beyond which the algorithm is fairly

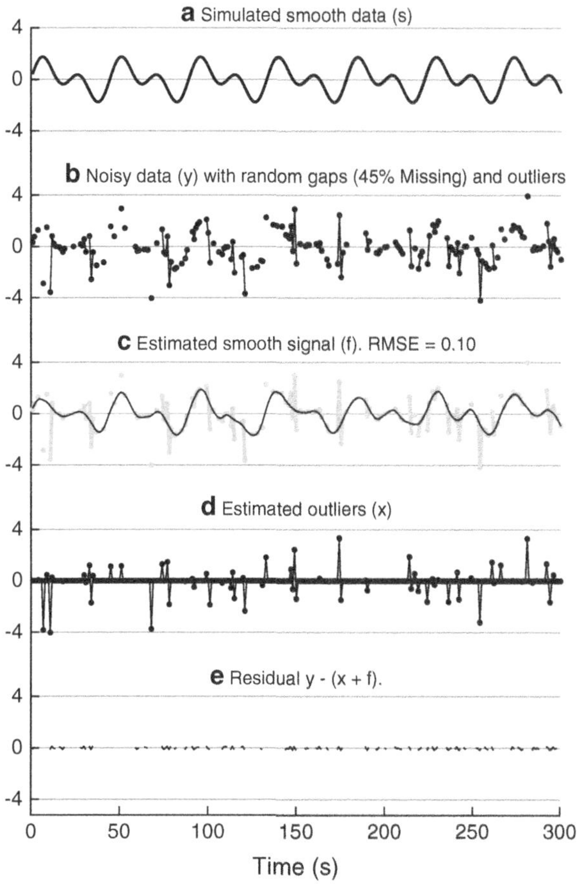

Fig. 3.3 Illustration of the proposed DRAGO method on simulated data s. The observed signal y shown in (**b**) contains missing data (random gaps) and outliers. DRAGO estimated smooth signal (f) is shown in (**c**). The outliers are shown in (**d**) with the residual values in (**e**)

unstable and the estimates cannot be obtained reliably. The noise level in this case was kept fixed at $\sigma = 0.25$.

Using the same simulated data s, we further assess the performance of the proposed DRAGO iterative algorithm across varying levels of noise. To this end, Fig. 3.7 shows the RMSE as a function of noise level σ with $0 \leqslant \sigma \leqslant 2$. Figure 3.7 shows the RMSE for several instances of the simulated data with varying percentages of missing data (0, 20, 40, and 50%). As expected, the error increases proportional to the level of noise (σ) as well as with increasing % missing data.

3.3.4 Parameter Selection

The proposed DRAGO iterative algorithm requires the selection of two regularization parameters λ_1 and λ_2. Recall that λ_1 influences the sparsity of the estimated

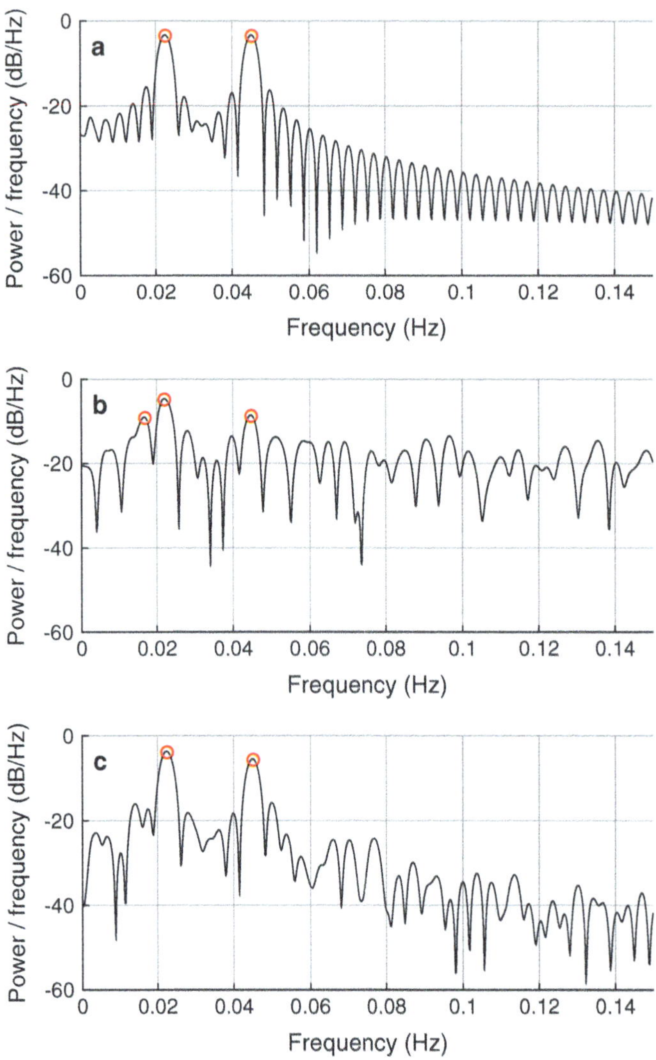

Fig. 3.4 Lomb-Scargle power spectral density estimates for the (**a**) simulated smooth data s, (**b**) noisy data y with random gaps and outliers, and (**c**) smooth signal estimate f using DRAGO. The signal s, y, and f are shown in Fig. 3.3

outliers x and λ_2 influences the smoothness of the estimate f. Here we detail a pseudo-analytic approach to set these parameters.

Consider the simpler problem wherein the input data y has no gaps or noise. In other words, we observe the underlying smooth signal with only outliers, but without random gaps or noise. Recall that in this case the matrix S, which is used to encode random gaps, reduces to the $N \times N$ identity matrix and the proposed optimization problem in (3.14) reduces to

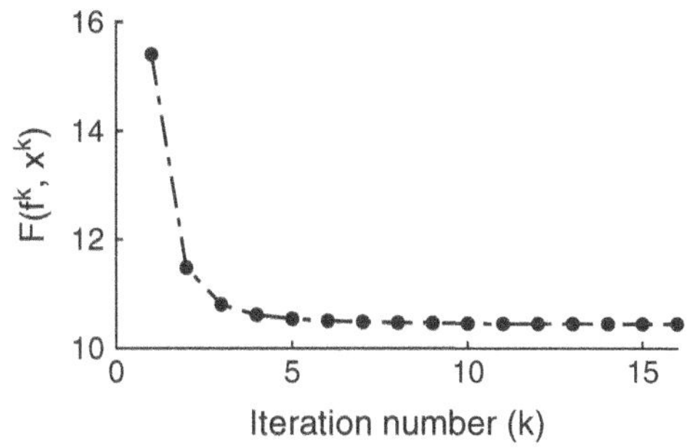

Fig. 3.5 Value of the objective function in (3.14) for every iteration using the simulated data in Fig. 3.3a as an example

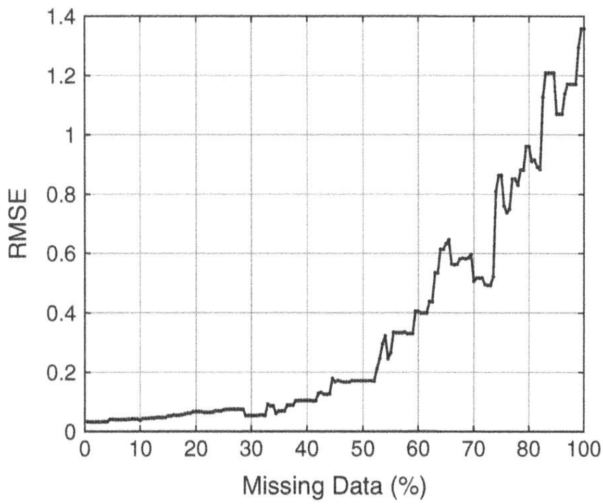

Fig. 3.6 Performance of DRAGO iterative algorithm across various levels of missing data. Shown here is the error (RMSE) as a function of % missing data for the simulated smooth data in Fig. 3.3 with $\sigma = 0.25$

$$\{\hat{f}, \hat{x}\} = \arg\min_{f,x} \left\{ F(f,x) := \frac{1}{2}\|y - f - x\|_2^2 + \frac{\lambda_1}{2}\|x\|_1 + \frac{\lambda_2}{2}\|Df\|_2^2 \right\}. \tag{3.37}$$

If the solution $\hat{f}$ were known, then $\hat{x}$ can be obtained by solving the optimization problem

$$\hat{x} = \arg\min_{x} \left\{ F_1(x) := \frac{1}{2}\|y - \hat{f} - x\|_2^2 + \frac{\lambda_1}{2}\|x\|_1 \right\}, \tag{3.38}$$

which is the sparse regularized least squares problem and whose solution is given explicitly by

$$\hat{x} = \text{soft}(y - \hat{f}, \lambda_1), \tag{3.39}$$

where soft$(\cdot, \cdot)$ is the soft-threshold function (Donoho 1995). If we assume that the solution $\hat{f}$ is sufficiently close to the true signal f, then $y - \hat{f}$ is the additive white

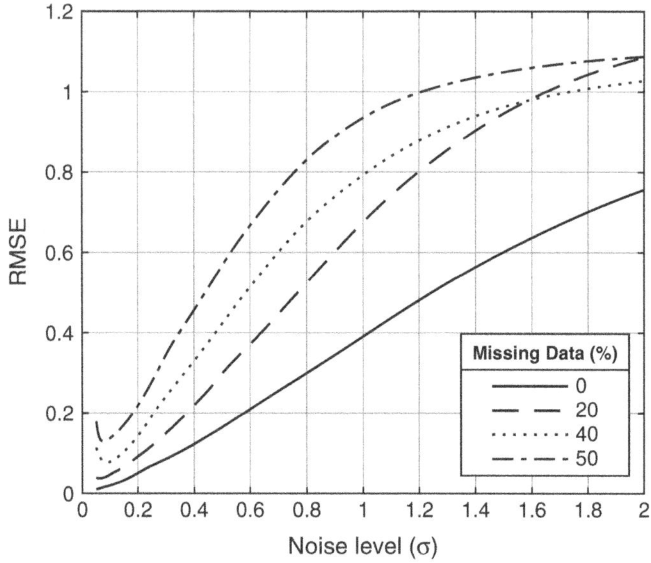

Fig. 3.7 Performance of DRAGO iterative algorithm across various levels of noise. Shown here is the error (RMSE) as a function of noise level (σ) for the simulated smooth data in Fig. 3.3. The different lines correspond to different levels of % missing data

Gaussian noise signal w. In this case, λ_1 should be chosen large enough so that $\hat{x}$ contains only true outliers. However, it should not be chosen arbitrarily large so as to exclude outliers from $\hat{x}$. As a result, it is reasonable to set λ_1 to three times the standard deviation of the noise (i.e., $\lambda_1 = 3\sigma$). Since we expect that for the additive white Gaussian noise signal with zero mean, 99.7% of the values will lie within 3σ. As a result, we suggest setting λ_1 as

$$\lambda_1 = c\sigma, \qquad c \in (2, 3). \tag{3.40}$$

In order to set λ_2, consider the simpler problem where in the observed data y does not contain any gaps or outliers. In other words, we observe a low-pass signal f with additive white Gaussian noise only. In this case, the optimization problem in (3.14) reduces to

$$\hat{f} = \arg\min_f \left\{ F_2(f) := \frac{1}{2}\|y - f\|_2^2 + \frac{\lambda_2}{2}\|Df\|_2^2 \right\}, \tag{3.41}$$

whose solution is given explicitly by

$$\hat{f} = \left(I + \lambda_2 D^T D\right)^{-1} y. \tag{3.42}$$

This solution for $\hat{f}$ can be interpreted as a linear time-invariant (LTI) filter H with a frequency response

$$H(\omega) = \frac{1}{1 + \lambda_2 |D(\omega)|^2}, \tag{3.43}$$

where $D(\omega)$ is given by

$$D(\omega) = (1 - e^{-j\omega})^2 \tag{3.44}$$

$$= -4e^{-j\omega} \sin^2(\omega/2). \tag{3.45}$$

Hence $H(\omega)$ can be written as

$$H(\omega) = \frac{1}{1 + 16\lambda_2 \sin^4(\omega/2)}. \tag{3.46}$$

The frequency response $H(\omega)$ is that of a low-pass filter with $H(0) = 1$, i.e., with a DC gain of unity. We can use this frequency response $H(\omega)$ to solve for λ_2 at some frequency ω_0. Thus, λ_2 can be expressed as

$$\lambda_2 = \frac{1}{16 \sin^4(\omega_0/4)} \left(\frac{1}{H_0 - 1} \right), \qquad H(\omega_0) = H_0. \tag{3.47}$$

As such λ_2 can be obtained using the pair (ω_0, H_0). In particular, we can set the filter so that its passband contains the spectrum (if known) of the signal f. For example, we may define the passband edge frequency as ω_p for which $H(\omega_p) = 0.98$.

Since the value of λ_2 determines the frequency response $H(\omega)$ of the filter, we propose to set λ_2 according to an appropriate choice of filter. In particular, if a segment of the input data is available, one that is not corrupted by random gaps or outliers, then this segment can be used to determine a suitable value of λ_2. In this case, we apply the low-pass filter prescribed by $H(\omega)$ to this data and vary λ_2 until the result is satisfactory (so that the output signal is smooth but not distorted).

It should be noted that the strategies described above for setting λ_1 and λ_2 make certain assumptions about the underlying signal which may not be true for real data. However, these values can be used as a starting point to then empirically set the parameters λ_1 and λ_2 so as to achieve the best estimate of the smooth signal f possible. Indeed, this was the approach used to set the regularization parameters for the simulated example in Fig. 3.3.

3.4 Estimating Circadian Rhythm Using DRAGO Processed Core Body Temperature Signal

We now illustrate the application of the DRAGO iterative algorithm for estimating circadian rhythm from raw CorTemp pill data. Figure 3.8a, c shows the raw data from two fully entrained subjects who participated in a parent study on orexin and tau pathology in cognitively normal elderly. The circadian rhythm, i.e., period of the CorTemp data, estimated using the Lomb-Scargle PSD estimate is shown in Fig. 3.9a, c for Subject 1 and 2, respectively. These subjects were fully entrained in a 24-h environment, confirmed with 7-day actigraphy, and had no complaints of circadian rhythm sleep disorders. Entrainment is defined as alignment of the circadian system to the 24-h day. As a result, these subjects are expected to demonstrate a roughly 24-h circadian rhythm. The subjects were administered the pill on the first night of their scheduled two-night in-lab polysomnography visits,

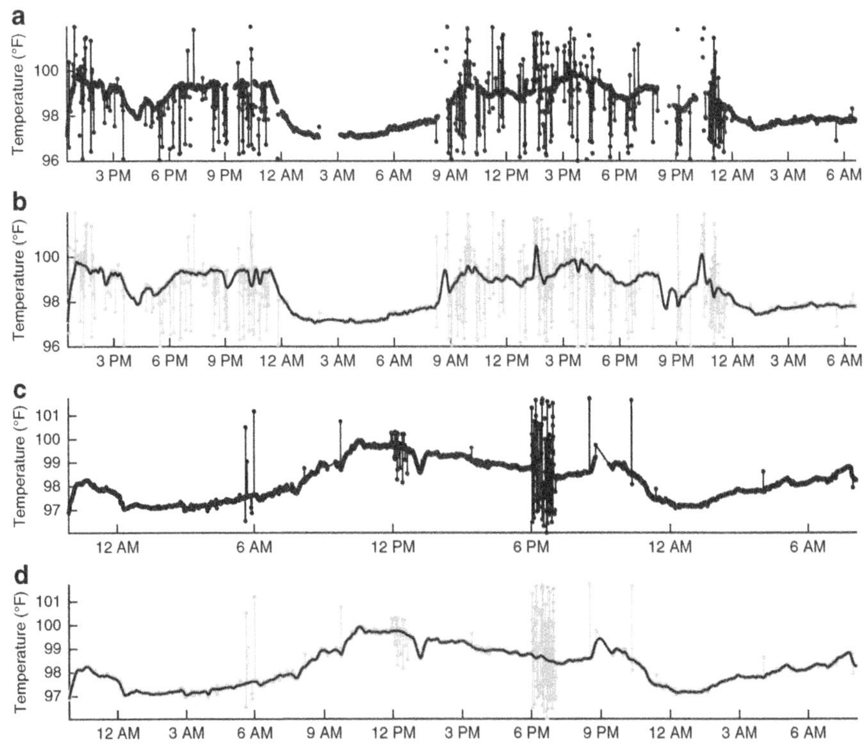

Fig. 3.8 Core body temperature data using CorTemp ingestible pill from fully entrained cognitively normal subjects is shown in (**a**) and (**c**). The DRAGO smoothed signal is shown (solid black line) in (**b**) and (**d**) for the two subjects, respectively. The gray background shows the original unprocessed signals

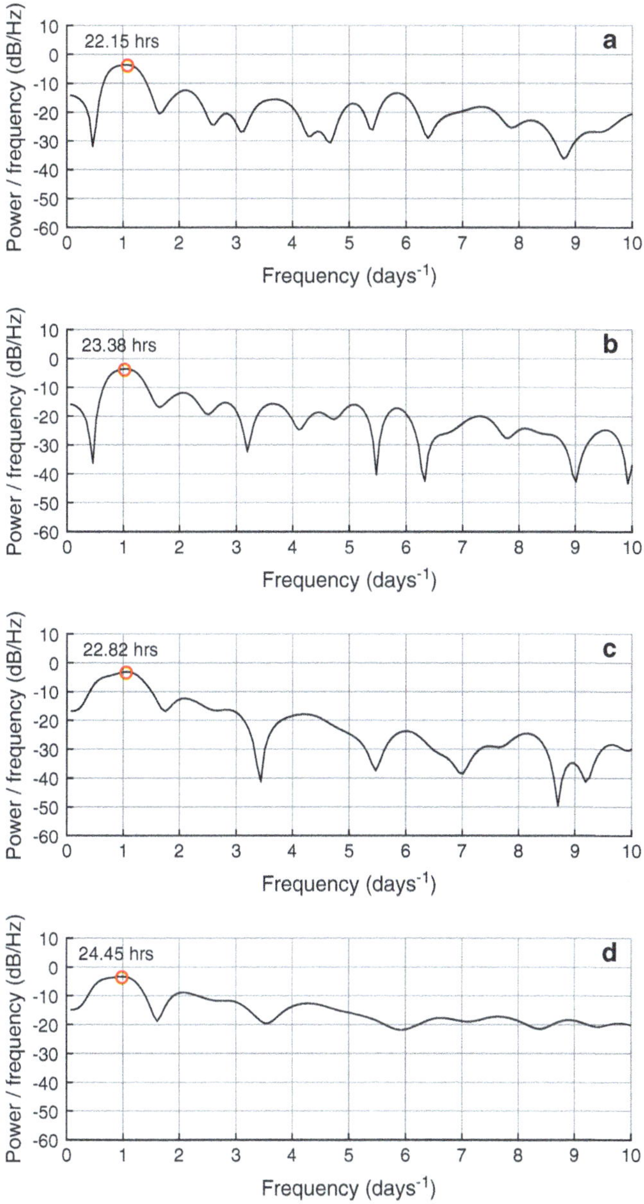

Fig. 3.9 Lomb Scargle PSD estimates for the corresponding data in Fig. 3.4. Note that the circadian rhythm calculated from the raw data in Fig. 3.4a and Fig. 3.4c is inaccurate as we expect a roughly 24-h circadian rhythm

and the data was collected until the pill was passed by the body (approx. 36–40 h). The sampling rate for the CorTemp data was fixed at 1 sample per 25 s. Note that the sampling rate is not uniform since datapoints are recorded when the subjects manually read the temperature data. All subjects signed informed consent documents, and the protocol for the study was approved by the NYU IRB and the Mount Sinai IRB.

Figure 3.8b, d shows the result of using the DRAGO iterative algorithm on the raw CorTemp data. Note that the data has been re-gridded to a sampling rate of 1 sample per second. It can be seen that the estimated smooth data contains no outliers (e.g., significant outliers in Fig. 3.8c around 6PM) and the missing data has been approximated with a smooth segment (e.g., the segment of missing data in Fig. 3.8a around 3AM on Night 1). It worth noting that estimates of the mean temperature from the smooth signal estimated using DRAGO are more accurate due to the absence of outliers. The estimated circadian rhythm using the smoothed CorTemp data for the Subjects 1 and 2 can be seen in Fig. 3.9b, d, respectively. Figure 3.6 shows the circadian rhythm estimated from the raw data and the DRAGO processed data for all the 18 subjects who participated in the parent study. It can be seen that processing the CBT signal using DRAGO provides better circadian rhythm estimates than using the raw signal alone. The DRAGO iterative algorithm takes on an average 0.67 ± 0.02 s for a CBT signal with a duration of approx. 45 h.

One of the limitations of the proposed DRAGO framework is that it requires the setting of two regularization parameters λ_1 and λ_2. For simulated data where the ground-truth is available, often the parameters are set so as to minimize the error criteria (RMSE). However, when no ground-truth data is available, a suggested method is to synthetically set a segment of raw data as missing and/or with outliers and tune the two parameters so as to obtain the lowest RMSE for that segment. We used this method for processing the CBT signals from the 18 participants shown in Fig. 3.10. In addition, as is seen often with imputation methods, when a significantly large segment of data is missing, the reconstructed signal using the proposed

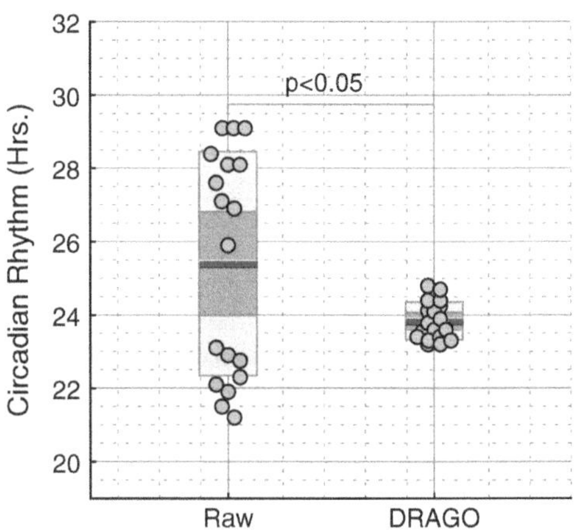

Fig. 3.10 Circadian rhythm estimates using Lomb-Scargle periodogram directly on the raw and on the DRAGO pre-processed CBT signal from N=18 participants. Median values are indicated by the solid red lines. Light colored patches represent

DRAGO framework may not be accurate. Our ongoing work is directed toward developing a theoretical framework for the setting of regularization parameters as well as deriving bounds on the length of missing data when the reconstructed signal using DRAGO may not be reliable.

3.5 Conclusion and Future Work

Ingestible pills allow feasible monitoring of core body temperature in a home-based ambulatory setting. However, the presence of random gaps and outliers hinders the assessment of circadian rhythm and its features. In this chapter we detail our principled convex optimization based framework for smoothing the core body temperature data with random gaps and outliers (DRAGO). We propose a convex objective function utilizing the sparsity of the outliers and the smoothness of the underlying signal. We derive a computationally efficient iterative algorithm using the majorization-minimization procedure and demonstrate its performance on simulated data as well as on actual data from fully entrained subjects with an expected 24-h circadian rhythm. We show that the proposed method can reliably estimate the underlying CBT signal and its features such as the period and phase.

Acknowledgments This work is partially supported by the NIH R21AG055002, R01AG056682, R21AG059179, AASM Foundation FP-199-18, BS-233-20, NSF CCF-1525398, and the Office of Postdoctoral Affairs at the Icahn School of Medicine at Mount Sinai.

References

H. Akima, A new method of interpolation and smooth curve fitting based on local procedures. J. ACM **17**(4), 589–602 (1970)

C. Byrne, C.L. Lim, The ingestible telemetric body core temperature sensor: a review of validity and exercise applications. Br. J. Sports Med. **41**(3), 126–133 (2007)

D. Donoho, De-noising by soft-thresholding. IEEE Trans. Inf. Theory **41**(3), 613–627 (1995)

G.A. Dowling, R.L. Burr, E.J. Van Someren, E.M. Hubbard, J.S. Luxenberg et al., Melatonin and bright-light treatment for rest-activity disruption in institutionalized patients with alzheimer's disease. J. Am. Geriatr. Soc. **56**(2), 239–246 (2008)

J.F. Duffy, D.J. Dijk, E.F. Hall, C.A. Czeisler, Relationship of endogenous circadian melatonin and temperature rhythms to self-reported preference for morning or evening activity in young and older people. J. Investig. Med. **47**(3), 141–50 (1999)

C.K. Enders, *Applied Missing Data Analysis* (Guilford Press, New York, 2010)

M.A.T. Figueiredo, J.M. Bioucas-Dias, R.D. Nowak, Majorization–minimization algorithms for wavelet-based image restoration. IEEE Trans. Image Process. **16**(12), 2980–2991 (2007)

P. Fulbrook, Core temperature measurement in adults: a literature review. J. Adv. Nurs. **18**(9), 1451–60 (1993)

D.A. Golombek, R.E. Rosenstein, Physiology of circadian entrainment. Physiol. Rev. **90**(3), 1063–1102 (2010)

M. Knight, M. Nunes, G. Nason, Spectral esti- mation for locally stationary time series with missing observations. Stat. Comput. **22**, 877–895 (2012)
T.L. Leise, Wavelet analysis of circadian and ultradian behavioral rhythms. J. Circadian Rhythms **11**(1), 5 (2013)
N.R. Lomb, Least-squares frequency analysis of unequally spaced data. Astrophys. Space Sci. **39**(2), 447–462 (1976)
T.H. Monk, D.J. Buysse, C.F. Reynolds, D.J. Kupfer, P.R. Houck, Circadian temperature rhythms of older people. Exp. Gerontol. **30**(5), 455–474 (1995)
C.R. Monnard, E.J. Fares, J. Calonne, J.L. Miles-Chan, J.P. Montani et al., Issues in continuous 24-h core body temperature monitoring in humans using an ingestible capsule telemetric sensor. Front Endocrinol (Lausanne) **8**, 130 (2017)
R. Refinetti, G.C. Lissen, F. Halberg, Procedures for numerical analysis of circadian rhythms. Biol. Rhythm Res. **38**(4), 275–325 (2007)
J.D. Scargle, Studies in astronomical time series analysis. II. statistical aspects of spectral analysis of unevenly spaced data. Astrophys. J. **263**, 835–853 (1982)
D.J. Skene, D.F. Swaab, Melatonin rhythmicity: effect of age and alzheimer's disease. Exp. Gerontol. **38**(1–2), 199–206 (2003)
J.T. VanderPlas, Understanding the lomb-scargle periodogram. arXiv:17030982, pp. 1–54 (2017)
R. Wever, The circadian multi-oscillatory system of man. Int. J. Chronobiol. **3**(1), 19–55 (1975)
P.C. Zee, H. Attarian, A. Videnovic, Circadian rhythm abnormalities. Continuum (Minneap Minn) **19**(1) Sleep Disorders 132–47 (2013)
P.C. Zee, M.V. Vitiello, Circadian rhythm sleep disorder: irregular sleep wake rhythm type. Sleep Med. Clin. **4**(2), 213–218 (2009)

Chapter 4
Wearable Smart Garment Devices for Passive Biomedical Monitoring

Chelsea Amanatides, Stephen Hansen, Ariana S. Levitt, Yuqiao Liu, Patrick O'Neill, Damiano Patron, Robert Ross, Daniel Schwartz, Jesse Stover, Md Abu Saleh Tajin, Genevieve Dion, Adam K. Fontecchio, Vasil Pano, William M. Mongan, and Kapil R. Dandekar

4.1 Introduction

Textile-based wearable systems have the potential to enable unobtrusive monitoring of ambulatory patients, improving Quality of life during critical care periods. Often, patients are immobilized while tethered to a medical device, increasing the risk of side effects such as bedsores, blood clots, and muscle atrophy. Wearable devices embedded in textile garments allow a patient to be monitored in specified ways and, potentially, to be actuated unobtrusively (e.g., via a noninvasive ventilator for respiratory therapy). We have developed a knitted textile antenna (Mongan et al. 2016) that deforms as the wearer moves and tunes near the 902–928 MHz Industrial, Medical, and Scientific (ISM) RFID frequency band in the United States. As RFID interrogation signals are reflected by the knitted antenna and passive RFID chip, the physical properties of the interrogation backscatter, such as the received signal strength indicator (RSSI), are perturbed in a controlled and predictable manner. We deploy biomedical sensors by fabricating knitted antenna and RFID chip assemblies on a wearable textile garment.

C. Amanatides · S. Hansen · A. S. Levitt · Y. Liu · P. O'Neill · D. Patron · R. Ross · D. Schwartz
J. Stover · Md. A. S. Tajin · G. Dion · A. K. Fontecchio · V. Pano · W. M. Mongan (✉)
K. R. Dandekar
Drexel University, Philadelphia, PA, USA
e-mail: cek56@drexel.edu; sph77@drexel.edu; ariana.sarah.levitt@drexel.edu; yl636@drexel.edu; po73@drexel.edu; des338@drexel.edu; js4677@drexel.edu; mt3223@drexel.edu; gd63@drexel.edu; af63@drexel.edu; vp93@drexel.edu; wmm24@drexel.edu; krd26@drexel.edu

I. Obeid et al. (eds.), *Biomedical Signal Processing*,
https://doi.org/10.1007/978-3-030-67494-6_4

These sensors can enable real-time, unobtrusive, passive patient monitoring in a number of settings, such as passive monitoring of uterine contractions in a pregnant woman or respiration for apnea detection in an infant. Several elements of this effort, including real-time capture, post-processing, and big data analytics of RFID data, rely on a software module to capture and store this data in real time from various hardware devices. However, this software module is dependent upon the type of chip being sensed and the type of interrogator being used. Moreover, it is necessary to compare this data to that collected by legacy medical equipment in a clinical trial setting in order to measure performance of and determine viability of the system. All of this necessitates a software framework for collecting data in real-time from heterogeneous medical devices and RFID sensors simultaneously, providing a consistent data representation for each.

RFID interrogation works by transmitting RF energy at a certain frequency to a small chip. The chip may contain a state machine capable of performing rudimentary collision avoidance to reduce the possibility that it responds at the same time as another chip, which would result in interference in the returned signal. The signal is then modulated and reflected back to the interrogator, either with the aid of an external battery source (an "active" tag), or using only the original interrogation signal as the energy source (a "passive" tag). The reflected signal modulation contains information about the chip; specifically, an identifier string is encoded into the response back to the interrogator. This chip is often embedded within an item, which enables a mapping of the identifier string to an item in space. This process is outlined in Fig. 4.4.

RFID has been used for localization or movement tracking of items in space by observing changes in the physical properties of the reflected signal energy during successive interrogations (Han et al. 2014; Nguyen et al. 2005; Yamanoi et al. 2004; Schloter 2006; Wang et al. 2017; Li et al. 2016). For example, the received signal strength indicator (RSSI) from successive interrogations may become stronger or weaker as the chip is moved closer or farther from the interrogation source. If the source or reference tags are in known locations, the movements of an RFID chip and the item to which it is attached can be tracked (Amendola et al. 2014; Montaser and Moselhi 2014; López et al. 2011; Dag and Arsan 2018; Truijens et al. 2014). In addition to observing changes in the observed signal strength of the energy reflected from the chip and received by the interrogator, changes in the phase angle (Qiu et al. 2017; López et al. 2017; Alsalih et al. 2014) and Doppler shift (Boyer 1963) have been observed for chip tracking and associated subject movements or activities.

We similarly exploit observable changes in physical backscattered signal properties to detect subject activity state. Specifically, we have knitted a smart garment "Bellyband" which embeds a small, passive RFID chip. Our aim is to detect fine movements such as respiratory patterns, uterine contractions at the abdominal wall, and electrical changes resulting from human heartbeats, by knitting an antenna around the chip that deforms as the subject moves. We will consider respiratory artifacts such as sleep apnea and respiratory rate as a case study here. For example, during inspiration, a subject's abdominal wall will expand, stretching the fabric antenna; during expiration, the knitted antenna contracts again with the abdomen or

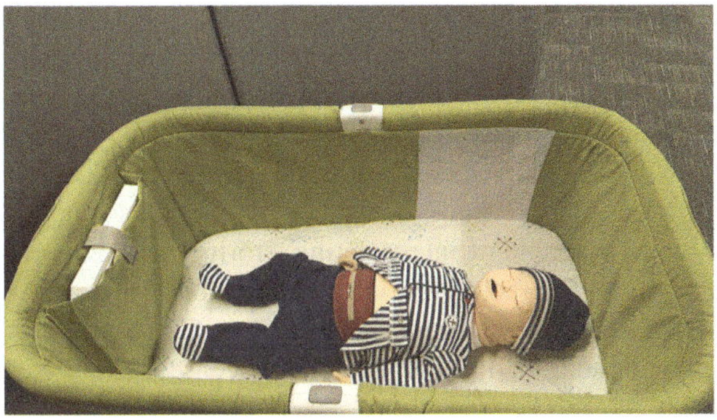

Fig. 4.1 A knitted smart-fabric Bellyband is worn about the abdominal area by a mannequin SimBaby (Laerdal), showing the knitted antenna as a gold rectangle of conductive yarn surrounding the chip in the center (O'Neill et al. 2019). ©2019 IEEE. Reprinted, with permission, from *An Adaptive Search Algorithm for Detecting Respiratory Artifacts Using a Wireless Passive Wearable Device*. IEEE Signal Processing in Medicine and Biology (SPMB)

chest wall. The antenna tunes across a frequency band during this movement, which perturbs the reflected physical signal to the interrogator. See Fig. 4.1 for an example of the Bellyband, including the knitted antenna, on a mannequin SimBaby (Laerdal).

In this chapter, we address several challenges in order to employ RFID technology for movement or activity monitoring and synthesize those solutions into an "end-to-end" system for generating, collecting, processing, and classifying signals from knitted antennas using RFID systems for biomedical applications. First, RF sheet antennas are usually made from solid conductive substrates such as copper sheets, rather than from knitted conductive materials; fabrication modeling systems must be synthesized with antenna modeling systems, and the resulting chip cannot be soldered to the antenna. The antenna must be modeled so as to mitigate signal loss due to its proximity to aqueous tissues of the human body. Commercial-off-the-shelf (COTS) RFID interrogators in the United States must comply with Federal Communication Commission (FCC) regulations that require spread-spectrum operation in the 900 MHz frequency band (U.S. Government Publishing Office 2018); this is implemented via frequency hopping, such that the interrogation frequency iterates every 200 ms over 50 channels, 500 kHz apart, between 902 and 928 MHz. Because COTS RFID interrogators are typically designed for chip inventory purposes, the repeated interrogation of those chips is intended to mitigate signal loss due to reflected interference in a dense tag environment. Unfortunately, changes in interrogation frequency perturb the observed physical properties in the backscattered signal.

Because the physical properties are perturbed as the interrogation frequency is changed, and because the tag identifier is more important in inventory applications than the RF physical attributes associated with the interrogation, the physical properties from successive tag reports are sometimes not retained in favor of merely reporting the tag identifier in each interrogation. To obtain these RF physical attributes for processing, it is necessary to configure the interrogator to send a single tag report for each interrogation, so that the physical backscatter signal properties are retained; however, this results in network inefficiencies that can push processing time beyond that conducive to real-time performance. To facilitate efficient communication with the interrogator, we have designed a software framework for communicating with heterogeneous Internet-of-Things sensor networks, including RFID-based systems, capable of interrogating, storing, processing, and communicating sensor readings for real-time classification. The software frameworks for data collection and communication,[1] and for sensor fusion and classification[2] are available on GitHub under a GPLv3 open-source license.

4.1.1 System Deployment

The Bellyband uses a Murata MAGICSTRAP RFID (Murata) chip, which we interrogate using an Impinj R420 (Impinj) RFID interrogator. We have also used an Intermec IP30 (Intermec) Bluetooth portable interrogator, an Impinj R1000 interrogator, and an Impinj XArray. The interrogator is placed at a distance from the human subject based on the FCC Maximum Permissible Exposure (MPE) of 0.6 mW/cm^2 (U.S. Government Publishing Office 2018). At our minimum separation of 50 cm and a maximum interrogation power of 1 W, the theoretical MPE is 0.03 mW/cm^2, which we confirmed via an RF power meter in the field. A minimum distance of 50 cm will limit the peak Specific Absorption Rate (SAR) below the maximum permissible 0.8 W/kg, as the SAR is 0.25 W/kg at 50 cm from a 1 W interrogator (Fiocchi et al. 2013). A software module (described in Sect. 4.3) drives the interrogator and stores or communicates sensor readings to a processing framework for classification. The workflow is summarized in Fig. 4.2, and a sample deployment can be seen in Fig. 4.3 and summarized by the block diagram in Fig. 4.4.

4.2 Functional Fabrics

We now describe two versions of the smart garment Bellyband that were produced and the design decisions that were taken into account. The first generation of the Bellyband was inductively coupled. However, in the second generation, the RFID chip is soldered on top of a PCB (printed circuit board) and inserted into a pocket, connecting two ports of the folded dipole structure.

---

[1] `iot-sensor-framework` (Mongan et al. 2020b) codebase: https://github.com/drexelwireless/iot-sensor-framework.

[2] `iot-processing-framework` (Mongan et al. 2020a) codebase: https://github.com/drexelwireless/iot-processing-framework.

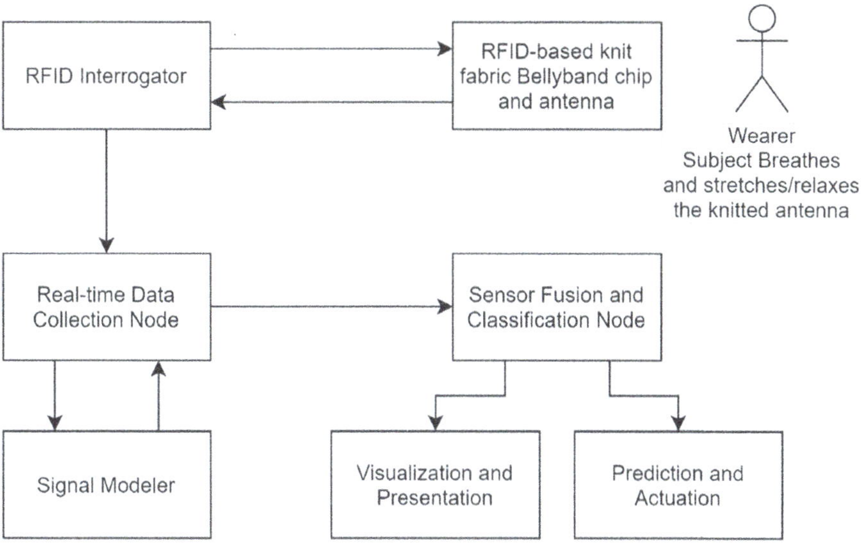

Fig. 4.2 A system-level block diagram of a deployed wearable RFID-based system. The subject wears a knitted fabric Bellyband (which could be unobtrusively integrated as part of a traditional garment), which responds to interrogations from an RFID interrogation antenna and stores data in a storage node for processing and classification. The results of this processing can be visualized, communicated to a predictive module, or forwarded for medical advice or for just-in-time wearable actuation therapy

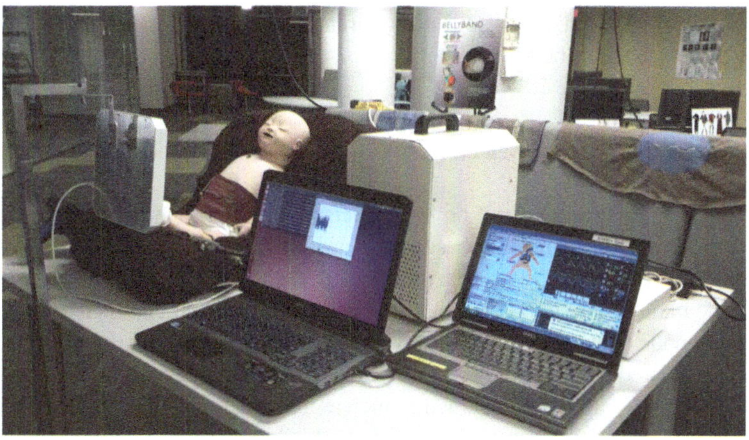

Fig. 4.3 A square RFID interrogator interrogates a knitted smart-fabric Bellyband (including an embedded passive RFID chip) with a respiratory visualization plot on the middle laptop screen (Patron et al. 2016). The laptop on the right and air compressor at the rear are used to control the SimBaby mannequin to create ground-truth respiratory movements for passive wireless monitoring. (©2016 IEEE. Reprinted, with permission, from *On the Use of Knitted Antennas and Inductively Coupled RFID Tags for Wearable Applications*. IEEE Transactions on Biomedical Circuits and Systems)

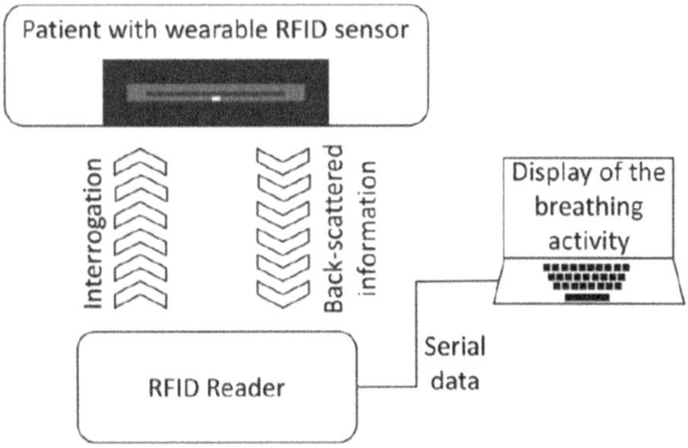

Fig. 4.4 Block diagram of the RFID interrogator system. The RFID reader antenna powers up the sensor over the air. The sensor replies to the reader in terms of RSSI. The continuous stretching and relaxation of the wearable sensor causes the RSSI to fluctuate over time (Patron et al. 2016). (©2016 IEEE. Reprinted, with permission, from *On the Use of Knitted Antennas and Inductively Coupled RFID Tags for Wearable Applications*. IEEE Transactions on Biomedical Circuits and Systems)

4.2.1 First Generation Knitted Antenna: Initial Prototype

The design procedure of the knitted strain sensor includes the selection of conductive and non-conductive yarns, the RFID chip/transponder, and the RF design (Patron et al. 2016). The design parameters for the first generation knitted antenna are now described.

4.2.1.1 Fabric Material Selection

The knitted antenna consists of both conductive and non-conductive knitted yarns. Since the sensing is performed based on periodic cycles of stretch and relaxation, it is imperative that the final structure would be flexible and comfortable to the user while maintaining good electrical performance. The non-conductive part of the antenna is made from a mix of wool and lycra yarn, and the conductive part is knitted with silver-coated nylon yarn. A polyethylene foam is used as a substrate support for non-human body-based measurements, such as a mannequin SimBaby (described in Sect. 4.5.1). The relative permittivity of the polyethylene form and the mix of wool and lycra is 1.2 and 1.5, respectively (both close to the relative permittivity of air, 1). Their loss tangents are 0.01 and 0.03, respectively, which is relatively low. The conductivity of the knitted fabric is dependent on the direction of the current flow in the fabric, knitting geometry, and loop density (Locher et al. 2006). The knitted antenna is washable and provides system level electrostatic discharge protection.

4.2.1.2 RFID Chip Selection

Unlike metal sheets, knitted conductive fabric cannot tolerate soldering. As a result, the seamless integration of RFID chip (with metal pads) and knitted fabric becomes a challenging task. On the other hand, the use of conductive epoxy and other solid compounds negatively affects the flexibility of the antenna. In this section, a novel approach is proposed to connect the RFID chip to the fabric antenna. A 2-port RFID chip (Murata MAGICSTRAP) Murata is inserted into a small pocket that enables the antenna ports to be inductively coupled to the chip pads. The advantage of this scheme is twofold. First, there is no need for soldering or conductive epoxy. Second, when the antenna is stretched, the distance between the antenna ports and the chip pads increases, resulting in a weaker coupling. The weakened coupling teams up with the impedance mismatch caused by the stretching and results in a higher degree of fluctuation (i.e., a greater dynamic range) in RSSI, which is convenient for the sensing purpose. The input impedance of the RFID chip is $25 - j200\ \Omega$. The negative reactance (capacitive) of the RFID chip plays an important role in the antenna design selection for conjugate matching.

4.2.1.3 Antenna Design

According to the theory of maximum power transfer, maximum power will be delivered when the input impedance of the antenna is the complex conjugate of the chip input impedance. Since the chip impedance is $25 - j200\ \Omega$, the antenna impedance is aimed to be $25 + j200\ \Omega$. A folded dipole structure is knitted that serves as the strain sensor antenna. The loop structure aims to achieve the inductive reactance needed for conjugate match impedance. The textile antenna is manufactured using fully automated industrial knitting machines. The antenna design is imported into the 2D software tool, then knitted in a single piece of fabric incorporating conductive and non-conductive yarns, a pocket for the RFID chip, and the rest of the surrounding structure required for use as a garment.

After selecting the antenna design, a simulation model is created. While conventional metal sheets (e.g., copper, silver, aluminum, etc.) can be easily modeled with electromagnetic simulators, the knitted fabrics pose new challenges in terms of electrical characteristics. Metal-coated yarns form loops to provide flexibility, leading to rough surface and irregular coating profile. The sheet conductivity of a knitted antenna highly depends from the density of the knitted loops. Furthermore, at high frequencies the skin depth of knitted fabrics is harder to model. To simplify the simulation process, complex sheet impedance is assigned to a 2D structure that resembles the conductive layout. The real part of the sheet resistance accounts for the ohmic losses in the structure, and the imaginary part is related to the antenna reactance. A parametric modeling of the sheet impedance may be necessary to fit the simulation model to the measured characteristics. Figure 4.5 shows the simulation of the knitted antenna in HFSS (High Frequency Structure Simulator) at 870 MHz.

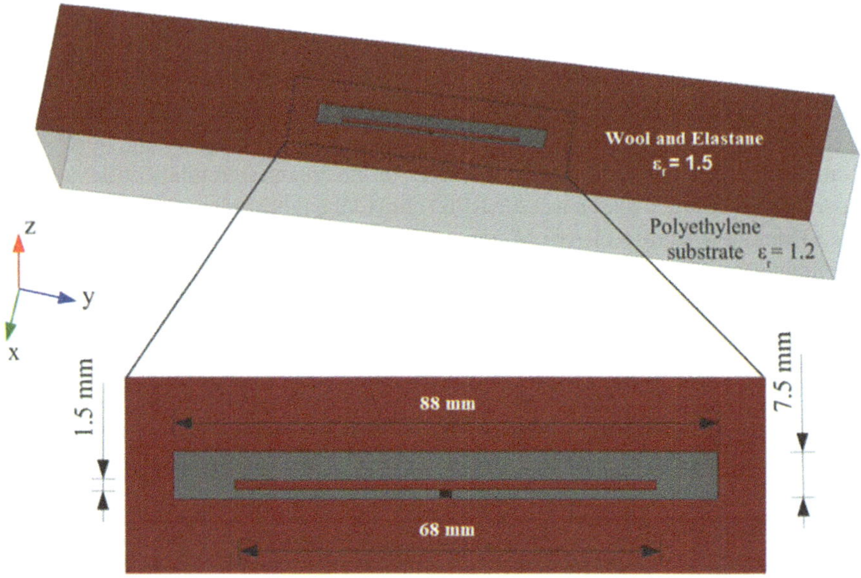

Fig. 4.5 HFSS simulation of the wearable knitted strain sensor. Instead of a standard 50 Ohm impedance, a lumped port with an impedance $Z_c = 25 - j200\ \Omega$ is used to design the RFID chip (Patron et al. 2016). (©2016 IEEE. Reprinted, with permission, from *On the Use of Knitted Antennas and Inductively Coupled RFID Tags for Wearable Applications*. IEEE Transactions on Biomedical Circuits and Systems)

The outer dimension of the antenna is 88 mm × 7.5 mm, with a 68 mm × 1.5 mm slot made from non-conductive fabric.

The return loss (S_{11}) of the antenna shows the range of tuning between the antenna and the RFID chip. Since antenna feed port is balanced, the return loss is measured with a differential RF probe (Fig. 4.8),

$$S_{11} = 10\ \log_{10}\left(1 - \frac{4R_aR_c}{|Z_a + Z_c|^2}\right) \tag{4.1}$$

where Z_a (Fig. 4.6), Z_c, R_a, and R_c indicate the antenna impedance, chip impedance, real part of the antenna impedance, and real part of the chip impedance.

The simulated return loss (Fig. 4.7) shows that the 10 dB bandwidth ranges from 870 to 915 MHz, covering most of the relevant ISM (Industrial, Scientific, and Medical) band 865–928 MHz. Additionally, the radiation pattern is omnidirectional, as expected by design (Fig. 4.8).

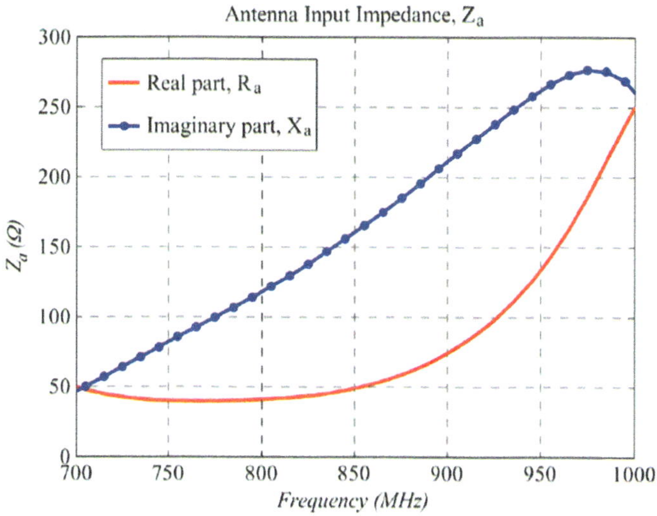

Fig. 4.6 Simulated input impedance *vs.* frequency plot with real and imaginary parts (Patron et al. 2016). (©2016 IEEE. Reprinted, with permission, from *On the Use of Knitted Antennas and Inductively Coupled RFID Tags for Wearable Applications*. IEEE Transactions on Biomedical Circuits and Systems)

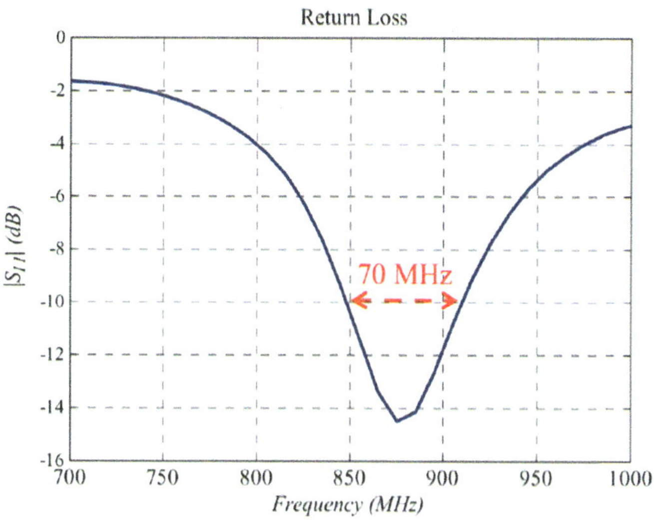

Fig. 4.7 Simulation of the return loss using equation 4.1 (Patron et al. 2016). (©2016 IEEE. Reprinted, with permission, from *On the Use of Knitted Antennas and Inductively Coupled RFID Tags for Wearable Applications*. IEEE Transactions on Biomedical Circuits and Systems)

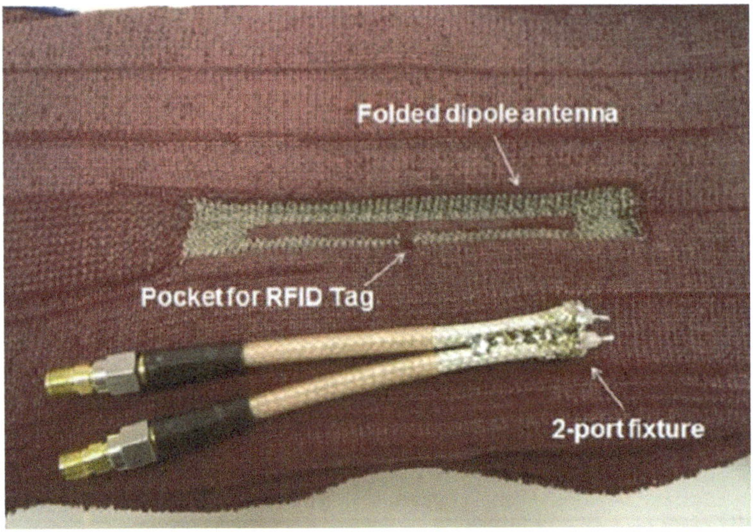

Fig. 4.8 Differential probe and knitted dipole antenna prototype (Patron et al. 2016). (©2016 IEEE. Reprinted, with permission, from *On the Use of Knitted Antennas and Inductively Coupled RFID Tags for Wearable Applications*. IEEE Transactions on Biomedical Circuits and Systems)

4.2.2 Second Generation Knitted Antenna: Improved Design Liu et al. (2016)

In the design of the first generational of the wearable strain sensor, inductively feeding method was used in order to avoiding physically soldering the RFID chip to the antenna arms. However, the coupling technology required less than 10 μm spacing between the chip pads and antenna arms, therefore, was proved to be difficult to control during fabrication.

The second version of design solves the coupling problem faced by previous versions of the strain sensor antenna by soldering the tag chip onto a small and thin Printed Circuit Board (PCB) ($10 \times 10\,mm^2$). Copper pads have been wrapped around the sides of the PCB or FPC to improve coupling. Conductive yarns are knitted into each side edge of a non-conductive pocket knit from elasticated yarn. This provides a compression-based connection between the conductive yarns and the RFID chip. The PCB or FPC is then inserted into an integrated pocket within the knit antenna. Conductive yarns are knitted into the pocket using tuck stitches, stitches produced when a knitting needle holds an original loop while receiving a new one, to improve the connection between the antenna arms and the RFID chip. The Bellyband is designed such that during the stretching of the antenna, the transmission coefficient and radiation efficiency significantly increase or decrease simultaneously. By designing an antenna with higher efficiency and good matching while it is being stretched and lower efficiency and poor matching while at rest, the

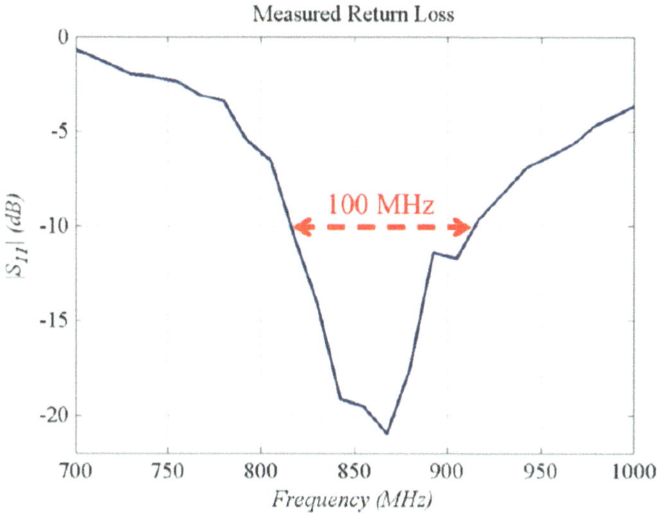

Fig. 4.9 Measured return loss of the folded dipole prototype (Patron et al. 2016). (©2016 IEEE. Reprinted, with permission, from *On the Use of Knitted Antennas and Inductively Coupled RFID Tags for Wearable Applications*. IEEE Transactions on Biomedical Circuits and Systems)

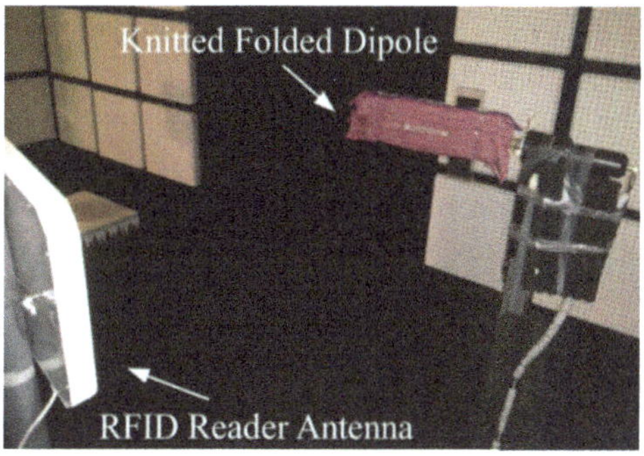

Fig. 4.10 Directional RFID reader antenna connected to Impinj Speedway reader and knitted folded dipole antenna with MAGICSTRAP tag attached to a 3D positioner (Patron et al. 2016). (©2016 IEEE. Reprinted, with permission, from *On the Use of Knitted Antennas and Inductively Coupled RFID Tags for Wearable Applications*. IEEE Transactions on Biomedical Circuits and Systems)

RSSI value will change according to the following equation (Liu et al. 2016):

$$RSSI = f(P_t, d)G_{\text{tag}}(1 - |S_{11}|^2) \tag{4.2}$$

where P_t is the transmitted power from the reader antenna, d is the distance from the reader antenna to the tag, G_{tag} is the tag gain, and S_{11} is the reflection coefficient defined in equation 4.1. $f(P_t, d)$ is a nonlinear function of the distance between the

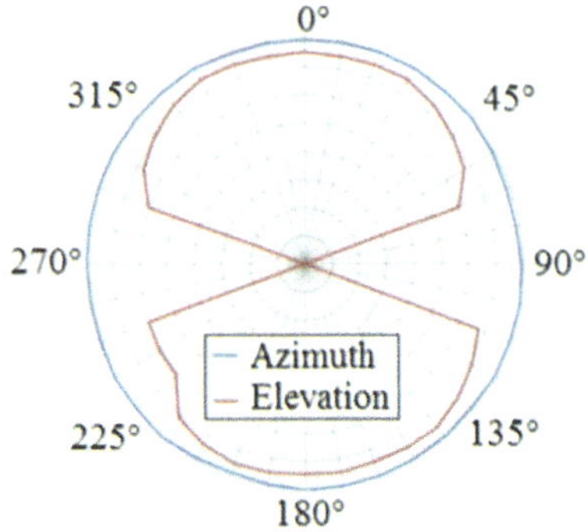

Fig. 4.11 Measured radiation pattern of the knitted folded dipole along the azimuth and elevation planes (Patron et al. 2016). (©2016 IEEE. Reprinted, with permission, from *On the Use of Knitted Antennas and Inductively Coupled RFID Tags for Wearable Applications*. IEEE Transactions on Biomedical Circuits and Systems)

reader and tag (d) and transmitted power (P_t). $f(P_t, d)$ is dependent on the RFID chip manufacturer. It can be obtained using the datasheet of the chip.

Due to the complexity of knit smart textiles arising from variables including yarn material properties and fabric properties such as stretch and relaxation, the sheet impedance is determined through a series of parametric simulations and compared with a measured prototype. The optimal sheet impedance value is $Z_s = 0.8 + j1.8\Omega/sq$. The dimension of the antenna is tuned for conjugated matching with the complex input impedance of Murata MAGICSTRAP $Z_c = 25 - j200\Omega$, while considering the radiation efficiency. Figure 4.12 shows the 3D antenna HFSS model for numerical simulations. In the stretching condition with good impedance matching and radiation efficiency, the outer dimension of the optimized antenna is $W = 30$ mm and $L = 100$ mm, while the internal slot dimension is $W_{\text{slot}} = 2$ mm and $L_{\text{slot}} = 25$ mm, as shown in Fig 6. When the antenna is at rest, the outer dimension is $W = 30$ mm and $L = 80$ mm, while the internal slot dimension is $W_{\text{slot}} = 2$ mm and $L_{\text{slot}} = 20$ mm. This results in larger return loss, lower radiation efficiency, and lower gain (Fig. 4.9).

4.2.2.1 Characteristics of Improved Bellyband

The antenna is first knitted with a PCB alone (without an RFID chip) to measure the reflection coefficient and radiation pattern using a vector network analyzer. Figure 4.13 demonstrates both the simulated reflection coefficient and measured results. While the antenna is being stretched, simulated, and measured, results match very well. Both show the return loss is lower than −8 dB within the UHF RFID band. At rest, we observe the frequency shift of the return loss curves, resulting in lower RSSI. However, simulated and measured results do not match as well because the sheet impedance of the knitted yarns is also a function of frequency and antenna size. Figure 4.14 demonstrates the radiation pattern of the antenna. The gain G_{tag} is

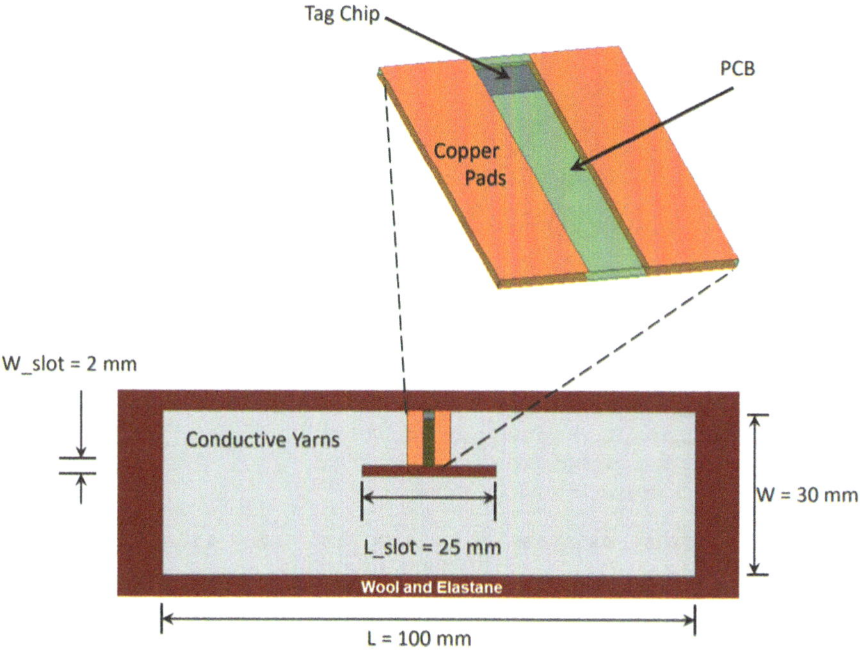

Fig. 4.12 Dimension when stretching with PCB in the pocket of improved Knitted antenna (Liu et al. 2016). (©2016 IEEE. Reprinted, with permission, from *An improved design of wearable strain sensor based on knitted RFID technology*, 2016 IEEE Conference on Antenna Measurements & Applications (CAMA))

about 3 dB greater in stretching condition than in the rest condition. The Bellyband antenna is then knitted with an RFID chip soldered onto the PCB. By using an Impinj Speedway RAIN RFID Reader, the variation of maximum RSSI value is verified and the maximum reading range is measured. Reader antenna is placed 3 feet away from the tag antenna. Figure 4.15 shows the measurement results of RSSI change *vs.* the change of antenna length L. Due to the contribution of both radiation efficiency (antenna gain) and impedance matching condition (reflection coefficient or return loss), RSSI changes from −58 to −48 dBm when stretched. The tag sensitivity to length change is about 1 dB/mm. The maximum reading range is up to 13 feet in the Line of Sight (LOS) indoor environment.

4.2.3 Antenna Characteristics

The folded dipole is a balanced structure, while the coaxial cable is an unbalanced feed. As a result, the conventional S-parameters do not apply. A differential probe (Fig. 4.8) is used to determine the input impedance of the balanced folded dipole antenna using Equation 4.3:

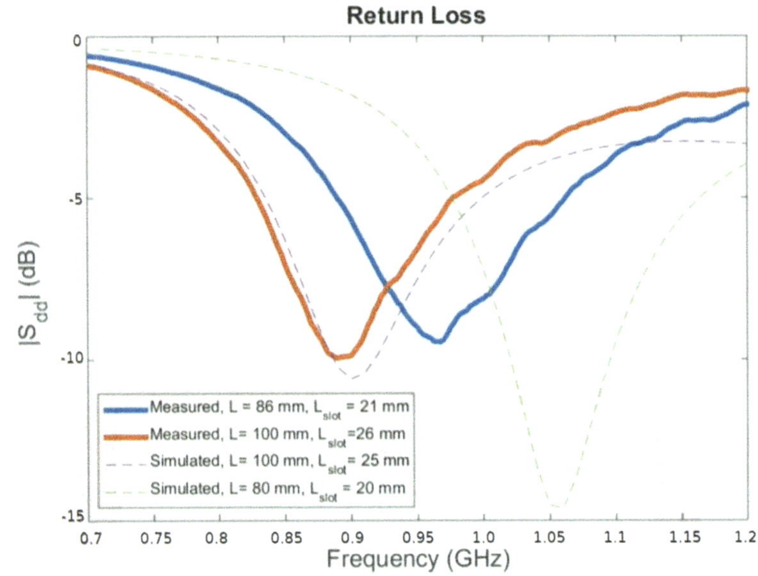

Fig. 4.13 Comparison of measured and simulated Reflection Coefficient *vs.* frequency when stretching and at rest (Liu et al. 2016). (©2016 IEEE. Reprinted, with permission, from *An improved design of wearable strain sensor based on knitted RFID technology,* 2016 IEEE Conference on Antenna Measurements & Applications (CAMA))

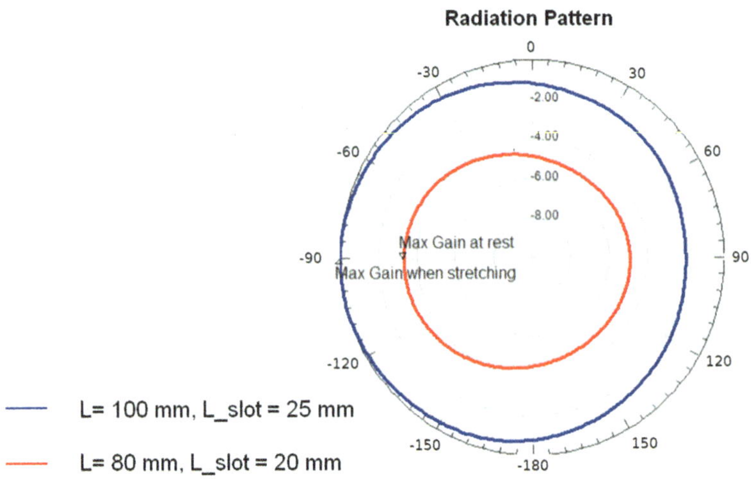

Fig. 4.14 Azimuth radiation pattern of Bellyband antenna showing the change of maximum gain while stretching at center frequency of 900 MHz (Liu et al. 2016). (©2016 IEEE. Reprinted, with permission, from *An improved design of wearable strain sensor based on knitted RFID technology,* 2016 IEEE Conference on Antenna Measurements & Applications (CAMA))

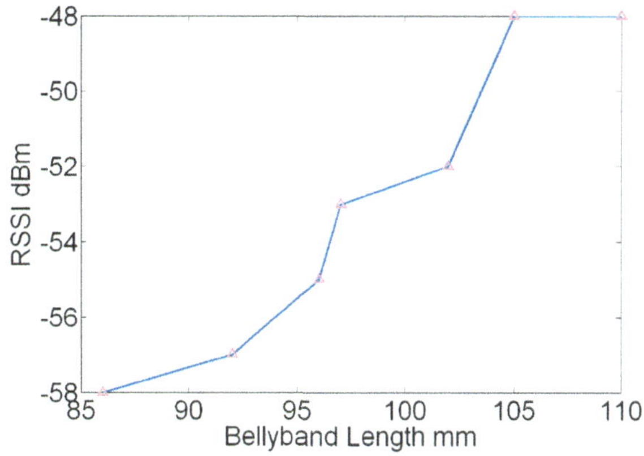

Fig. 4.15 RSSI *vs.* antenna length plot. The slope of the curve is the sensitivity of the sensor (Liu et al. 2016). (©2016 IEEE. Reprinted, with permission, from *An improved design of wearable strain sensor based on knitted RFID technology*, 2016 IEEE Conference on Antenna Measurements & Applications (CAMA))

$$Z_a = R_a + jX_a = 2Z_0\frac{(1 - S_{11}^2 + S_{21}^2 - 2S_{12})}{(1 - S_{11})^2 - S_{21}^2} \tag{4.3}$$

4.2.4 Radiation Pattern

The radiation pattern of folded dipole antennas is omnidirectional. The radiation pattern is measured in an anechoic chamber where a directional RFID reader antenna is connected to Impinj Speedway reader (Impinj) and the folded dipole antenna with MAGICSTRAP tag is attached to a 3D positioner (Fig. 4.10). The radiation pattern of the antenna is measured in an anechoic chamber along the azimuth and elevation planes (Fig. 4.11).

4.2.5 Fabrication and Sheet Resistance Extraction Tajin et al. (2020b)

The use of HFSS simulation is crucial to the design of wearable knitted antennas. Unlike metals, conductive fabrics do not have fixed electrical properties (e.g., conductivity). The knitting and handling of the silver-coated nylon yarns introduce exfoliation of silver coating. The effect of exfoliation is addressed by extracting sheet resistance from transmission line measurements. Sheet resistance helps us compare multiple sets of fabrics with different coating profile (thickness), knitting pattern, coating material (e.g., copper, silver, etc.). If pure silver plates were used, exfoliation would not be a concern; however, this is not conducive to a knitted wearable application. Gradual exfoliation during use would lead to increased conductor loss. As a result, the radiation efficiency (and gain) of the antenna would

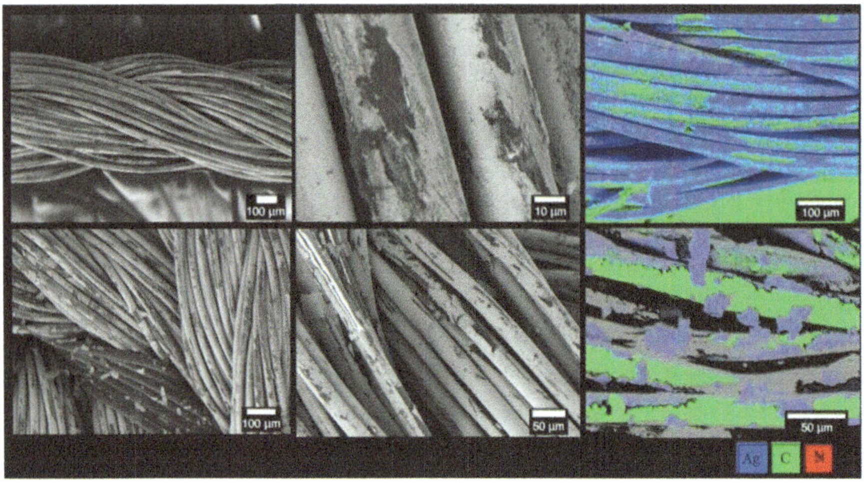

Fig. 4.16 (top) SEM (FESEM Zeiss VP5 Supra) images and EDS (Oxford EDS with INCA software) hypermaps prior to knitting; (bottom) silver-coated nylon yarns after knitting

gradually decrease. Consequently, the read range would be reduced. Nevertheless, the sensor would be functioning since we are comparing inhalation and exhalation state RSSI values. From our observation, silver-coated nylon is very robust, and the moisture study supports the claim. Moreover, antenna tuning (with chip) is a strong function of the antenna dimensions, rather than the sheet resistance. As a result, with gradual increase in sheet resistance, the sensor remains functioning, with minuscule decrease in the read range.

Moreover, oxidation of silver coating plays an important role. Scanning Electron Microscope (SEM) images (Fig. 4.16) show the silver flakes around nylon yarn. In HFSS, a complex sheet impedance is assigned to a 2D structure resembling the Bellyband antenna geometry. Previously the designer went through repeated trial-and-error stages to extract effective sheet impedance by matching the simulation and measurement results. This is a time-consuming process and excessive amount of materials are consumed. The real part of the sheet impedance is called the sheet resistance. The behavior of the knitted antenna is strongly determined by sheet resistance, compared to its complex counterpart. DC sheet resistance can be measured using four-probe method; however, this method does not work for radio frequencies. Radiofrequency sheet resistance of knitted conductive fabric can be extracted from S-parameter measurements of two-port fabric transmission lines (Fig. 4.17) (Tajin et al. 2020b,c). The top layer of a two-port microstrip transmission line (Fig. 4.17) is constructed with conductive knitted fabric, while the ground is made of copper and the substrate is FR4. Two-port S-parameters ($s_{i,j}$; $i, j = 1, 2$) are measured with a network analyzer. ABCD parameters are calculated from measured S-parameters using Equations 4.4(a–d) (Kiirgad et al. 1991):

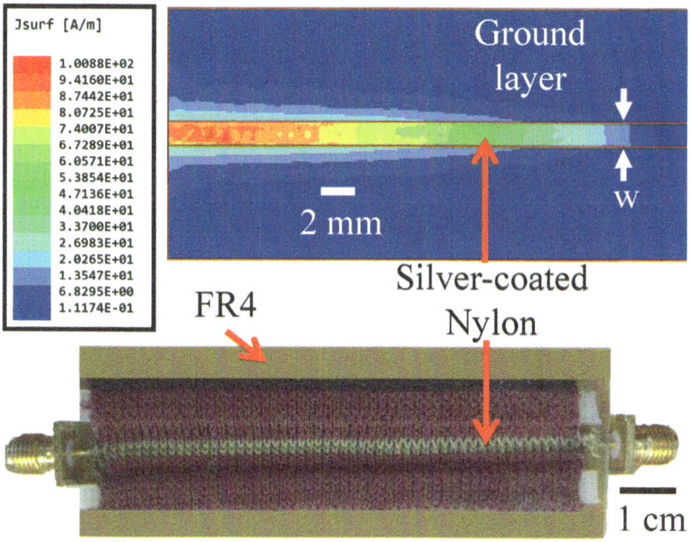

Fig. 4.17 (top) Simulated surface current density at the top (conductive fabric) and bottom (copper) layer, (bottom) conductive fabric-based microstrip transmission line structure (Tajin et al. 2020b). (©2020 IEEE. Reprinted, with permission, from *On the Effect of Sweat on Sheet Resistance of Knitted Conductive Yarns in Wearable Antenna Design*. IEEE Antennas and Wireless Propagation Letters)

$$A = \frac{(1+s_{11})(1-s_{22})+s_{12}s_{21}}{2s_{21}} \quad C = \frac{1}{Z_0}\frac{(1-s_{11})(1-s_{22})-s_{12}s_{21}}{2s_{21}}$$
$$B = Z_0\frac{(1+s_{11})(1+s_{22})-s_{12}s_{21}}{2s_{21}} \quad D = \frac{(1-s_{11})(1+s_{22})+s_{12}s_{21}}{2s_{21}} \tag{4.4}$$

where Z_0 is the normalizing impedance (50 Ω). Characteristic impedance (Z_c) and propagation constant (γ) of the transmission line can be derived from the ABCD parameters according to Equation 4.5:

$$Z_c = \sqrt{\frac{B}{C}}\ ; \ \gamma = \frac{1}{l}\cosh^{-1}(A) \tag{4.5}$$

where l is the length (80mm) of the transmission line. As the extraction of RLGC parameters is an ill-posed mathematical problem, ripples are observed in Z_c, while γ is free from ripples (Papazyan et al. 2004). So we accept γ and reconstruct Z_c by optimization (Papazyan et al. 2004).

A transmission line can be represented by an equivalent electrical circuit (Fig. 4.18) with distributed parameters (R, L, G, and C). The per unit length distributed parameters can be found:

$$R = Re(\gamma Z_c)\ ; \ L = Im(\gamma Z_c)/\omega \tag{4.6a}$$

$$G = Re(\gamma / Z_c)\ ; \ C = Im(\gamma / Z_c)/\omega \tag{4.6b}$$

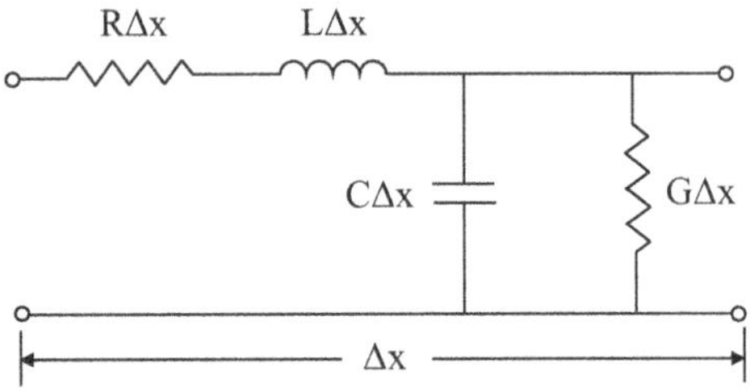

Fig. 4.18 Distributed RLCG parameter model of a transmission line (Tajin et al. 2020b). (©2020 IEEE. Reprinted, with permission, from *On the Effect of Sweat on Sheet Resistance of Knitted Conductive Yarns in Wearable Antenna Design*. IEEE Antennas and Wireless Propagation Letters)

where $\omega = 2\pi f$, f being the frequency of interest (913MHz). To validate the process, S-parameters are reconstructed with the extracted RLGC parameters. Total resistance (Ω) between the two ports of the transmission line is $R_{\text{total}} = (\frac{l}{1000})R \enspace ; l = 80mm$. The total conductor loss in the transmission line is the summation of the losses occurring in the top (fabric) layer (R_{fab}), bottom (copper) layer ($R_{\text{gnd}} = 0.05\Omega$), and radiation resistance (Balanis 2005; Faraji-Dana and Chow 1990), as shown in Equation 4.7. Finally, sheet resistance (R_s, Ω/sq) of the conductive fabric is given in Equation 4.8, where w is the width (4 mm) of the top layer of the transmission line.

$$R_{\text{total}} = R_{\text{fab}} + R_{\text{gnd}} + R_{\text{rad}} \tag{4.7}$$

$$R_s = \left(\frac{w}{l}\right) R_{\text{fab}} \tag{4.8}$$

Figure 4.19 demonstrates the extracted R-parameters *vs.* frequency plot. The R-parameters for different transmission line samples increase with frequency. The calculated sheet resistance of the fabric transmission line at 913 MHz is 0.4 Ω/sq.

4.2.6 Mitigating On-Body Effects and Signal Degradation

The maximum allowable distance between the reader antenna and the RFID tag/sensor is called the read range. The read range of the Bellyband antenna is reduced in human body proximity. The two factors responsible for this limiting phenomenon are the antenna radiation pattern and the water-dense structure of human body tissues. The relative permittivity of water is 81 times higher than that of air ($\epsilon_{\text{air}} = 1$). The Bellyband antenna has an omnidirectional radiation pattern in free space. However, in the presence of the human body, the radiation pattern becomes directional with reduced maximum gain. To investigate the effect of body-proximity, the radiation efficiency η_{rad} (see Equation 4.9) of the Bellyband

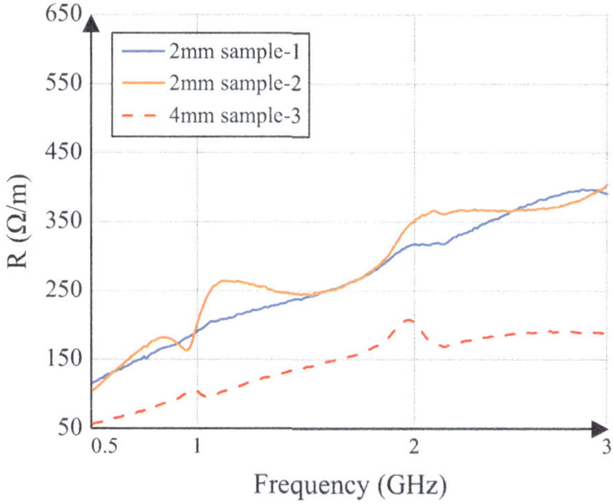

Fig. 4.19 Extracted per unit length resistance (R-parameter) of three fabric-based transmission line samples before the introduction of sweat (Tajin et al. 2020b). (©2020 IEEE. Reprinted, with permission, from *On the Effect of Sweat on Sheet Resistance of Knitted Conductive Yarns in Wearable Antenna Design*. IEEE Antennas and Wireless Propagation Letters)

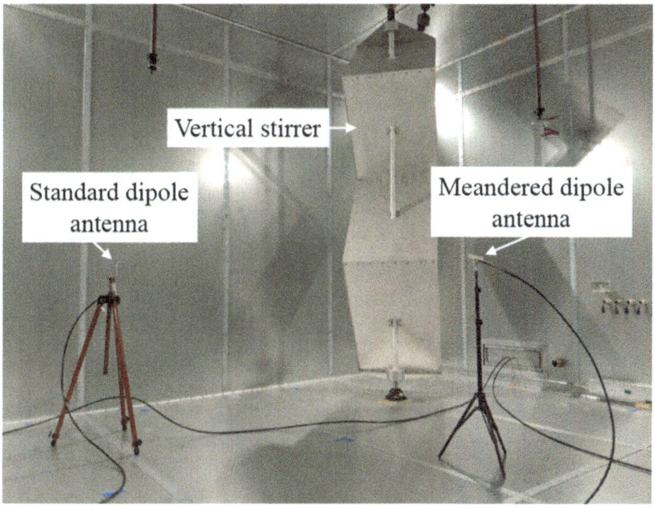

Fig. 4.20 Reverberation chamber setup for radiation efficiency measurement

is measured in a reverberation chamber at different antenna orientations (free-space/on-body, relaxed/stretched) (Tajin et al. 2020a).

$$\eta_{\text{rad}} = \frac{\text{Power radiated by the radiator}}{\text{Power delivered to the radiator}} \tag{4.9}$$

The reverberation chamber is a metal cavity equipped with horizontal and/or vertical metal stirrers/paddles. Reverberation chambers are gaining popularity for antenna radiation pattern measurement, mostly due to brief measurement time and convenience for on-body measurement. The reverberation chamber used for Bellyband antenna radiation efficiency measurement is a 5 m × 5 m × 3.5 m chamber with a vertical stirrer (Fig. 4.20). The measured radiation efficiency results

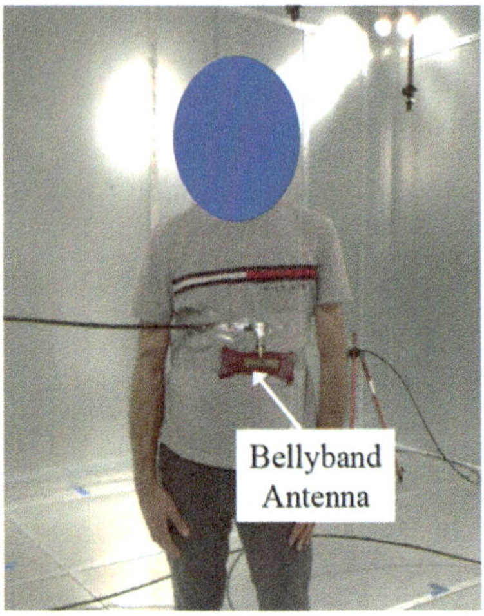

Fig. 4.21 On-body radiation efficiency measurement in the reverberation chamber

Table 4.1 Radiation efficiency measured in different methods at 900 MHz

Antenna orientation	HFSS Radiation efficiency (%)	Reverberation chamber radiation efficiency (%)	Anechoic chamber radiation efficiency (%)
Unstretched and not attached to body	22.4	24.4	20.5
Stretched and not attached to body	44	41.5	40.9
Unstretched and On-body	2.8	2.9	N/A
Stretched and On-body	5.9	7.3	N/A

Table 4.2 Comparison of Bellyband read range

Antenna orientation	Predicted read range (m)	Measured read range (m)
Free-space	1.61	1.6
On-body	0.7	0.6

are validated with anechoic chamber measurements and HFSS (High Frequency Structure Simulator) simulations. Figure 4.21 shows the on-body antenna under test in the reverberation chamber. The radiation efficiency results are as follows:

Table 4.1 shows that the free space radiation efficiency of the unstretched/relaxed (81 mm × 20 mm) Bellyband antenna is 24.4%. The radiation efficiency jumps to 41.5% when the flexible antenna is stretched (100 mm × 20 mm) along its length. When the antenna is worn by a human subject around the abdomen, the radiation efficiency sharply drops to 2.9%. On-body stretching increases the radiation efficiency to 7.3%. The interpretation of the results is that radiation efficiency is another important factor that dictates the RSSI (received signal strength indicator) fluctuation due to periodic stretching and relaxation of the antenna. This is true for both free-space and on-body cases. Body proximity limits the read range of the antenna, but the antenna does not lose sensing capabilities. Table 4.2 shows how the read range is affected due to body proximity:

4.2.7 Effect of Sweat and Moisture on Antenna Performance

As a wearable knitted antenna, the Bellyband is supposed to undergo cycles of sweat, moisture, washing, and drying. To understand their effects on the performance of the antennas, artificial sweat is applied to the top fabric layer of fabric-based microstrip transmission lines. The sweat solution is rinsed with distilled water and dried. This cycle is repeated for 7 days. Sheet resistance (at 913 MHz) of the knitted conductive fabric is extracted for each day.

With the introduction of sweat, the sheet resistance of the fabric shows an increasing trend. This is likely due to the silver coating delaminating from the surface of the nylon fibers upon exposure to sweat, washing, and drying. Consequently, the resistive loss in the antenna increases. This increase in internal loss mainly affects the fabric antenna in two ways. First, the radiation efficiency declines with increased loss. HFSS simulation of the fabric-based Bellyband antenna shows that after undergoing cycles of sweat-immersion, washing and drying for 6 days, the radiation efficiency of the antenna decayed from 32.7% to 24% (Fig. 4.22, sample-1). At 913 MHz this degradation in radiation efficiency represents a reduction in

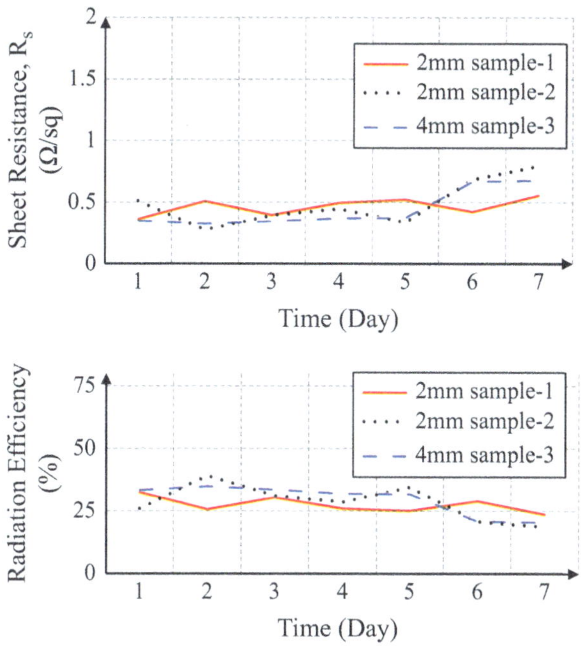

Fig. 4.22 Extracted sheet resistance and simulated radiation efficiency of the fabric antennas at 913 MHz *vs.* time. The samples are separated by the width of transmission line top layer (Tajin et al. 2020b). (©2020 IEEE. Reprinted, with permission, from *On the Effect of Sweat on Sheet Resistance of Knitted Conductive Yarns in Wearable Antenna Design*. IEEE Antennas and Wireless Propagation Letters)

read range by 0.17 m (10% of initial value 1.6 m (Tajin et al. 2020a)). Additionally, the impedance match between the RFID chip and the antenna might be affected due to a change in antenna input impedance. However, HFSS simulation shows that over 7 days of experimentation, the input impedance of the antenna changed from $(12.6 + j176.02)\ \Omega$ to $(17.1 + j175.95)\ \Omega$. Compared to the reduction in radiation efficiency, this small variation in impedance mismatch does not result in any significant change in read range.

4.3 A Software Framework for Signal Collection and Processing in the Internet-of-Things

The data typically reported by an RF interrogator includes the RSSI, Doppler shift, phase angle, interrogation frequency, antenna port, among other measurements. Unlike inventory applications which must successfully interrogate a tag at least once, we rely on repeated interrogations of the same tag in order to observe small differences in these measurements over time to infer state changes in the knitted textile antenna and, thus, changes in the state of the subject wearing the garment.

In order to facilitate repeated experimentation across signal processing algorithms, it is useful to provide a software framework for collecting, storing, and transmitting interrogator data for processing (Mongan et al. 2020b) (see Sect. 4.3.1). This framework extracts features from these measurements; for example, we compute the received power (P_{rx}) from the RSSI that accounts for changes caused by interrogation frequency hopping required in the United States by FCC regulations (U.S. Government Publishing Office 2018). Data collected is encrypted, and access is logged per Health Insurance Portability and Accountability Act (HIPAA) guidance. Specifically, we implement an audit table, and encryption using AES in Counter Mode (CTR) for use with streaming interrogations. Because this stream is likely to contain repetitive data, we use a counter derived from the timestamp of the interrogation itself (Mongan 2018; View et al. 2011), and this is combined with a user password to form the key. We organize a modular database layer so that the database engine can be rotated according to usage requirements, balancing ease of portability of data with the need for high-performance data collection and storage. Software to drive the interrogators are modular and are architected to enable real-time storage and processing. Finally, a RESTful interface is provided to facilitate adaptation with processing clients; we have developed connectors to the REDCap (Vanderbilt University) human subjects research data system as well as to external processing systems developed in-house (Mongan et al. 2020a) (see Sect. 4.3.2). These software frameworks are available as open-source projects for download and modification (Mongan et al. 2020a,b).

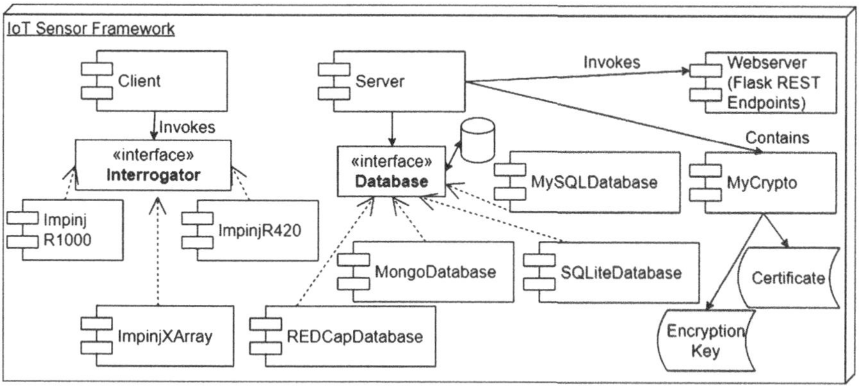

Fig. 4.23 A high-level design of the IoT Sensor Framework software

4.3.1 A Sensor Data Framework for Heterogeneous Sensor Communications in the Internet-of-Things

The IoT Sensor Framework is a Python-based adaptor that connects a heterogeneous suite of interrogators to a modular choice of database engine. Data collected can be retrieved "live" as it arrives or in "simulated" mode (which "plays back" a database from the beginning as if it were being collected in real-time), via a RESTful web service interface. This approach facilitated repeated experimentation on existing datasets with different algorithms, different parameterizations on those algorithms, and various fusion approaches carried out using those algorithms. It has also enabled the rapid generation of new synthetic datasets probabilistically generated from existing ones, to simulate environmental effects such as multipath fading and shadowing. The high-level design of the IoT Software Framework, which we detail in this section, is shown in Fig. 4.23.

4.3.1.1 Interrogator Drivers

The interrogator drivers are designed by creating a generic `Interrogator` interface that defines the minimal base functionality required to communicate data collected from an interrogator to a database engine or server. It defines the starting time, the timestamp of the most recent interrogator data collection, the number of interrogations (used to compute the interrogation rate), and connection information to a database engine. Additionally, a "dispatch sleep" time specifies an interval by which data is packaged and communicated with the server; this is offered in order to reduce network overhead resulting from sending each received interrogation packet individually to the database (Mongan et al. 2017a).

4.3.1.2 Modular Database

Like the `Interrogator` drivers, the database engine layer provides modular drivers that accept data from an interrogator driver and store them in a database for live or future retrieval by a processing module. The `Database` interface provides for the minimal base functionality for such a database engine driver and stores an SSL key, an encryption/decryption module, interface methods to connect, initialize, store, and retrieve data from the underlying database engine, and common data functionality such as categorizing data into sliding time windows or according to their tag identifier. This interface is implemented for specific databases, such as Sqlite, MySQL, MongoDB, REDCap, and others. Like the interrogator layer, the database implements a Producer/Consumer pattern, in which the Producer listens on a RESTful service endpoint for new data to arrive and enqueues it; this approach separates the I/O functionality from the data processing functionality in order to reduce latency. The corresponding Consumer thread retrieves data from the queue and inserts it into the database; the Consumer also retrieves records in batches when able to reduce the I/O latency of inserting the data into a possibly disk- or cloud-based database. As records are inserted, they are encrypted by the database class (they are subsequently decrypted when they are retrieved, but transmitted via SSL between the interrogator, the database, and the subsequent processor); as records are retrieved, a log entry is made in a corresponding `Audit` table within the database for HIPAA control purposes.

4.3.2 A Signal Processing, Multisensor Fusion and Visualization Framework

The IoT Processing Framework provides a Visualizer, a live Detector processing module, and a Multisensor Fusion processing module; each operates by polling the IoT Sensor Framework (described in Sect. 4.3.1) via its RESTful interface for data. If the software is being run in "live" mode, the software polls for the most recent n seconds of data (i.e., $n = 1$). If the software is run in "simulated" mode (i.e., on an existing dataset not populated in real-time by an interrogator), then the software polls for a window of data starting at time $n = 0$ and iterating until it reaches the end of the dataset. In both cases, the records are passed to the processing module(s) and appear to the algorithm as if they are arriving from a "live" interrogator in real time. The high-level design of the IoT Processing Framework is shown in Fig. 4.24.

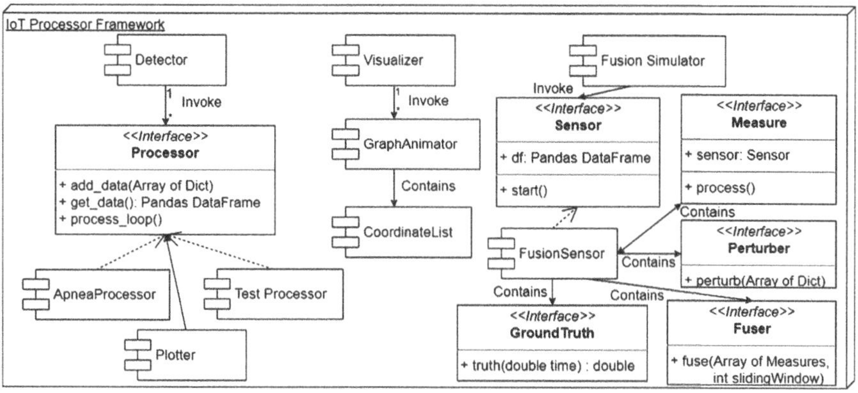

Fig. 4.24 A high-level design of the IoT Processing Framework software

4.3.2.1 Visualization

The `Visualizer` module is a matplotlib animated plot (Vanderplas) that refreshes itself at an interval. The records are grouped by their Electronic Product Code (EPC) tag and antenna number and plotted according to a data field (i.e., RSSI or phase).

4.3.2.2 `Detector` Processing Module

The `Detector` is built upon a similar foundation as the `Visualizer`, in that it polls the server for data in "live" or "simulated" mode. However, to support easy interchangeability of processing algorithms, a `Processor` superclass is provided. The class provides basic underlying functionality, including spawning threads to manage and plot the data. Two methods are required to implement the superclass interface: `process_loop()`, which is called automatically by the thread, and `get_data()`, which is called automatically by the `Plotter`.

4.3.2.3 Sensor Fusion and Experimental Protocols with Semi-synthetic Data

The `Fusion Framework` module is an extension of the `Detector` which allows for manipulation of the data, comparison to ground truth for error calculation, and fusion of multiple processing measurements while preserving the general structure of the `Processor`. Here, the processor is referred to as a `Sensor` superclass and implementing subclass. The `Sensor` operates like the `Processor` from the `Detector` module, but instead of implementing processing algorithms directly, it creates an array of objects that specify how to perturb the data to generate new synthetic datasets, how to process the data, and how to compare against ground truth for deeper experimental reporting. When the `Sensor` is started, it invokes each of these modules to automate processing.

4.4 Signal Processing for Sensing and Actuation

As discussed in Sect. 4.1 and shown in Fig. 4.4, an RFID interrogation signal is modulated with a tag identification string called an EPC. This EPC is decoded by the interrogator and used traditionally for tag inventory purposes. However, the interrogator antenna can also sense physical properties of the reflected and modulated RF signal, including the RSSI, phase angle, Doppler shift, and time of arrival. We model features extracted from the small changes in these signal properties over time as the wearable RFID-based smart garment is queried repeatedly by the interrogator at a variable rate (typically approximately 90 Hz) that we resample for spectral analysis to 25 Hz.

In this section, we process sensor inputs from an RFID interrogator using the knitted Bellyband antenna, perform filtering with a reference tag (if available, when knitted on the fabric on a relatively stationary part of the body) and without, extract features from the filtered data, and perform temporal, spectral, and fusion analysis to generate one or more estimates of the wearer's state (e.g., to estimate respiratory rate, to detect an apnea condition, to detect muscle movements consistent with a uterine contraction, or to detect the absence of muscle movements in the extremities that could indicate risk of blood clotting). An overview of our algorithmic approach is shown in Fig. 4.25.

4.4.1 RF Signal Model for Biomedical Monitoring

The strength of a reflected RF signal is defined by Friis Transmission Formula (Su et al. 2010), and the phase is defined in terms of the interrogation frequency and Doppler shift over successive interrogations (Impinj). The tag velocity and signal strength are shown in Equations 4.10 and 4.12, respectively, where: $P_{Rx,\text{reader}}$ is the calculated power received at the interrogator given a constant environment $P_{Tx,\text{reader}}$ is the interrogator transmit power (configured to be 1 Watt) G_{reader} is the reader gain (assumed to be constant) G_{tag} is the tag gain (which can change over time with the shape of the knit antenna) λ is the interrogation wavelength ($\frac{1}{f}$, given an interrogation frequency f) r is the interrogation radius (which can change as the subject moves in space with the tag) R is the return loss over the interrogation path v is the tag velocity c is the speed of light in a vacuum f_m is the Doppler shift, or change in phase angle, observed in two successive tag interrogations α is the interrogation angle (which can change over time as the tag moves in space)

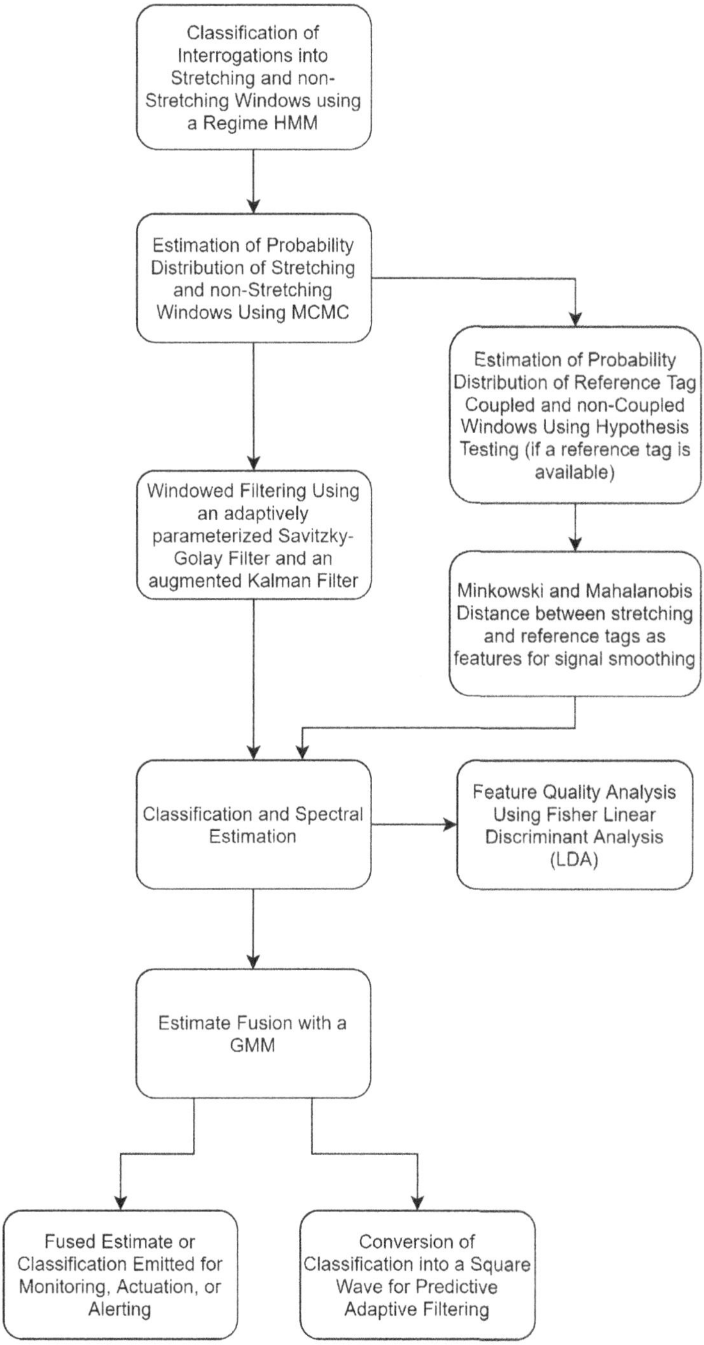

Fig. 4.25 A flowchart indicating the data flow and algorithmic processing of RFID data into features and, ultimately, state estimation or classification

$$v = \frac{c \times f_m}{2f \times cos(\alpha)} \tag{4.10}$$

$$v \times cos(\alpha) = \frac{c \times f_m}{2f} \tag{4.11}$$

Of these terms, r, G_{tag}, R, v, and α may change over time as the wearer moves about, inhales, exhales, etc. Our goal, then, is to observe signal changes that are compounded within those terms and infer wearer state changes from them. These velocity-based and received signal strength features are given in Equations 4.11 and 4.13, respectively. Substituting for $G = 4\pi A\lambda^{-2}$ (relating the tag gain G to the effective antenna aperature A) in Equation 4.13 (Su et al. 2010), we obtain the relationship for received power ζ with respect to the interrogation frequency in Equations 4.14 through 4.15 (Mongan 2018).

$$P_{Rx,\text{reader}} = P_{Tx,\text{reader}} \times G^2_{\text{reader}} \times G^2_{\text{tag}} \times \left(\frac{\lambda}{4\pi r}\right)^4 \times R \tag{4.12}$$

$$\hat{\zeta} = \frac{r^4}{G^2_{\text{tag}} \times R} = \frac{P_{Tx,\text{reader}} \times G^2_{\text{reader}}}{P_{Rx,\text{reader}}} \times \left(\frac{\lambda}{4\pi}\right)^4 \tag{4.13}$$

$$\hat{\zeta} = \frac{r^4}{(4\pi\lambda^{-2}A_{\text{tag}})^2 \times R} = \frac{P_{Tx,\text{reader}} \times (4\pi\lambda^{-2}A_{\text{reader}})^2}{P_{Rx,\text{reader}}} \times \left(\frac{\lambda}{4\pi}\right)^4 \tag{4.14}$$

$$\hat{\zeta} = \frac{r^4\lambda^4}{(4\pi A_{\text{tag}})^2 \times R} = \frac{P_{Tx,\text{reader}} \times (4\pi A_{\text{reader}})^2}{\lambda^4 \times P_{Rx,\text{reader}}} \times \left(\frac{\lambda}{4\pi}\right)^4 \tag{4.15}$$

$$\hat{\zeta} = \frac{r^4}{A^2_{\text{tag}} \times R} = \frac{P_{Tx,\text{reader}} \times A^2_{\text{reader}}}{\lambda^4 \times P_{Rx,\text{reader}}} \tag{4.16}$$

Finally, we compute ζ from $\hat{\zeta}$ by removing a residual sawtooth artifact that results from quantization of the reported RSSI that mitigates part of the compensation for interrogation frequency when computing $\hat{\zeta}$.

4.4.2 Signal Filtering and Denoising

There are two potential approaches to signal denoising in this medium. If the noise is somewhat observable out-of-band via a reference tag, which is an RFID knitted antenna worn on a relatively stationary area of the body (and thus not subject to stretching artifacts), we can extract higher order features by fusing this reference signal and the signal received from the primary worn antenna as it interacts with the body during cardiorespiratory activity. This is discussed in Sect. 4.4.2.2. This approach requires a second tag; although the knitted antennas are small enough to support multiple deployments on a body, it is advantageous to explore statistical filtering approaches that do not assume the presence of a reference tag in order to improve SNR on the primary band signal. Statistical filtering algorithms exist for this purpose, but one challenge is that they must be parameterized and configured for use. In Sect. 4.4.2.1, we explore automatic and dynamic parameterization of such a statistical filter for use in real-time respiratory applications. We outline each of these two pre-processing steps in this section.

4.4.2.1 Filtering with an Adaptively Parameterized Savitzky-Golay Filter

It is necessary to determine certain parameters in order to configure a Savitzky-Golay (SG) filter (Savitzky and Golay 1964; Schafer 2011) for a biomedical application like respiratory monitoring, including how high a peak must be to be considered the point of maximum inhale, how large a window over which to calculate respiratory rate, etc. For this application, we chose to fit a polynomial of degree three ($k = 3$) to the data which represents a single breath. The difficulty is that we do not know beforehand the number of data points which represent a single breath and so we don't know how to set n. If we did, we would already know the respiratory rate. Further, a person's respiratory rate changes through time, so no constant value for n will suffice. Instead, we modify the SG filter so that the n used in the current time window is chosen based upon the respiratory rate detected in the previous time window. Thus, the SG filter adapts, harnessing the intuition that the current respiratory rate will be close enough to the previous respiratory rate that an SG filter which uses an n value equal to the n value found in the previous window will be able to correctly smooth the signal in the current window. In one of our experiments, a test subject varied their respiration wildly (moving from 10 breaths per minute (BPM) to 70 bpm instantaneously), and the adaptive SG filter was able to smooth the signal so that the algorithm could count the peaks. The equation for converting from the respiratory rate for the ith window to the n value to use in the $(i + 1)$th window is $n_{i+1} = \frac{s \times 60}{r_i}$, where s is the system's sample rate in Hz and r_i is the respiratory rate detected in the current window in breaths per minute.

4.4.2.2 Denoising with a Reference Tag

In addition to the challenge of quantization to the nearest integer unit of RSSI, RFID is susceptible to noise artifacts related to the environment and multipath effects. One method of isolating and removing environmental noise is by placing a second tag on the patient as a reference, then fusing the data from the two tags together.

Using sensor fusion, non-respiratory artifacts in the Bellyband's signal can be filtered irrespective of their source. We outline the algorithm below which improves the signal quality with an increase in signal-to-noise ratio (SNR). For this algorithm (Hansen et al. 2020), we describe the Bellyband as a main antenna, where a fixed relaxed state describes when it is in phase with the interrogator during exhalation, and so has a higher RSSI. A second stationary tag is introduced to the system, which we define as a reference antenna. The reference antenna is never physically altered and at every moment is either coupled or non-coupled with the main antenna. When coupled, the reference antenna has low RSSI; otherwise, the reference antenna signal is similar to the main antenna's fixed relaxed state and has high RSSI.

First, the RSSI and Doppler shift are observed for each RFID antenna. We compute the antenna velocity according to Equation 4.11. Next, for each antenna, we separate each interrogation feature into "stretching" (breathing) and "relaxed" (non-breathing) states as described in Sect. 4.4.3.1. A Metropolis random walk using a Markov Chain Monte Carlo simulation (MCMC), similar to that employed in Sect. 4.4.3.1, is used to predict posterior distributions of these hidden states without needing to train with a large dataset.

Since both tags may be coupled as a result of close proximity, we leverage a z-test to separate each signal's data, assigning every point to the distribution it is closest to. The points belonging to the distributions that describe the main antenna's fixed-relaxed state and the reference antenna's coupled state are ignored, resulting in two separate non-coupled signals. Sliding window sampling is applied to the resulting time series such that main antenna's signal has a set of windowed distributions concurrent with those of the reference antenna. RSSI values have relatively small changes during respiration, resulting in a singular covariance matrix for these distributions. To resolve this, a multidimensional covariance matrix is built from higher-order features (the Mahalanobis Distance and the Minkowski Distance measures), induced by the L_p norm, between each window's RSSI and Doppler values.

Sensor fusion is accomplished by measuring a Mahalanobis Distance, a multi-dimensional generalization of standard deviation, between the main and reference distributions for each window. The windowed Mahalanobis distance is interpolated over the dataset, outputting a final "transformed" signal. We compute the increase in SNR by calculating a delta of the SNRs for the raw input signal and the transformed signal. High-frequency components and other non-respiratory artifacts present in the Bellyband's raw signal decrease the signal's quality and SNR. After transformation, these artifacts are filtered out, resulting in a clear sinusoidal respiratory signal and higher SNR.

4.4.3 Biomedical Applications

The applications of the Bellyband within the biomedical signal domain are broad. In the past, our lab has used the Bellyband to detect bio-signals as diverse as uterine contractions in pregnant women (Mongan et al. 2016), risk factors of deep vein thrombosis (Gentry et al. 2019), and heart rate (Vora et al. 2017). In this section, we explore respiratory monitoring in detail (Mongan et al. 2017b, 2016), specifically: apnea detection (Sect. 4.4.3.1) and respiratory rate estimation (Sect. 4.4.3.2).

4.4.3.1 Activity Classification and Apnea Detection

Infant respiration results in small movements of the abdominal wall, and, thus, only small stretches of the knitted textile antenna on the Bellyband. Sleep apnea is defined by a 95% reduction in respiratory activity for at least 10 s (Begg and Palaniswami 2006); our hypothesis test identifies 95% outliers from the sample collected during a brief semi-supervised period (20 s), during which no explicit labeling is required but only that normal respiration is taking place. Using the fundamental features defined in Equations 4.11 and 4.15, we seek to emit a square-wave signal that represents a binary classification of band-stretching activity over time (i.e., stretched or unstretched), for purposes of wearer state detection such as sleep apnea. This activity can be mapped to biomedical applications such as respiration or a uterine contraction. For example, we used a pumping air-bladder to simulate abdominal movement due to a uterine contraction, and measured the change in pressure using a gold standard tocodynamometer (a Philips 50XM Philips) and simultaneously with the RFID-based Bellyband; a plot of these observed actuations is shown in Fig. 4.26.

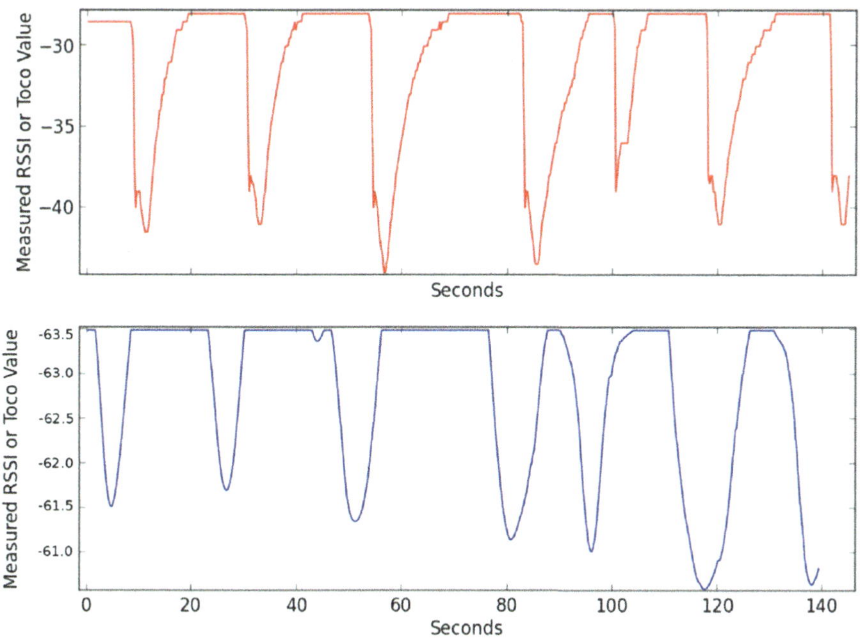

Fig. 4.26 Visualization of data collected from a tocodynamometer (top) and RFID (bottom), measured in dB, with a Gaussian filter and saturation point applied (Mongan 2018) (note a short time latency between the two devices which is attributable to their startup times)

Hypothesis Testing

We begin by performing a t-test against a null hypothesis which posits that respiration is taking place at the current time window. We then collect a short time window of recent RFID interrogations, compute their signal strength per Equation 4.15, and extract a set of samples for the hypothesis test. We investigated several statistical features on which to perform hypothesis testing, including the mean, extrema, average frequency component, and maximum spectral magnitude after computing the Fast Fourier Transform (FFT) on a window of data. Features were compared using Fisher Linear Discriminant analysis (LDA) (Fisher 1936), which compares the ratio of the difference of the means to the sum of the variances of the feature as collected across two classes (i.e., breathing *vs.* non-breathing). A high LDA score indicates that the means of the samples have a large difference across the two classes, with relatively small variances within each class; thus, features with a high LDA score are good candidates for hypothesis or other classification approaches. The mean and maximum spectral magnitude were somewhat separable feature, and we selected the spectral magnitude which enabled shorter 0.5 s FFT windows to compute these spectral densities.

Unsupervised Classification of Individual "Stretching" and "Non-stretching" Interrogations

One challenge in performing a hypothesis test is the need to compare the spectral magnitude against a reference in order to classify potential apnea conditions. This reference is obtained by assuming that a brief period at the start of monitoring is populated with normal respiratory activity. However, even during respiratory periods, there is a duration in-between inspiration and expiration (and subsequent inspiration) during which relatively little abdominal activity takes places. As a result, non-stretching data are intermixed with stretching data even during these samples. We observed an increase in the LDA score for the FFT magnitude feature from 0.49 to 3.85 when considering only data collected during the band's stretching periods. Classification of each RF interrogation as "stretching" or "non-stretching" would enable better unsupervised training of the hypothesis test classifier for sleep apnea detection and would enable finer-grained detection of uterine contractions or interbreath intervals, which require knowledge of the start and duration of each artifact.

To perform point-by-point classification, we construct a Hidden Markov Model (HMM), again with a brief period of unlabeled, semi-unsupervised data assumed to contain "normal" activity (i.e., respiratory activity). By computing correlation of the signal strength ζ and the tag velocity, and taking a rolling Root-Mean-Squared (RMS) calculation on sliding windows of this resulting correlation feature, we can identify the magnitudes of strain movements resulting from band stretching activity (Mongan et al. 2017b). As a result of the observed relationship between the signal strength and Doppler- or phase-based tag velocity, we constructed a feature tuple for the HMM consisting of the Doppler, the received signal strength, and the tag velocity (Mongan 2018).

Square-Wave Classification

To generate a square wave of point-by-point classification estimates, we begin with the Hidden Markov Model point-by-point estimate of each data point into a stretching distribution and a non-stretching distribution. An augmented Kalman Filter is employed to remove noise artifacts from the window using a voting classifier that fuses logistic regression, decision tree, Naive Bayes, and similarity classification (Acharya et al. 2019). This filter was augmented by modeling the measurement noise as an Autoregressive Moving Average (ARMA) process, to capture temporal correlations observed in the measurement noise (Acharya et al. 2019). To correct for high-frequency spikes in this square wave, k-means classification is performed on the data in the window with varying threshold levels for classification. A voting classifier determines which of the two distributions best fits each data point, and a resulting smoothed square wave is emitted that indicates the start time and duration of each detected artifact from the RFID-based input features on a point-by-point basis (O'Neill et al. 2019).

Activity-State Classification Using a Monte Carlo Simulation

For subject activity classification, we initialize an MCMC simulation using the rough but generally unsupervised estimate of each data point's classification (i.e., band stretching or stationary states). Specifically, the MCMC model is initialized to assume that the data in the window is comprised of two distinct distributions: one representing band stretching activity, and the other representing a stationary band. Each distribution is initially defined by the mean and variance of the states identified by the HMM, and the MCMC iterates to converge upon parameters of one or two distributions in the window (Mongan 2018).

By inverting the activity classes, we can consider a similar approach to classification of uterine activity during labor and delivery. We perform hypothesis testing on the distribution of data identified by the Markov Chain Monte Carlo process, with the null hypothesis asserting that the band is stationary. If the band is stationary, only a single distribution should exist in the data, and so the hypothesis tests that the window consists of one of the distributions identified by the MCMC process. Similarly, if only a single distribution is observed during respiratory monitoring, we infer that a potential apnea condition has commenced because the band is no longer stretched by the wearer.

Fusion with a Voting Classifier

The MCMC simulation yields useful features for classification and estimation. Specifically, we observe properties of the two distributions identified by the MCMC simulation to classify changes in wearer state. For example, if the mean of the distribution representing motion artifacts (the band stretching class) increases, we can infer that the band itself is being stretched further during that window. Symmetrically, we can infer that the band is being relaxed as this distribution mean decreases, until the MCMC-estimated distribution population has become small or disappears because the band has become stationary again. It is assumed that a single distribution corresponds to a "non-stretching" classification, with no "stretching" distribution present. Finally, we initialize a voting classifier that observes changes in the MCMC stretching distribution mean, the proportion of data samples assigned to each MCMC distribution, a change in variance of the stretching distribution, the original HMM classifications, and the hypothesis test z-score using the maximum spectral magnitude. Voting yields the classification of band state activity (Mongan 2018).

4.4.3.2 Respiratory Rate Estimation

Dominant Frequency Extraction via the Fourier Transform

The classification approach taken in Sect. 4.4.3.1 can be useful for classifying anomalies such as cessation of breathing or detecting a uterine contraction. However, it is also useful to determine the rate of the observed activity, using peak-frequency analysis via a Fourier Transform. Frequency-domain analysis suffers from spectral leakage, which is more pronounced as the window size becomes smaller. Unfortunately, it is desirable to use a small window to compute a more precise instantaneous respiratory rate. To balance these constrains, we utilized Quinn's interpolation method (Quinn 1994) to estimate the dominant frequency between discrete Fourier Transform magnitude coefficients. To select the dominant frequency in the potential presence of non-stationary motion artifacts, we applied Giovannelli's algorithm to track the respiratory frequency as a Markov chain over successive time window samples (Giovannelli et al. 2002). This approach applies the Baum-Welch Forward-Backward algorithm as a Bayesian approach to identify the most likely frequency given not only the current sample but the recent history of samples (referred to as a frequency "track").

Savitzky-Golay Smoothing

In Sect. 4.4.2.1, we described the method of smoothing the oscillatory, varying frequency, signal which comes from the Bellyband when it is attached to the subject's abdomen and the subject breathes. Once the signal is smoothed with a Savitzky-Golay (SG) filter, the extrema are counted. In our application, we calculated the respiratory rate over a 15 s window and returned that value as the instantaneous respiration rate for the moment at the end of the 15 s window. We used a sliding window with $\Delta_t = 0.5$ s.

The equation for converting from the number of extrema detected in the current window to the respiratory rate for the current window is $r = \frac{\frac{1}{2}(z-1)}{t_f - t_i} \times 60$, where z = the number of extrema in the window, t_f = either the time (in seconds) of the final extremum or the time (in seconds) of the final point in the window, as observed by that point's time of arrival, and t_i = either the time (in seconds) of the initial extremum or the time (in seconds) of the initial point in the window, as observed by that point's time of arrival.

Fusion of Respiratory Rate Estimates

Each rate detection algorithm is subject to estimation error: spectral analysis is subject to leakage and variance, especially when the window is small, Bayesian tracking approaches can drift and "lose" the primary frequency, requiring re-initialization, and time-domain approaches may misclassify spurious peaks. We have addressed these challenges in this section, but can apply fusion techniques on these estimates to reduce the variance of these estimates over time. We constructed a Gaussian Mixture Model (GMM) using the recent history of our rate estimation algorithms and interpreted the relative variance among those histories as a measure of uncertainty within each sensor estimate (Mongan et al. 2017b). The current point estimates from the sensors is taken as the mean of each distribution and is weighted according to its corresponding likelihood constructed from its history variance.

4.5 Experimental Setup, Results, and Discussion

4.5.1 Experimental Setup

The Bellyband has been tested on three platforms: (1) a robotic mannequin that mimics various bio-signals, including respiration and heartbeat, (2) human test subjects in a controlled lab environment, and (3) a synthetic channel emulator. To simulate an experimental environment in preparation for human study, we use the Laerdal Simbaby (Laerdal) as a simulator for apnea detection and a pregnant mannequin as a simulator for uterine monitoring, each containing an air bladder, and each wearing a tocodynamometer and an RFID Bellyband. The SimBaby is programmed to execute several respiratory scenarios for detection purposes. The Bellyband and tocodynamometer are each monitored using a thread spawned by the software, and they are plotted together with optional data filtering techniques. The mannequin is actuated using a peristaltic pump that fills the bladder with either water or air to a predefined and programmable pressure or duration. We also gathered respiration rate data from human test subjects.[3] The humans wore two sensors: the Bellyband and a Vernier Go Direct Respiration Belt (Vernier) (used to establish ground truth respiration rate). In some tests, subjects were instructed to breathe at a constant rate while listening to a metronome. In other tests, subjects were instructed to instantaneously double their respiration, from, for example, 15 to 30 breaths per minute, again listening to a metronome for assistance. In all, 22 min of data were collected in this way. Finally, an Echo Ridge DYSE (DYnamic Spectrum Environment Emulator) (Dandekar et al. 2019; Echo Ridge) is used to emulate two channels for sensor fusion. One channel represents the realized gain fluctuation of Bellyband, while the other channel represents a reference tag with static gain. Non-respiratory artifacts such as fading can be added to each channel by randomly sampling from a statistically modelled noise profile. We generate this model by fitting Rayleigh, Rician, and Normal distributions to a static signal with non-respiratory features present. Chi squared and KS tests are then leveraged to choose which of the resulting parameterized distributions best describe the non-respiratory features present in this signal. A value randomly sampled from the chosen distribution is used as a factor to scale each channel output by the DYSE.

4.5.2 Results and Discussion

4.5.2.1 Semi-unsupervised Classification

In simulation, we observed significant improvement in respiratory event classification (i.e., inspiration) using a mannequin SimBaby using the tag velocity feature over the signal strength alone (RMS error of 0.56 s *vs.* 1.22 s, $p = 0.0001$) (Mongan et al. 2017b). As a result, tag velocity was fused with signal strength as a feature via a GMM as described in Sect. 4.4.3.2 (Mongan et al. 2017b). Initializing an MCMC simulation using a semi-unsupervised HMM classifier, we constructed a voting classifier using features extracted from the distributions (one for a stationary band, or two if stationary band interrogations are mixed with stretching interrogations in the data window) detected by the simulation, as described in Sect. 4.4.3.1.

A human subject was instructed to breathe at a rate of 30 breaths per minute, with cessations at 30 and 90 s. As shown in Fig. 4.27, the cessations were identified by the voting classifier at 34 and 98 s, with no false positives (false apnea detections). These experiments were repeated at different breathing rates (10, 15, 20, 30 breaths per minute) (Mongan 2018); in each trial, the cessations were detected within 15 s, with at most one false positive occurring generally around the boundary of a state change from breathing to non-breathing or vice versa. These datasets were

[3]Human subjects testing was approved by the Drexel University IRB under protocol numbers 1504003601, 1504003602, and 1604004440.

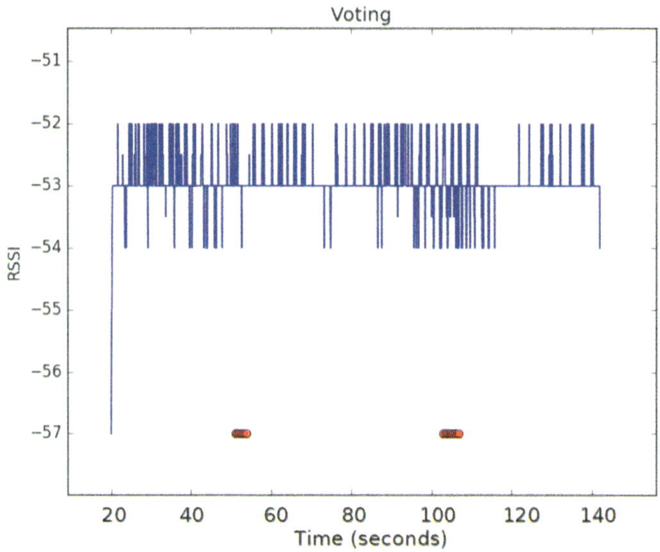

Fig. 4.27 RFID signal strength plotted over time during a human trial of a subject breathing at a rate of 30 breaths per minute with brief cessations at 30 and 90 s (denoted by red dots near the x-axis) (Mongan 2018)

typically collected for a period of 2 to 5 min.[4] The MCMC simulation features allowed voting that eliminated two false positives that would have been identified by hypothesis testing alone. A similar experiment using the SimBaby mannequin and depicting the internal classifier features is shown in Fig. 4.28. Individual point-by-point classification of each interrogation was achieved through an augmented Kalman Filter, which improved classification accuracy from 76.7% (F-Score: 0.56) without the augmented Kalman Filter to 91.8% accuracy (F-Score: 0.87) using the augmented Kalman Filter (Acharya et al. 2019).

4.5.2.2 Respiratory Rate Estimation

Using hypothesis testing (Mongan et al. 2016), we performed peak detection as depicted by the oscillations between classification states over time, resulting in a RMS error of 9 respirations per minute overall, as shown in Fig. 4.29, for a SimBaby mannequin programmed to breathe during 1-min intervals at rates of 31, 15, 0, 15, and 30 breaths per minute. Using our spectral estimator and the same experimental data collection setup, we estimated an average rate over each 30 s period of 28.6 (time 0–30), 39.9 (time 30–60), 18.9 (time 60–90), 18.9 (time 90–120), 0.3 (time

[4]Non-human datasets are available at: https://github.com/drexelwireless/bellyband-datasets.

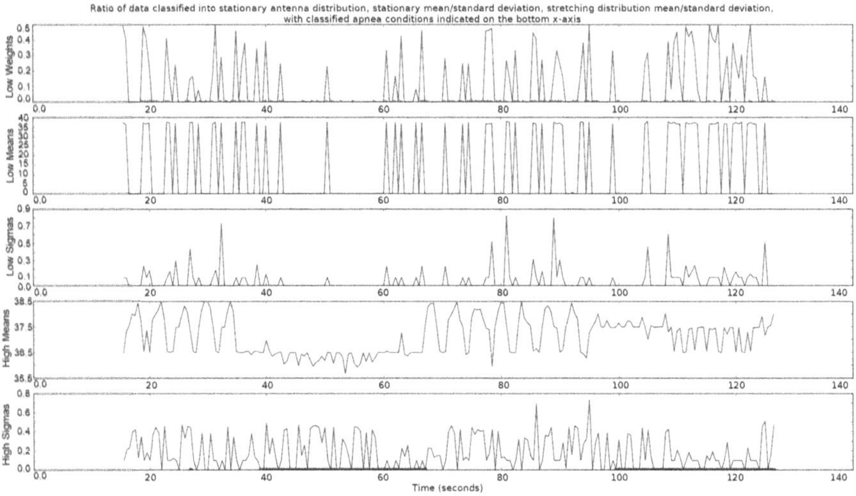

Fig. 4.28 A plot depicting respiratory data collected from the Bellyband worn on a SimBaby mannequin, programmed to breathe at a rate of 15 breaths per minute, with periodic cessations in breathing (from times 30–60 s and 90–120 s). The plots include (from top to bottom) the percentage of interrogations classified in the "low mean" distribution by the MCMC simulation, the mean and variance of each "low mean" distribution, and, finally, the mean and variance of the "high mean" distribution (Mongan 2018). Blue dots along the x-axis of the bottom plot indicate the voting classifier classification of cessation periods. Additional dots indicate the results of individual classification votes along the x-axes of the remaining graphs

120–150), 0.0 (time 150–180), 15.9 (time 180–210), 17.2 (time 210–240), 22.6 (time 240–270), and 25.2 (time 270–300) breaths per minute. Respiratory rate estimation RMS error was reduced from 9 (using hypothesis testing) to 6 breaths per minute by utilizing HMM frequency tracking (Giovannelli et al. 2002; Mongan et al. 2017b). Our estimators were fused using Expectation Maximization on a GMM constructed on the estimator history with Quinn interpolation (Quinn 1994) applied to the Fourier frequency bins, and with relative variance (uncertainty). An example result is shown in Fig. 4.30.

4.5.2.3 Square-Wave Generation for Artifact Prediction

Using the dynamic k-means voting classifier for square wave generation using a Hidden Markov Model, we detected all but one breath in a SimBaby simulation, within 0.38 s on average and within 0.92 s in the worst case (O'Neill et al. 2019). This square wave can be integrated with an adaptive respiratory artifact prediction algorithm using Maximum Likelihood analysis on an autoregressive model using the observed interbreath interval times (Indic et al. 2013; Barbieri et al. 2005).

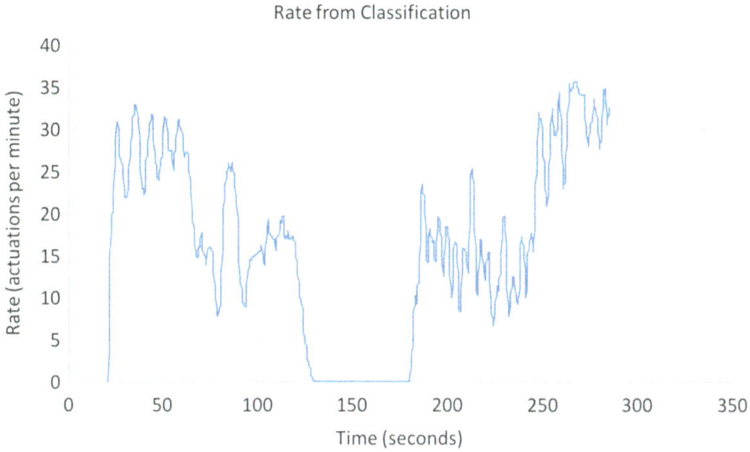

Fig. 4.29 Respiratory rate estimation using hypothesis testing for a SimBaby trial programmed to breathe at 31 breaths per minute, 15 breaths per minute, no breathing, 15 breaths per minute, and 30 breaths per minute, for 1 minute each. The first 20 s are omitted since this is used for the semi-unsupervised training period (Mongan et al. 2016). (©2016 IEEE. Reprinted, with permission, from *Real-Time Detection of Apnea via Signal Processing of Time-Series Properties of RFID-Based Smart Garments*. IEEE Signal Processing in Medicine and Biology (SPMB))

4.6 Conclusion and Future Work

Using passive RFID technology, we have developed an unobtrusive wearable garment using conductive yarns that interact with the human body to communicate biometric data for ongoing ambulatory monitoring. These yarns stretch and contract as the wearer moves naturally in space, and the resulting changes in reflected RF signal properties about the deforming antenna are monitored to estimate the wearer's state. This technology enables monitoring outside of the hospital setting or for more comfortable monitoring as an alternative to tethered sensors. Our novel approach required fusion of technical innovations in knitted conductive textile-based antennas, design and manufacturing, and semi-supervised machine learning. We have developed and released an open-source software framework that uses a modular architecture and lightweight communications mechanism to enable rapid integration of heterogeneous IoT sensors such as our wearable smart garments.

In the future, we seek to integrate our ubiquitous sensors across the medical pipeline, to support real-time therapy devices such as ventilation, and to develop an adaptive filtering algorithm to refine predictive strategies for inferring the onset of artifacts in time for actionable response using our classification algorithms.

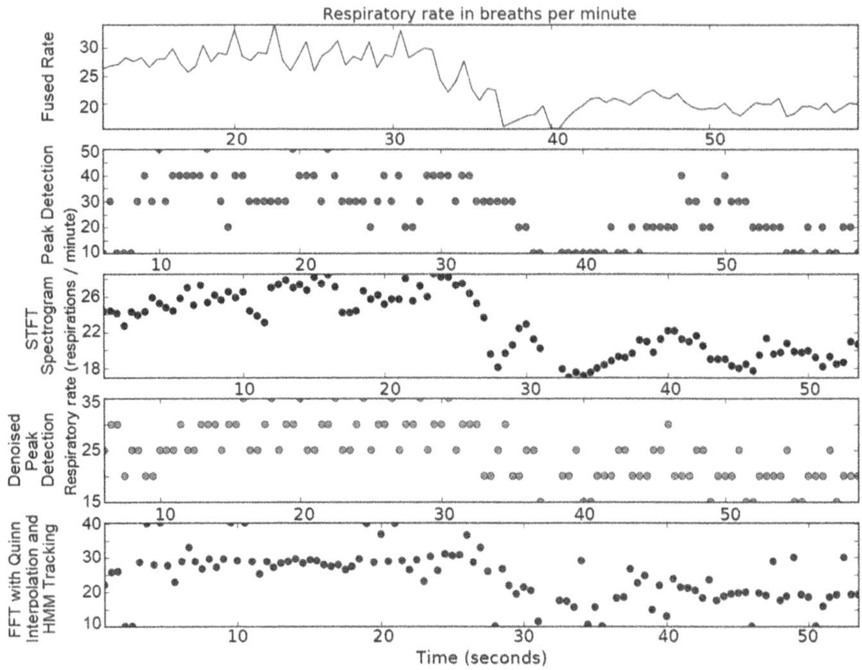

Fig. 4.30 Respiratory rate estimation using estimate fusion for a human subject breathing at a rate of 30 per minute for 30 s, followed by a rate of 15 per minute for 30 s (Mongan et al. 2017b). The bottom four subplots indicate point-by-point estimates using temporal and spectral algorithms, with the GMM fused result shown in the top subplot. (©2017 IEEE. Reprinted, with permission, from *Data Fusion of Single-Tag RFID Measurements for Respiratory Rate Monitoring*. IEEE Signal Processing in Medicine and Biology (SPMB))

Acknowledgments Our research results are based upon work supported by the National Science Foundation Division of Computer and Network Systems under award number CNS-1816387 and award number CNS-1711773. Any opinions, findings, and conclusions or recommendations expressed in this material are those of the author(s) and do not necessarily reflect the views of the National Science Foundation. Research reported in this publication was supported by the National Institutes of Health under award number R01 EB029364-01. The content is solely the responsibility of the authors and does not necessarily represent the official views of the National Institutes of Health.

Conflict of Interest Statement The authors declare that they have no conflict of interest.

References

S. Acharya, W.M. Mongan, I. Rasheed, Y. Liu, E. Anday, G. Dion, A. Fontecchio, T. Kurzweg, K.R. Dandekar, Ensemble learning approach via Kalman filtering for a passive wearable respiratory monitor. IEEE J. Biomed. Health Inform. **23**(3), 1022–1031 (2019). https://doi.org/10.1109/JBHI.2018.2857924

W. Alsalih, A. Alma'aitah, W. Alkhater, RFID localization using angle of arrival cluster forming. Int. J. Distrib. Sens. Netw. **10**(3), 269596 (2014). https://doi.org/10.1155/2014/269596

S. Amendola, R. Lodato, S. Manzari, RFID technology for IoT-based personal healthcare in smart spaces. Internet Things **1**(2), 144–152 (2014). http://ieeexplore.ieee.org/xpls/abs_all.jsp?arnumber=6780609

C.A. Balanis, *Antenna Theory: Analysis and Design* (Wiley-Interscience, Hoboken, 2005), p. 81

R. Barbieri, E.C. Matten, A.A. Alabi, E.N. Brown, A point-process model of human heartbeat intervals: new definitions of heart rate and heart rate variability. Am. J. Physiol. Heart Circ. Physiol. **288**(1), H424–H435 (2005). https://doi.org/10.1152/ajpheart.00482.2003. PMID: 15374824

R. Begg, M. Palaniswami, *Computational Intelligence for Movement Sciences: Neural Networks and other Emerging Technologies* (Idea Group Publishing, Hershey, 2006)

W.D. Boyer, A Diplex, Doppler phase comparison radar. IEEE Trans. Aerosp. Navig. Electron. **ANE-10**(1), 27–33 (1963). https://doi.org/10.1109/TANE.1963.4502075

T. Dag, T. Arsan, Received signal strength based least squares lateration algorithm for indoor localization. Comput. Electr. Eng. **66**, 114–126 (2018). https://doi.org/https://doi.org/10.1016/j.compeleceng.2017.08.014. http://www.sciencedirect.com/science/article/pii/S0045790617308509

K.R. Dandekar, S. Begashaw, M. Jacovic, A. Lackpour, I. Rasheed, X.R. Rey, C. Sahin, S. Shaher, G. Mainland, Grid software defined radio network testbed for hybrid measurement and emulation, in *2019 16th Annual IEEE International Conference on Sensing, Communication, and Networking (SECON)*, pp. 1–9 (2019)

Echo Ridge: DYSE – DYnamic Spectrum Environment Emulator. https://www.echoridgenet.com/products/dyse. Accessed 25 Jan 2021 Philips: Accessed 10 Oct 2016

R. Faraji-Dana, Y.L. Chow, The current distribution and AC resistance of a microstrip structure. IEEE Trans. Microwave Theory Tech. **38**(9), 1268–1277 (1990). https://doi.org/10.1109/22.58653

S. Fiocchi, I.A. Markakis, P. Ravazzani, T. Samaras, SAR exposure from UHF RFID reader in adult, child, pregnant woman, and fetus anatomical models. Bioelectromagnetics **34**(6), 443–452 (2013). https://doi.org/10.1002/bem.21789

R.A. Fisher, The use of multiple measurements in taxonomic problems. Ann. Eugenics **7**(7), 179–188 (1936)

A. Gentry, W. Mongan, B. Lee, O. Montgomery, K. Dandekar, Activity segmentation using wearable sensors for DVT/PE risk detection, in *2019 IEEE 43rd Annual Computer Software and Applications Conference (COMPSAC)*, vol. 2, pp. 477–483. IEEE (2019)

J.F. Giovannelli, J. Idier, R. Boubertakh, A. Herment, Unsupervised frequency tracking beyond the nyquist frequency using Markov chains. IEEE Trans. Signal Process. **50**(12), 2905–2914 (2002). https://doi.org/10.1109/TSP.2002.805501

J. Han, H. Ding, C. Qian, D. Ma, W. Xi, Z. Wang, Z. Jiang, L. Shangguan, CBID: A customer behavior identification system using passive tags, in *Proceedings – International Conference on Network Protocols, ICNP*, pp. 47–58 (2014). https://doi.org/10.1109/ICNP.2014.26

S. Hansen, D. Schwartz, J. Stover, Tajin, M.A.S., W.M. Mongan, K.R. Dandekar, Fusion learning on multiple-tag RFID measurements for respiratory rate monitoring, in *2020 IEEE International Conference on Bioinformatics and Biomedical Engineering (BIBE)* (2020). (To Appear)

Impinj: Application Note – Low Level User Data Support. https://support.impinj.com/hc/en-us/article_attachments/200774268/SR_AN_IPJ_Speedway_Rev_Low_Level_Data_Support_20130911.pdf

Impinj: SPEEDWAY R420 RAIN RFID READER. https://www.impinj.com/platform/connectivity/speedway-r420/. Accessed 04-May-2020

P. Indic, D. Paydarfar, R. Barbieri, Point process modeling of interbreath interval: a new approach for the assessment of instability of breathing in neonates. IEEE Trans. Biomed. Eng. **60**(10), 2858–2866 (2013). https://doi.org/10.1109/TBME.2013.2264162

Intermec: IP30 Handheld RFID Reader User Guide. https://www.honeywellaidc.com/en-au/-/media/en/files-public/data-sheets/ip30-rfid-handheld-reader-en-a4.pdf. Accessed 25-Jan-2021

I. Kiirgad, S. Member, N. Dagli, G.L. Matthaei, L. Fellow, S.I. Long, S. Member, Experimental analysis of transmission line parameters in high-speed GaAs digital circuit interconnects **39**(8), 1361–1367 (1991)
Laerdal: Laerdal SimBaby and Linkbox. https://www.laerdal.com/us/products/simulation-training/obstetrics-pediatrics/simbaby/. Accessed 17-May-2020
X. Li, Y. Zhang, I. Marsic, A. Sarcevic, R.S. Burd, Deep learning for RFID-based activity recognition, in *Proceedings of the 14th ACM Conference on Embedded Network Sensor Systems CD-ROM – SenSys '16*, pp. 164–175 (2016). https://doi.org/10.1145/2994551.2994569. http://dl.acm.org/citation.cfm?doid=2994551.2994569
Y. Liu, A. Levitt, C. Kara, C. Sahin, G. Dion, K.R. Dandekar, An improved design of wearable strain sensor based on knitted rfid technology, in *2016 IEEE Conference on Antenna Measurements Applications (CAMA)*, pp. 1–4 (2016)
I. Locher, M. Klemm, T. Kirstein, G. Trster, Design and characterization of purely textile patch antennas. IEEE Trans. Adv. Packag. **29**(4), 777–788 (2006). https://doi.org/10.1109/TADVP.2006.884780
Y.Á. López, M.E. de Cos Gómez, J.L. Álvarez, F.L.H. Andrés, Evaluation of an RSS-based Indoor Location System. Sens. Actuators A Phys. **167**(1), 110–116 (2011). https://doi.org/10.1016/j.sna.2011.02.037. http://www.sciencedirect.com/science/article/pii/S0924424711000999
Y.Á. López, M.E. de Cos Gómez, F.L.H. Andrés, A received signal strength RFID-based indoor location system. Sens. Actuators A Phys. **255**, 118–133 (2017). https://doi.org/10.1016/j.sna.2017.01.007. http://www.sciencedirect.com/science/article/pii/S0924424716309153
W. Mongan, E. Anday, G. Dion, A. Fontecchio, K. Joyce, T. Kurzweg, Y. Liu, O. Montgomery, I. Rasheed, C. Sahin, S. Vora, K. Dandekar, A multi-disciplinary framework for continuous biomedical monitoring using low-power passive RFID-based wireless wearable sensors, in *2016 IEEE International Conference on Smart Computing (SMARTCOMP)*, pp. 1–6 (2016). https://doi.org/10.1109/SMARTCOMP.2016.7501674
W. Mongan, I. Rasheed, K. Ved, S. Vora, K. Dandekar, G. Dion, T. Kurzweg, A. Fontecchio, On the use of radio frequency identification for continuous biomedical monitoring, in *2017 IEEE/ACM Second International Conference on Internet-of-Things Design and Implementation (IoTDI)*, pp. 197–202 (2017a). https://doi.org/10.1145/3054977.3055002
W. Mongan, R. Ross, I. Rasheed, Y. Liu, K. Ved, E. Anday, K. Dandekar, G. Dion, T. Kurzweg, A. Fontecchio, Data fusion of single-tag RFID measurements for respiratory rate monitoring, in *2017 IEEE Signal Processing in Medicine and Biology Symposium (SPMB)*, pp. 1–6 (2017b). https://doi.org/10.1109/SPMB.2017.8257028
W.M. Mongan, Predictive analytics on real-time biofeedback for actionable classification of activity state. Ph.D. thesis, Drexel University, Philadelphia (2018)
W.M. Mongan, K.R. Dandekar, A.K. Fontecchio, drexelwireless/iot-processing-framework: Public release 1.1 (2020a). https://doi.org/10.5281/zenodo.3786930
W.M. Mongan, I. Rasheed, E. Segun, H. Dang, V.S. Cushman, C.R. Chiccarine, K.R. Dandekar, A.K. Fontecchio, drexelwireless/iot-sensor-framework: Public release 1.0 (2020b). https://doi.org/10.5281/zenodo.3786932
W.M. Mongan, I. Rasheed, K. Ved, A. Levitt, E. Anday, K. Dandekar, G. Dion, T. Kurzweg, A. Fontecchio, Real-time detection of apnea via signal processing of time-series properties of RFID-based smart garments, in *2016 IEEE Signal Processing in Medicine and Biology Symposium (SPMB)*, pp. 1–6 (2016). https://doi.org/10.1109/SPMB.2016.7846871
A. Montaser, O. Moselhi, RFID indoor location identification for construction projects. Autom. Constr. **39**, 167–179 (2014). https://doi.org/10.1016/j.autcon.2013.06.012. http://www.sciencedirect.com/science/article/pii/S092658051300109X
Murata: Murata MAGICSTRAP UHF Tag [Online]. http://www.murata.com/en-us/campaign/ads/americas/rfid/. Accessed 04-May-2020
X. Nguyen, M.I. Jordan, B. Sinopoli, A Kernel-based learning approach to ad hoc sensor network localization. Trans. Sensor Networks (TOSN **1**(1), 134–152 (2005). https://dl.acm.org/doi/10.1145/1077391.1077397

P. O'Neill, W. Mongan, R. Ross, S. Acharya, A. Fontecchio, K.R. Dandekar, An adaptive search algorithm for detecting respiratory artifacts using a wireless passive wearable device, in *2019 IEEE Signal Processing in Medicine and Biology Symposium (2019)*. http://par.nsf.gov/biblio/10118763

R. Papazyan, P. Pettersson, H. Edin, R. Eriksson, GäU. fvert, Extraction of high frequency power cable characteristics from s-parameter measurements. IEEE Trans. Dielectr. Electr. Insul. **11**(3), 461–470 (2004)

D. Patron, W. Mongan, T.P. Kurzweg, A. Fontecchio, G. Dion, E.K. Anday, K.R. Dandekar, On the use of knitted antennas and inductively coupled RFID tags for wearable applications. IEEE Trans. Biomed. Circuits Syst. **10**(6), 1047–1057 (2016). https://doi.org/10.1109/TBCAS.2016.2518871

Philips: Series 50 Fetal Monitors, Design Interface Protocol Specifications: Programmer's Guide. http://www.frankshospitalworkshop.com/equipment/documents/ecg/service_manuals/Philips_Series_50_-_Programmers_guide.pdf. Accessed 10-Oct-2016

L. Qiu, X. Liang, Z. Huang, PATL: A RFID tag localization based on phased array antenna. Sci. Rep. **7**, 1–12 (2017). https://doi.org/10.1038/srep44183

B.G. Quinn, Estimating frequency by interpolation using Fourier coefficients. IEEE Trans. Signal Process. **42**(5), 1264–1268 (1994). https://doi.org/10.1109/78.295186

A. Savitzky, M.J. Golay, Smoothing and differentiation of data by simplified least squares procedures. Anal. Chem. **36**(8), 1627–1639 (1964). https://doi.org/10.1021/ac60214a047

R.W. Schafer, What is a Savitzky-Golay filter? IEEE Signal Process. Mag. **28**(4), 111–117 (2011). https://doi.org/10.1109/MSP.2011.941097

C.P. Schloter, H. Aghajan, Wireless symbolic positioning using support vector machines. In Proceedings of the 2006 international conference on Wireless communications and mobile computing (IWCMC '06). Association for Computing Machinery, New York, NY, USA, 1141–1146 (2006). https://doi.org/10.1145/1143549.1143778

Z. Su, S.C. Cheung, K.T. Chu, Investigation of radio link budget for UHF RFID systems, in *Proceedings of 2010 IEEE International Conference on RFID-Technology and Applications, RFID-TA 2010 (June)*, pp. 164–169 (2010). https://doi.org/10.1109/RFID-TA.2010.5529938

M.A.S. Tajin, O. Bshara, Y. Liu, A. Levitt, G. Dion, K.R. Dandekar, Efficiency measurement of the flexible on-body antenna at varying levels of stretch in a reverberation chamber. IET Microwaves, Antennas Propag. **14**(3), 154–158 (2020a)

M.A.S. Tajin, A.S. Levitt, Y. Liu, C.E. Amanatides, C.L. Schauer, G. Dion, K.R. Dandekar, On the effect of sweat on sheet resistance of knitted conductive yarns in wearable antenna design. IEEE Antennas Wirel. Propag. Lett. **19**(4), 542–546 (2020b)

M.A.S. Tajin, A.S. Levitt, Y. Liu, C.E. Amanatides, L. Schauer, G. Dion, K.R. Dandekar, Extraction of knitted RFID antenna design parameter from transmission line measurements (2020c). To appear

M. Truijens, X. Wang, H. de Graaf, J.J. Liu, C. Wu, Evaluating the performance of absolute RSSI positioning algorithm-based microzoning and RFID in construction materials tracking, in *Optimization in Industrial Systems* (2014)

U.S. Government Publishing Office: Electronic Code of Federal Regulations, Title 47, Chapter I, Subchapter A, Part 15.247 (2018). http://www.ecfr.gov/cgi-bin/text-idx?node=pt47.1.15&rgn=div5#se47.1.15_1247

U.S. Government Publishing Office: FCC OET Bulletin 65 (2018). https://www.fcc.gov/Bureaus/Engineering_Technology/Documents/bulletins/oet65/oet65.pdf

Vanderbilt University: Project REDCap. http://project-redcap.org/

J. Vanderplas, Matplotlib Animation Tutorial. https://jakevdp.github.io/blog/2012/08/18/matplotlib-animation-tutorial/

Vernier: Go Direct Respiration Belt. https://www.vernier.com/product/go-direct-respiration-belt/#tab-specifications. Accessed 17-May-2020

M. View, J. Rydell, M. Pei, S. Machani, TOTP: Time-Based One-Time Password Algorithm. RFC 6238 (2011). https://doi.org/10.17487/RFC6238. https://rfc-editor.org/rfc/rfc6238.txt

S.A. Vora, W.M. Mongan, E.K. Anday, K.R. Dandekar, G. Dion, A.K. Fontecchio, T.P. Kurzweg, On implementing an unconventional infant vital signs monitor with passive RFID tags, in *IEEE RFID* (2017)

C. Wang, Z. Shi, F. Wu, Intelligent RFID indoor localization system using a Gaussian filtering based extreme learning machine. Symmetry **9**(3) (2017). https://doi.org/10.3390/sym9030030

K. Yamanoi, K. Tanaka, M. Hirayma, E. Kondo, Y. Kimuro, Self-localization of mobile robots with RFID system by using support vector machine. Iros 3756–3761 (2004). https://doi.org/10.1109/IROS.2004.1389999

Chapter 5
Spatial Distribution of Seismocardiographic Signals

Md Khurshidul Azad, John D'Angelo, Peshala T. Gamage, Shehab Ismail, Richard H. Sandler, and Hansen A. Mansy

5.1 Introduction

Cardiovascular diseases are one of the leading causes of disability and death in the United States (Virani et al. 2020). Hence, improved means for early detection of cardiovascular disease is of great significance to engineering and medicine. Modern clinical techniques of measuring heart function most frequently involve history and physical examination (including stethoscope auscultation), electrocardiograms (ECG), echocardiogram imaging, and various blood tests. While these techniques provide valuable electrophysiological, acoustic, structural, and hemo-chemical/hormonal information, additional potentially diagnostically useful information may be gleaned from measurements of the mechanical vibrations induced by cardiac movements. Seismocardiography (SCG) relies on accelerometers to measure vibrations on the chest wall surface and can be used in ambulatory settings to measure heart function along with other modalities. SCG also offers significant

Md. K. Azad (✉) · P. T. Gamage · S. Ismail
Biomedical Acoustic Research Lab, University of Central Florida, Orlando, FL, USA
e-mail: khurshid@knights.ucf.edu

J. D'Angelo
Biomedical Acoustic Research Lab, University of Central Florida, Orlando, FL, USA

College of Medicine, University of Central Florida, Orlando, FL, USA

R. H. Sandler
Biomedical Acoustic Research Lab, University of Central Florida, Orlando, FL, USA

College of Medicine, University of Central Florida, Orlando, FL, USA

Biomedical Acoustics Research Company, Orlando, FL, USA

H. A. Mansy
Biomedical Acoustic Research Lab, University of Central Florida, Orlando, FL, USA

Biomedical Acoustics Research Company, Orlando, FL, USA

I. Obeid et al. (eds.), *Biomedical Signal Processing*,
https://doi.org/10.1007/978-3-030-67494-6_5

potential to provide additional information about cardiac function as it detects low frequency vibrations that are infrasonic which may offer unique insights into heart muscle and other cardiac functions. Phonocardiography (PCG), which is equivalent to stethoscope auscultation, uses microphones to detect sounds due to valve closure, abnormal blood flow, and pathological ventricular filling, but it does not always detect low frequency sounds such as S3 and S4 heart sounds (Siejko et al. 2013; Hosenpud and Greenberg 2007; Glower et al. 1992). SCG provides this information as it detects low frequency vibrations with good resolution, and it can also be used to detect cardiac events such as isovolumetric contraction, aortic opening, and mitral opening (Crow et al. 1994; Tavakolian 2016). Despite this, SCG signals are subject to noise as they pick up respiratory activity, abdominal sounds, and body movement. In addition, SCG signals vary based on the sensor's position on the chest, and an ideal position to detect cardiac activity has not yet been adequately studied.

As previously mentioned, SCG provides information about infrasonic vibrations of the chest wall surface, and Taebi et al. (Taebi and Mansy 2017; Taebi et al. 2019) examined the various frequencies that compose SCG signals in healthy human adults. Taebi found that SCG signal intensities reached maximal values during two portions of a cardiac cycle that roughly correspond to S1 and S2 sounds of PCG (referred to as SCG 1 and SCG 2, respectively). The SCG 1 signal provided greater signal intensity compared to SCG 2, and analysis of SCG 1's power spectral density (PSD) showed that the PSD consisted of three dominant frequencies at 9 Hz, 25 Hz, and 50 Hz. Taebi speculated that the lowest dominant frequency corresponds to ventricular contraction, while the larger frequency corresponds to atrioventricular valve closure.

In the past, the problem of identifying an ideal location to listen for heart sounds was also encountered in the realm of PCG, even though common auscultation sites have now been identified. Okada (1982) used 36 spatially distributed PCG microphones to acquire heart sounds, and their results showed that sounds specifically associated with closure of the aortic and pulmonic valves were loudest at the cardiac apex and 2nd intercostal space along the right parasternal border, respectively. Cozic et al. (1998) expanded on this by placing 22 spatially distributed PCG microphones on the chest surface and found that the highest amplitude were associated with the S1 heart sound (corresponding to mitral and tricuspid valve closure) at the mid-clavicular 5th ICS location and tricuspid auscultation location. Kompis et al. (1998, 2001) placed PCG sensors at the neck, 3rd ICS, 5th ICS, and 7th ICS and found that heart sounds with the highest intensity were detected at the neck bilaterally and parasternally in the 3rd ICS on the left. However, this result was likely due to detection of the carotid pulse in the neck and not of valvular activity. In addition, the neck has little muscle and fat compared to the chest wall, and this makes it easier to detect sound. More recently, Sapsanis et al. (2018) used a vest with 12 embedded PCG sensors to record heart sound and suggested that the loudest signals were associated with S1 along the left parasternal border especially near the 4th ICS.

This century, there have been pilot studies on the SCG genesis from cardiac activity and its propagation across the chest wall surface with a limited number of subjects. Kawamura et al. (2007) used 64 accelerometers to measure cardiac activity over the left anterior chest wall. Kawamura postulated that vibration waves due to cardiac activity stem from a source and then spread over a plane. He suggested that SCG peak associated with aortic opening achieves a maximal value near the right upper sternal border and propagates down toward the apex. By doing a cross-correlation of adjacent SCG signals and determining the shortest path of propagation using the Dijkstra method (1959), Kawamura et al. (2007) created surface contour maps of SCG signal propagation over the chest surface that showed how the loudness of SCG 1 peak moved away from the apex, while the SCG 2 peaks loudness moved away from the aortic valve. Based on this, they speculated that the SCG wave associated with mitral opening initially reaches its maximal value near the apex and moves up toward the right upper sternal border. Using this, Kawamura et al. (2007) estimated that the SCG signal propagation speed across the chest wall surface was approximately 11 m/s. Nogata et al. (2010, 2014) used an identical set up to Kawamura et al. with 64 SCG sensors to study the propagation of the chest wall vibrations, and they concluded that the SCG signal high-frequency peaks associated with the traditional S1 sound of cardiac auscultation started in the apex and the traditional S2 sound started near the aortic valve of the right upper sternal border. Nogata speculated that these SCG signals were due to both valve closure and chamber contraction, and not just valve closure

While SCG is measured on different locations on the chest surface (i.e., xiphoid process, 4th intercostal space, mid-sternum), most studies have placed SCG sensors on the sternum (Taebi et al. 2019). Pandia et al. (2012) suggested that larger amplitude of SCG 2 peak were observed at the left mid-sternal, mid-clavicular location. While this location was noted for louder SCG 2 signal compared to the mid-sternal location, variations in the SCG waveform relative to other positions were not examined. Given the reported differences in SCG signal intensity between the sternum and the left mid-sternal, mid-clavicular location, it becomes apparent that understanding SCG signal variations across the chest wall surface is critical for precise feature extraction. A detailed study of the spatial distribution of SCG feature variations on the chest surface has not yet been reported. The objective of the current study is to:

(a) Document spatial SCG signal variability over the chest surface
(b) Understand effects of sensor location on different SCG signal features
(c) Document signal quality over sensor placement

5.2 Methods

Figure 5.1 summarizes the methodology employed in this study. More details are provided in following sections.

5.2.1 Accelerometer Calibration

The current study used 36 uniaxial accelerometers (Model: 352C65, PCB Piezotronics, Depew, NY) to acquire the SCG on the chest surface. Prior to human subject

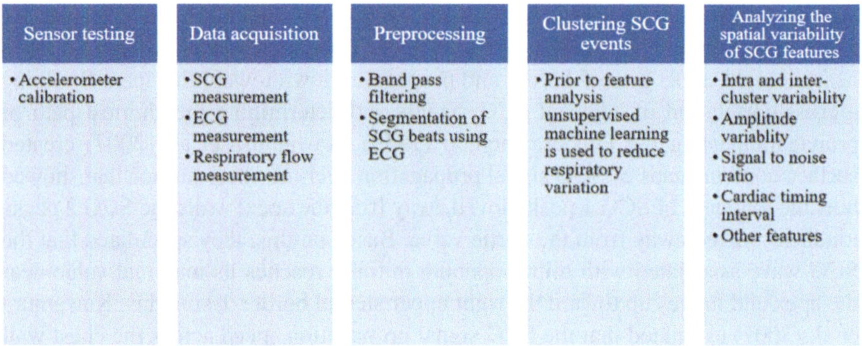

Fig. 5.1 Methodology workflow

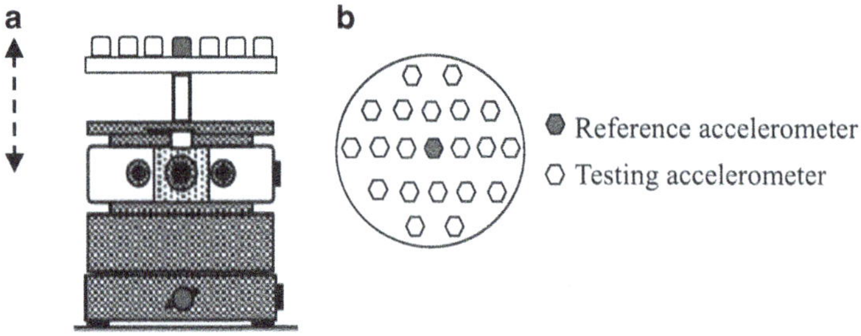

Fig. 5.2 Accelerometer calibration showing (**a**) accelerometer placed on the metal disc attached to the mechanical wave driver, (**b**) top view of the metal disc showing accelerometer arrangement on the disc. Arrow indicates the direction of wave driver movement

experiment, all 36 accelerometers were calibrated using a pre-calibrated reference accelerometer and a mechanical wave driver (model: SF-9324, Pasco, Roseville, CA) moving with a reference signal. In addition, the waveform variability of each accelerometer was compared relative to the reference accelerometer output. A metal disc was attached on the driver stinger to attach the accelerometers. Figure 5.2 shows the accelerometer calibration setup.

Due to limited space on the disc, the accelerometers were separated into a group of 16 and a group of 20 accelerometers. The first group of accelerometers were then attached using double-sided medical-grade tape (B205-1, 3M, Minneapolis, MN) on the driver disc. An artificial SCG signal (Taebi and Mansy 2017) having similar characteristics of a typical SCG signal were then employed to drive the disc. All accelerometer outputs were recorded. The experiment was repeated for the remaining 20 accelerometers. The accelerometer output is shown in Fig. 5.3.

Waveform morphological variability (later discussed in Sect. 5.2.5.3) was calculated for each accelerometer output relative to the waveform of the reference accelerometer. The mean variability with standard error of the 36 sensors was found to be 0.16±0.04 mg which is approximately 10–15 times lower than the SCG variability observed at the chest surface (later discussed in Sect. 5.3.4).

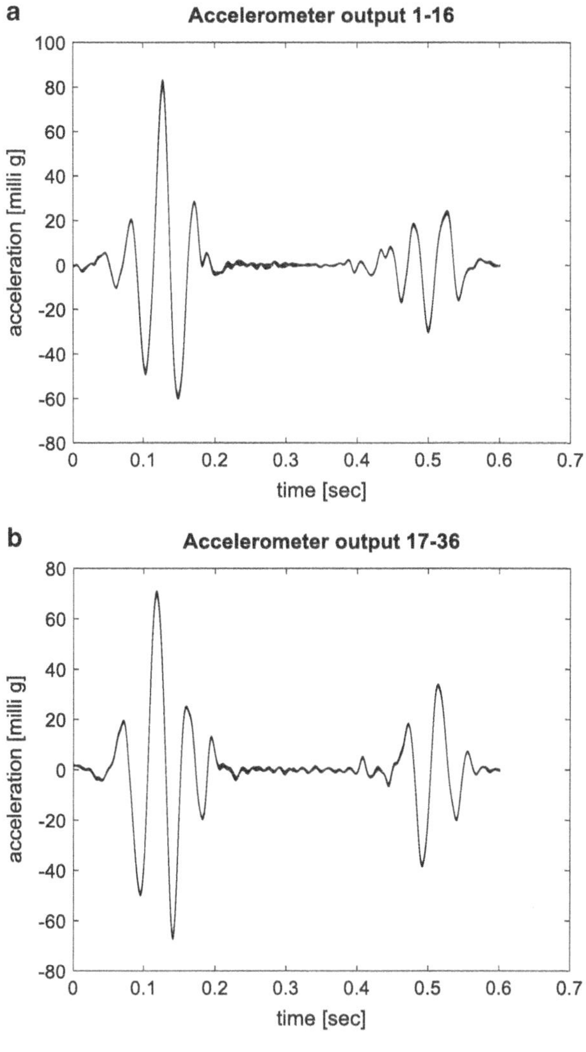

Fig. 5.3 Accelerometer output recorded from (**a**) accelerometer 1–16 (**b**) accelerometer 17–36 are shown. The waveforms are plotted on top of each other showing significant similarity between accelerometer outputs

The calibrated sensitivity of an accelerometer is given by Eq. 5.1:

$$\text{Calibrated sensitivity}_i = \frac{\text{Amp}_i}{\text{Amp}_{\text{ref}}} * \text{Sensitivity}_{\text{ref}} \tag{5.1}$$

where Calibrated sensitivity$_i$ and Amp$_i$ are the calibrated sensitivity and amplitude of ith accelerometer, while Sensitivity$_{\text{ref}}$ and Amp$_{\text{ref}}$ are the sensitivity and amplitude of reference accelerometer.

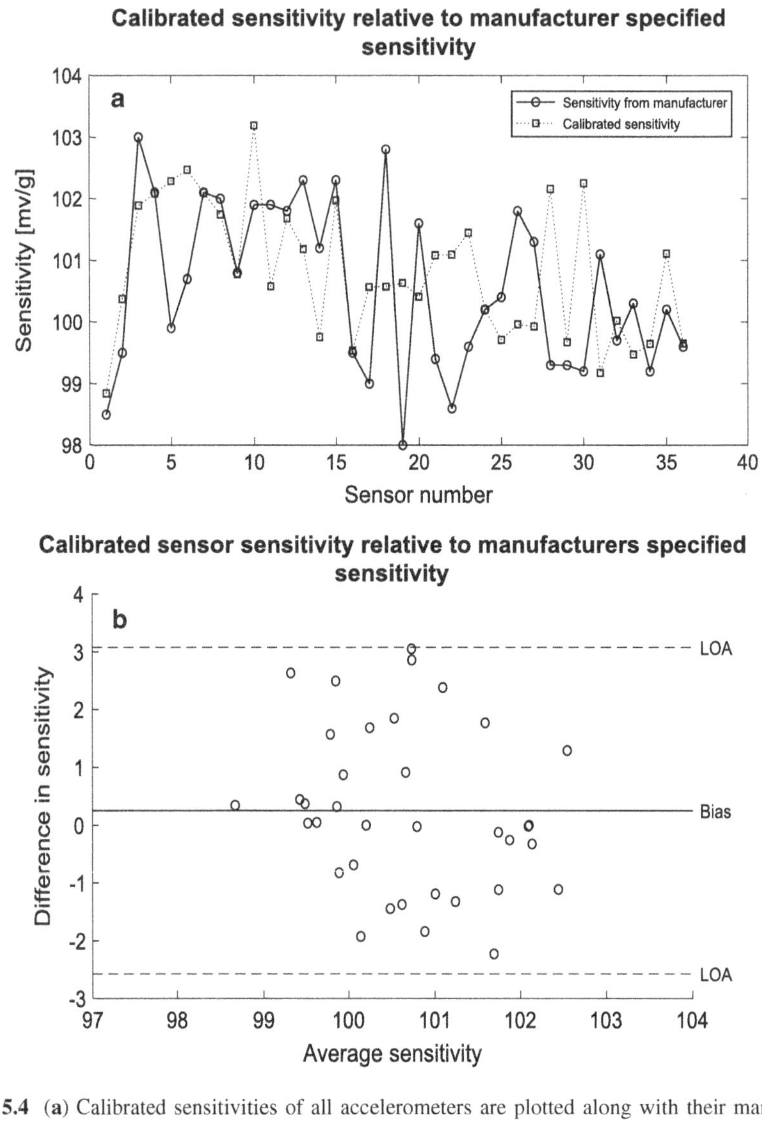

Fig. 5.4 (**a**) Calibrated sensitivities of all accelerometers are plotted along with their manufacturer's sensitivity (**b**) Bland-Altman analysis of calibrated sensitivity and manufacturer specified sensitivity. The difference in sensitivity values is within the limit of agreement (±1.96*SD)

The sensitivities of all 36 accelerometer are plotted with their manufacturer's sensitivity and compared using Bland-Altman analysis (1999) in Fig. 5.4.

Figure 5.4 suggests that the calibrated sensitivities of the sensors are approximately 1–2% of manufacturer specified value and are within the limit of agreement (±1.96*SD). There is a small positive bias (~ 0.2 mV/g) between the calibrated sensitivity and the manufacturer's specified sensitivity values. Peak-to-peak amplitude

Table 5.1 Subject characteristics

Age (years)	26± 4.4
Height (cm)	174.1 ± 8.9
Weight (kg)	75.7 ± 14.5
BMI	24.9 ± 3.2

differences between sensors are within 1% of peak to peak amplitude of reference accelerometer.

5.2.2 Experimental Measurements

SCG signals were acquired from 15 healthy male subjects after Institutional Review Board (IRB) approval. Subject characteristics are listed in Table 5.1.

A diagram of the experimental setup along with sensor locations is shown in Fig. 5.5. Eight accelerometers were placed in each of the parasternal 2nd, 3rd, 4th, and 5th intercostal spaces (ICS) bilaterally. Two additional accelerometers were placed on the left and right clavicle along the mid clavicular line. In addition, two accelerometers were placed at mid-sternum and xiphoid process, respectively. The signal from the accelerometers were amplified using a charge amplifier (Model: 482C, PCB Piezotronics, Depew NY) and then acquired using a data acquisition module (Model: NI-USB-6255, National Instruments, Austin, TX). The utilized SCG sensor is sensitive to chest wall movement due to respiration. While this movement is an artifact that can corrupt SCG, that artifact has a much lower frequency (0.1–0.4 Hz). This makes it easy to remove that artifact by low pass filtering, which is the approach implemented in this study.

Two other signals were simultaneously acquired. These include ECG (in the lead two arrangement, Model: AD 8232, SparkFun Electronics, Niwot, CO) and respiratory flow signal (via a mouthpiece using a with a pressure transducer, Model: CXLdp, Ashcroft Inc, Stratford, CT). Subjects were asked to avoid food and drinks and heavy exercise approximately 4 h prior to experiment to help exclude potential effects of activity on SCG signal. The subjects laid supine on an exam table for approximately 10 min prior to data acquisition. The data was then acquired for approximately 5–10 min at a sampling rate of 10 kHz.

5.2.3 Preprocessing

5.2.3.1 Filtering

The signal processing steps were implemented in MATLAB (2017b. The MathWorks, Inc., MA). To reduce the background noise and baseline wondering (i.e., variation) due to respiration, SCG and ECG signals were forward-backward filtered

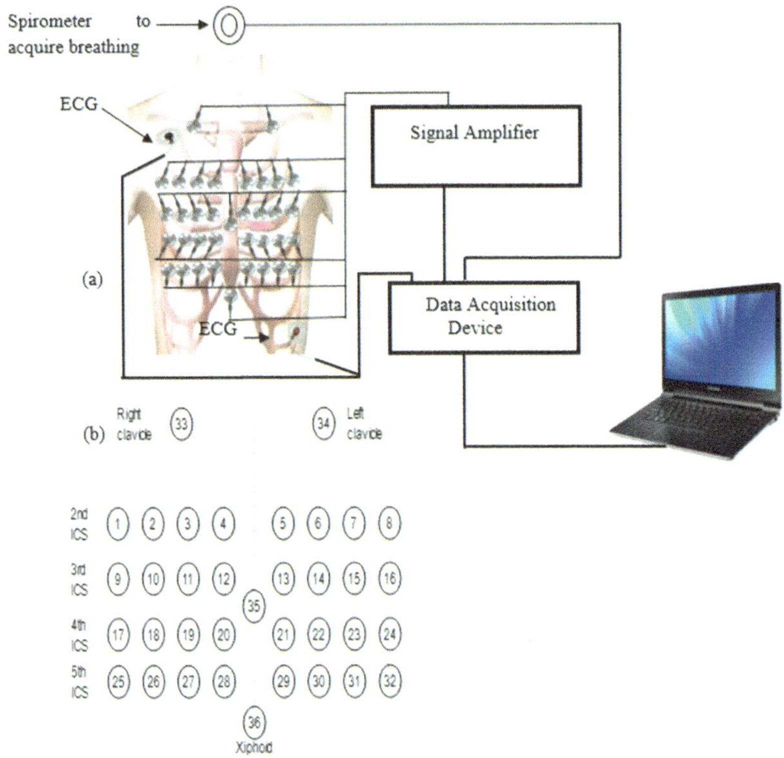

Fig. 5.5 (**a**) Setup for SCG spatial distribution measurement (**b**) sensor location with index

using a fourth-order Chebyshev 2 type band-pass filter (0.5-50 Hz) to remove respiratory sounds and low-frequency noise (typically lower than 0.5 Hz) and other high-frequency noise (typically higher than 50 Hz, e.g., 60 Hz come from electrical connections) described in previous studies (Azad et al. 2019; Gamage et al. 2020). In addition, a moving average filter of order 5 (low pass with cut-off ~ 2 kHz) was employed to further smooth the signal (Azad et al. 2019; Gamage et al. 2020). A similar method was used to filter SCG and ECG signals in previous studies (Azad et al. 2019; Gamage et al. 2020).

5.2.3.2 SCG Segmentation

R peaks of the ECG signal were used to segment the SCG signal into SCG beats (also called events in this manuscript). Here, Pan Tomkins algorithm (1985) was used to detect R peaks. Each SCG beat was selected to start 0.1 s before the R peak of the corresponding ECG, while the end point of SCG beat was selected 0.1 s before the R peak of the following ECG complex (Fig. 5.6). Since the R-R interval varies over time, this approach resulted in SCG beats with varying duration. Similar

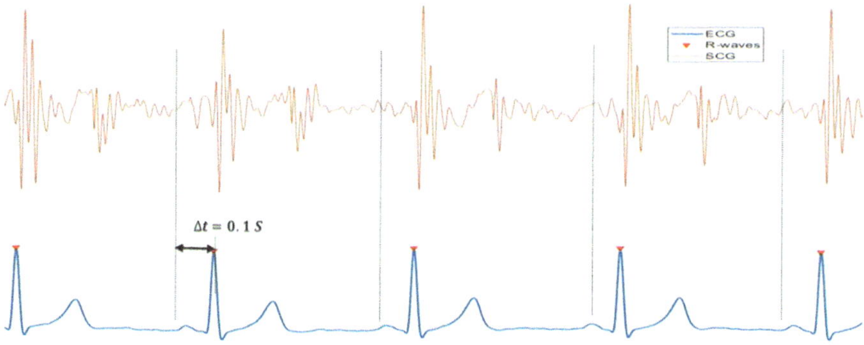

Fig. 5.6 Segmentation of the SCG signal using ECG beats (Gamage et al. 2020)

approach of segmenting the SCG signal is used in previous studies (Azad et al. 2019; Gamage et al. 2020).

5.2.4 *Reducing SCG Variability Using Unsupervised Machine Learning*

The effect of respiratory variation on the SCG signal may lead to inaccurate estimation of SCG features. Previous studies (Gamage et al. 2020; Sandler et al. 2019) have shown that the SCG morphology can be optimally clustered in to two groups which have coherent relations with the respiratory phases and such clustering allows precise estimation of SCG features. Hence, SCG events were clustered based on their morphology using unsupervised machine learning as suggested in previous studies (Azad et al. 2019; Gamage et al. 2018, 2020) which used k-medoid clustering with dynamic time warping (DTW) as a variability measure. This clustering method has shown higher accuracies over other methods for shape-based (i.e., morphology-based) clustering of time series (Paparrizos and Gravano 2017). After clustering, the cluster morphologies can be represented by the medoid SCG beat (i.e., the median beat) of each cluster (Gamage et al. 2020). Figure 5.7 shows an example of the distribution of SCG clusters relative to respiration cycle.

Figure 5.7 shows that SCG events don't cluster entirely based on respiratory flow or lung volume phases. The results suggest that most cluster 1 events happen from the late LLV-INSP phase to early HLV-EXP phase in the respiratory cycle while cluster 2 events happen from late HLV-EXP phase to early LLV-INS phase. To estimate SCG features, medoids of these clusters are considered to be the representative waveforms of these clusters (Gamage et al. 2020). Figure 5.8 shows an example of SCG waveform medoids of cluster 1 and 2 from a single measurement session.

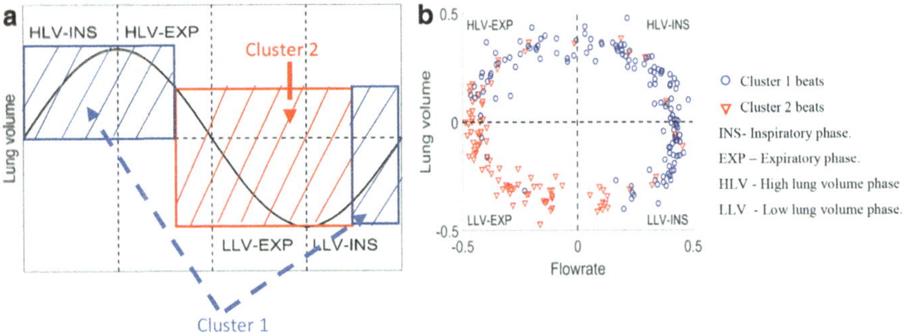

Fig. 5.7 (**a**) SCG clusters occurrence in a respiratory cycle (Lung volume). (**b**) SCG cluster assignment in a lung volume and respiratory flow rate space. SCG beats are represented by blue circles and red triangles showing their respiratory phase suggesting the clusters separate at LLV-INS and HLV-EXP phase

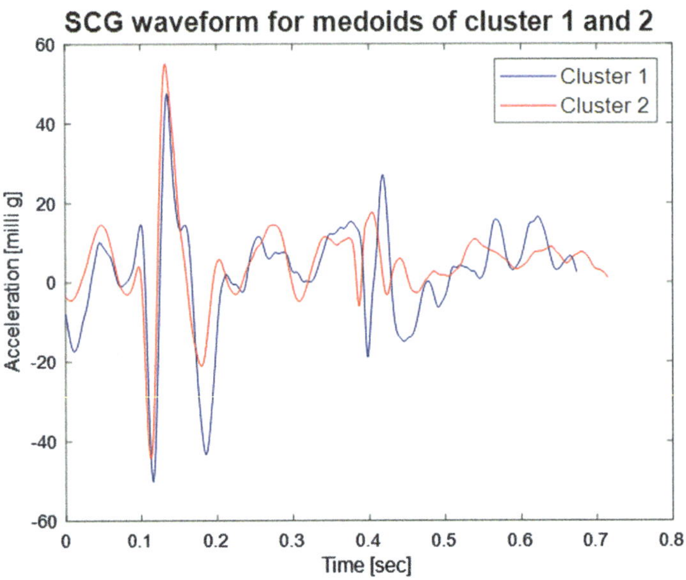

Fig. 5.8 An example of SCG waveform for medoid of cluster 1 and 2. There is noticeable morphological variability between the two cluster medoids due to respiratory variation

5.2.5 SCG Features

After reducing the SCG variability using clustering, the spatial distribution of different SCG features (or attributes) over the chest surface were analyzed. The analyzed features (or attributes) include SCG amplitude, signal-to-noise ratio, morphological variability, cardiac timing intervals (CTIs), and few other time and frequency domain SCG features.

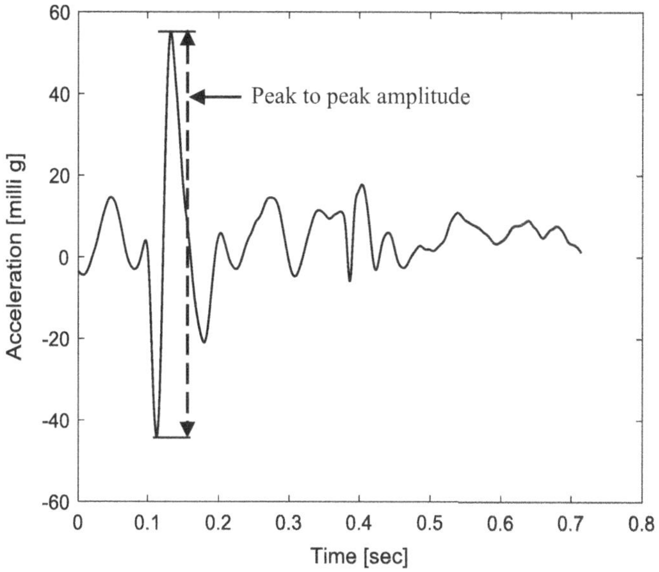

Fig. 5.9 An example of SCG waveform. The arrow indicates the peak to peak (i.e., max-min) amplitude of SCG waveform

5.2.5.1 SCG Peak-to-Peak Amplitude

Peak-to-peak amplitude of SCG waveform can be an important SCG feature which indicates the loudness of SCG signal. The spatial variability of SCG peak-to-peak amplitude would allow us estimate signal strength at different locations on the chest surface. Figure 5.9 illustrates the peak-to-peak amplitude of a SCG waveform.

5.2.5.2 SCG Signal-to-Noise ratio

Signal-to-noise ratio (SNR) is defined as the ratio between the signal energy and energy of background noise. SNR is regarded as a metric to estimate the signal quality over the background noise. The background noise is typically acquired in absence of the signal of interest. With regard to the signal quality of SCG signal, use of SNR is challenging because the signal of interest here is the SCG signal due to cardiac activity and is measured on the chest surface of a live human subject. Hence measurement of chest surface background noise is difficult. A previous study (Luu and Dinh 2018) suggested to use cardiac quiescent phase (T-P interval of ECG) as a period to measure noise, since the heart chambers in this period are at a relaxed phase and comparatively lower acceleration is observed during this period. Figure 5.10 illustrates the waveform window considered for the systolic and cardiac quiescent period to calculate relative SNR.

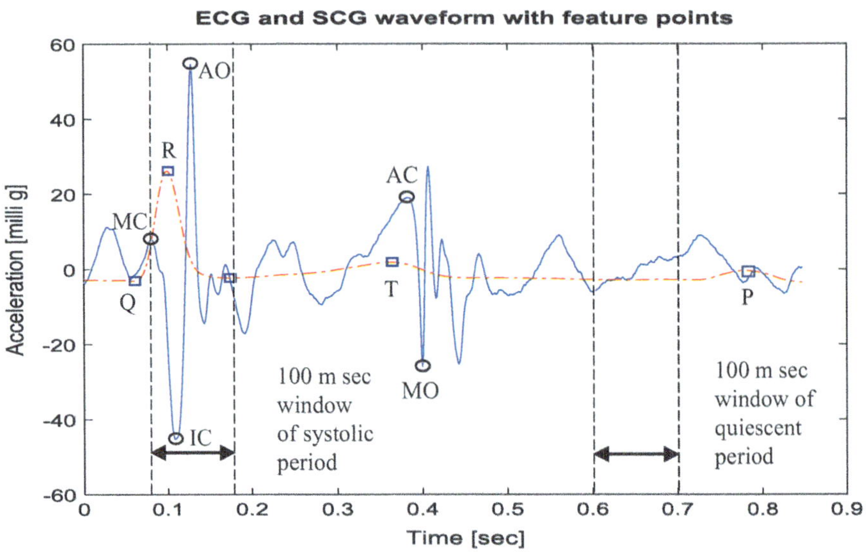

Fig. 5.10 SCG and simultaneously recorded ECG waveform showing SCG waveform window considered during systolic and quiescent period

The relative signal-to-noise ratio is calculated by the following equation.

$$\text{Relative SNR} = \frac{(\text{rms}\ (100\ \text{ms window of SCG waveform during systolic period}))}{(\text{rms}\ (100\ \text{ms window of SCG waveform during cardiac quiescent period}))} \tag{5.2}$$

5.2.5.3 SCG Morphological Variability

SCG morphological variability was quantified using intra-cluster variability and inter-cluster variability. These measures are indicative of beat-to-beat variation of SCG and may contain useful information about respiratory effects on the SCG signal due to the coherent relationships of clusters and respiratory phases (Azad et al. 2019; Gamage et al. 2020). The following equations were used to calculate the intra and inter-cluster variabilities. Similar variability measures are used in previous studies (Azad et al. 2019).

$$\text{Intra} - \text{cluster variability} = \frac{1}{n_1 + n_2}\left[\sum\nolimits_{i=1}^{n_1} dtw\,(C_1, X_{i1}) + \sum\nolimits_{i=1}^{n_2} dtw\,(C_2, X_{i2})\right] \tag{5.3}$$

$$\text{Inter} - \text{cluster variability} = \frac{1}{n_1 + n_2}\left[\sum_{i=1}^{n_1} dtw\,(C_2, X_{i1}) + \sum_{i=1}^{n_2} dtw\,(C_1, X_{i2})\right] \tag{5.4}$$

Here, X_{i1} , X_{i2} are the ith SCG event belonging to cluster 1 and cluster 2, respectively, while C_1 and C_2 are the respective cluster medoids. And n_1, n_2 are the total number of events belonging to cluster 1 and 2, respectively.

In Eqs. 5.3 and 5.4, the function *dtw* is used to calculate the morphological difference between two SCG beats using dynamic time warping (DTW) dissimilarity measure. DTW is an estimate of the similarity between two time series. Initially, DTW was used for automatic speech recognition (Sakoe and Chiba 1978) specifically to identify the same word spoken at different speeds. DTW calculates the optimal "global alignment" between two-time sequences (i.e., SCG beats) by identifying the temporal distortions between them (Sakoe and Chiba 1978; Silva and Batista 2016) and nonlinearly "warps," the two time series to determine a quantitative measure of their dissimilarity (Sakoe and Chiba 1978). Recent studies (Gamage et al. 2020; Paparrizos and Gravano 2017) used this measure in similar time series clustering. The steps for calculating the DTW distance between two time series with different lengths, X and Y, are as follows:

$$X = \{x_1, x_2, \ldots x_i, \ldots .x_n\} \tag{5.5}$$

$$Y = \left\{y_1, y_2, \ldots y_j, \ldots .y_m\right\} \tag{5.6}$$

where n and m are the lengths of the two signals.

This distance matrix is recursively filled using following formula,

$$D\,(i, j) = \delta\left(x_i, y_j\right) + \min\begin{cases} D\,(i, j-1) \\ D\,(i-1, j) \\ D\,(i-1, j-1) \end{cases} \quad \text{where } \delta\left(x_i, y_j\right) = \left(x_i - y_j\right)^2 \text{ or } \left|x_i - y_j\right| \tag{5.7}$$

An optimal alignment (warping path) $W = \{w_1, w_2, \ldots.\ w_k, \ldots, w_N\}$ is to be found where $w_k = (i, j)$ represent the alignment between i^{th} point of X and j^{th} point of Y.

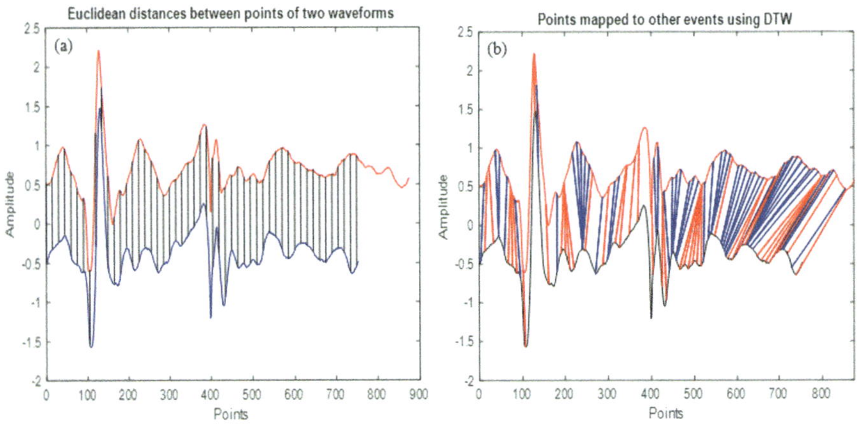

Fig. 5.11 An illustration of distance measure using (**a**) Euclidean distance and (**b**) DTW distance between two SCG signals. For convenience few points in each signal that corresponds to other signal are shown here

The optimal warping path is found such that it minimizes

$$DTW\,(X, Y) = \text{argmin} \sum_{k=1}^{k=N} D(w) \tag{5.8}$$

where the warping path should satisfy the following three conditions.

Boundary constraint: $w_1 = (1, 1)$, $w_N = (n, m)$
Monotonicity constraint: $w_k = (i,j)$, $w_{k+1} = (i^{'},j^{'})$ where $i^{'} \geq i$ and $j^{'} \geq j$
Continuity constraint: $w_k = (i,j)$, $w_{k+1} = (i^{'},j^{'})$ where $i^{'} \leq i + 1$ and $j^{'} \leq j + 1$

The computed *DTW*(*X*, *Y*) reflects the morphological dissimilarity between *X* and *Y*. Figure 5.11 shows the difference between using Euclidean distance and DTW as a dissimilarity measure.

Figure 5.11 shows the associated points between two SCG beats when measuring the dissimilarity between them. As can be seen in Fig. 5.11, associated points are concurrent for Euclidean distance and portion of one SCG beat is not considered due to length difference. In DTW, associated points are related nonlinearly in time based on the morphological similarity of the SCG beats.

5.2.5.4 Cardiac Timing Intervals (CTIs)

Cardiac timing intervals are important parameters in assessment of cardiac health (Crow et al. 1994; Tavakolian 2010; Shafiq et al. 2016). In the current study, the spatial variability of pre-ejection period (PEP) which is typically defined as the time duration between the Q wave location of ECG signal and aortic opening (AO) peak

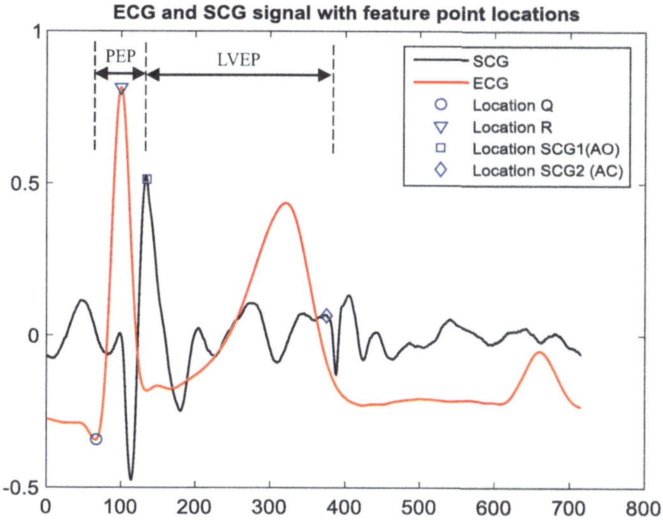

Fig. 5.12 An illustration of pre-ejection period (PEP) and left ventricular ejection period (LVEP) along with ECG and SCG signal

of SCG signal while left ventricle ejection period (LVEP) is defined as the time period between aortic opening (AO) peak and aortic closure (AC) peak in SCG signal are analyzed. Figure 5.12 shows the identification of cardiac timing intervals using simultaneously captured SCG and ECG waveforms.

5.2.5.5 SCG 3 Amplitude

Previous studies (Glower et al. 1992; Abrams 1978) suggested that the presence of the third heart sound (S3) detected in PCG measurements may indicate left ventricular dysfunction. The corresponding high energy region in the SCG signal is called SCG 3 in this paper. A recent study (Siejko et al. 2013) employed an accelerometer to record precordial vibrations located S3 (i.e., similar to SCG 3) by finding the peak of the signal envelop in the frequency band (5-60 Hz) within a window of 100–200 ms after S2 peak location. A similar approach was used to locate SCG 3 in the current study. Here, SCG 1, SCG 2, and SCG 3 were located by seeking for high energy peaks of the SCG signal. The energy signal of SCG waveform was calculated using polynomial chirplet transform (PCT) as it showed better accuracy in a previous study (Taebi and Mansy 2017). An example of located SCG 1, SCG 2, and SCG 3 locations and respective high-energy regions in the PCT distribution is shown in Fig. 5.13.

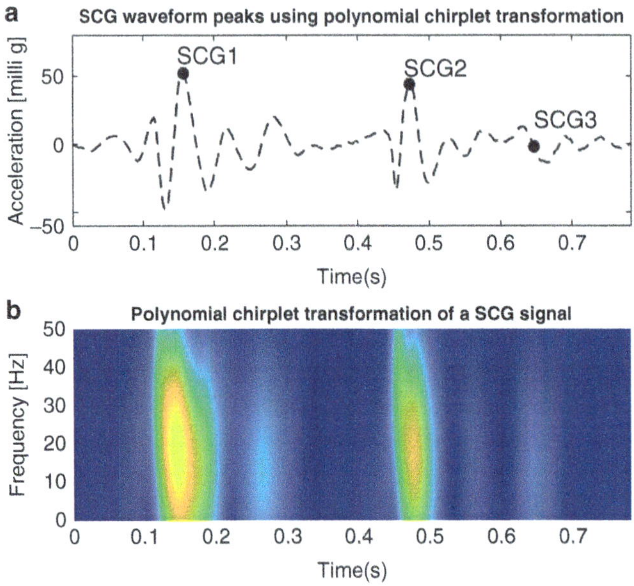

Fig. 5.13 (**a**) SCG 1, SCG 2, and SCG 3 located on the SCG waveform. (**b**) Time frequency distribution of SCG waveform using PCT showing high-energy regions corresponds to SCG 1, SCG 2, and SCG 3

5.2.5.6 Maximum Instantaneous Frequency Around SCG 1 and SCG 2 Peak

The instantaneous frequency (IF) is a transient parameter that corresponds to the average of the frequencies present in a signal at a given time as the signal morphology varies in time. The IF signal of SCG may provide important features related to cardiac mechanical movements such as myocardial movements (correspond to low frequency) and valve fluctuations (correspond to relatively higher frequencies) (Taebi and Mansy 2017). The instantaneous frequency was calculated using the following equation.

$$f_{\text{ins}}(t) = \frac{\int_{0.5}^{50} f.PCT\,(t,\,f)\,df}{\int_{0.5}^{50} PCT\,(t,\,f)\,df} \tag{5.9}$$

Here, f is the frequency and $PCT(t,f)$ is the energy in the time frequency distribution using PCT. An example of located maximum instantaneous frequencies around SCG 1 and SCG 2 in the instantaneous frequency signal is shown in Fig. 5.14.

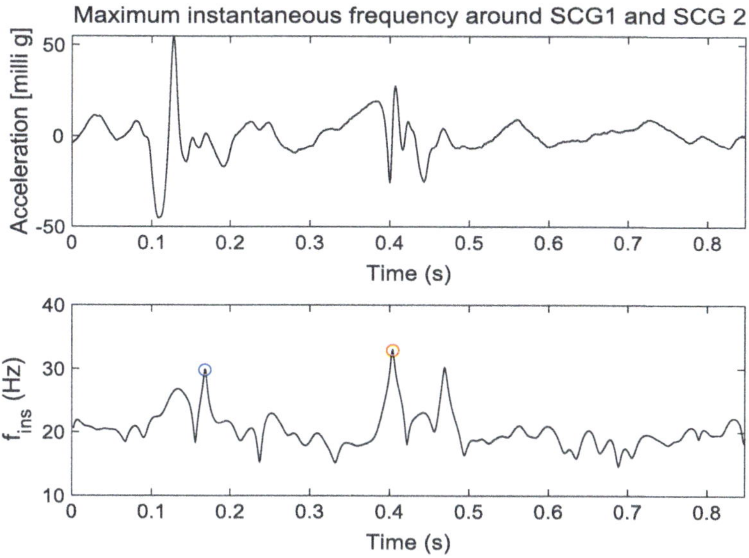

Fig. 5.14 Maximum instantaneous frequency around SCG 1 and SCG 2

5.3 Results

For each sensor location, two medoid SCG beats were calculated after clustering. These medoids were used to calculate the SCG features presented in the following parts of this section. Figure 5.15 shows an example of the derived two medoid SCG beats plotted on top of each other at each sensor location in one subject. In general, for all subjects, louder acceleration signals with prominent SCG feature points (i.e., clear peaks and nadirs) were observed near the left sternal border in the precordial region. In contrast, low-amplitude SCG with less clear SCG features were seen on the right side of the sternum. Also, the clarity of the SCG features diminished toward the lateral direction away from the left sternal boarder. As a whole, these results suggested that attaching a sensor on the precordium near left sternal border would deliver a strong SCG signal with prominent features.

The study focused further on evaluating the optimum sensor locations (or regions) for estimating particular SCG features based on their amplitudes and localized spatial variability. The color map plots representing the feature amplitudes and pairwise t-test connectivity graphs indicating the statistical significance of feature variations between neighboring locations are presented in the following sections. For simplicity, when calculating a feature value for a sensor location, the average feature value of the two SCG medoid beats were used in the presented results.

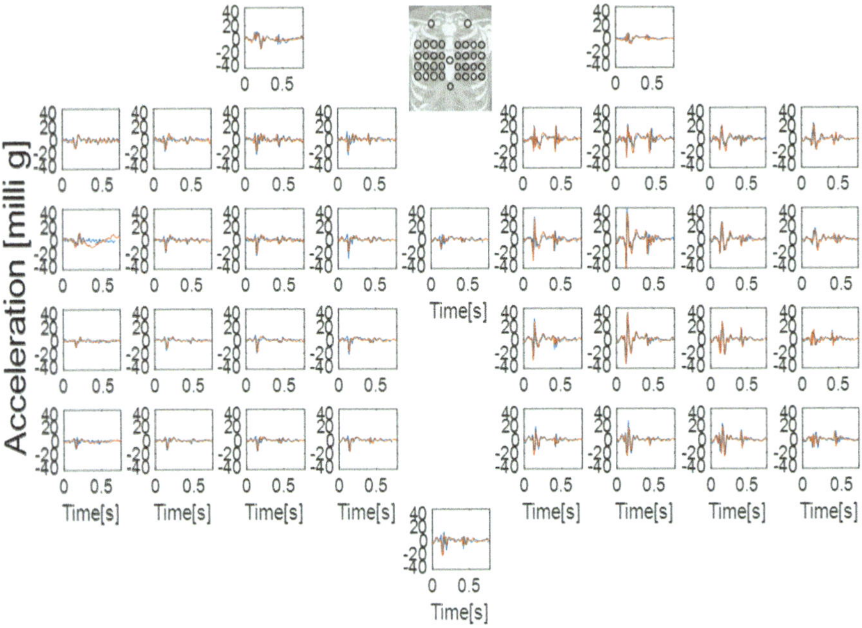

Fig. 5.15 Medoid SCG beats from cluster 1 and 2 plotted on top of each other at different sensor location. Magnitude of acceleration is louder around the left sternal border. Feature points are also prominent closer to the sternal border. Signal amplitude and feature point clarity diminish as the sensor location move laterally away from the left sternal border increasing error in feature point identification

5.3.1 SCG Peak-to-Peak Amplitude

Figure 5.16 shows the peak-to-peak amplitude variation with respect to sensor location.

While SCG amplitude varied from subject to subject, for most subjects, the region with high SCG amplitudes were concentrated at an approximately 3-cm-wide region near left sternal border ranging from 3rd ICS to 5th ICS. SCG amplitude varied significantly at the right lateral border (50~80%) compared to left sternal border (LSB). For some subjects, relatively high SCG amplitudes were seen on the xiphoid region.

5.3.2 Signal-to-Noise Ratio

The relative SNR as described in Sect. 5.2.5.2 with respect to sensor locations are illustrated in Fig. 5.17.

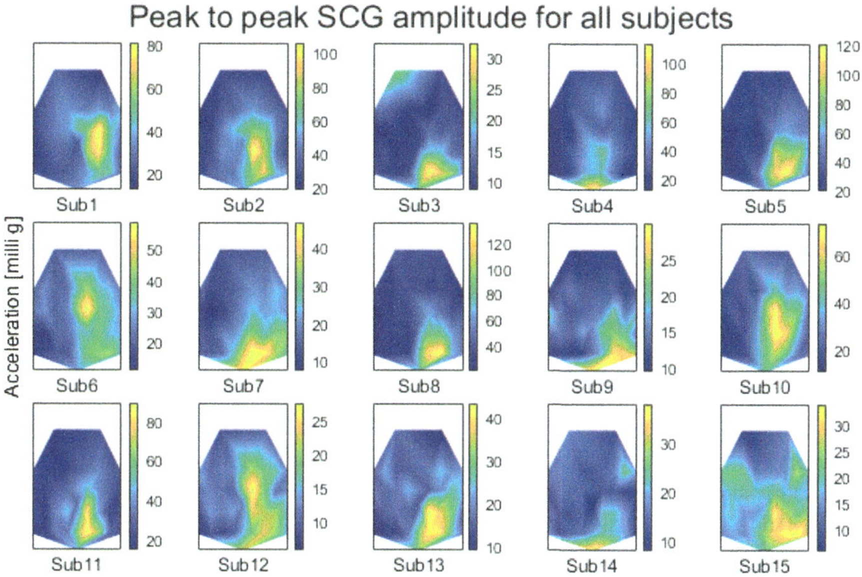

Fig. 5.16 Peak-to-peak SCG amplitude variation visualized by color map. Amplitude of the waveform tends to increase as the sensor move toward left sternal border for most cases. A few subjects showed higher amplitude around xiphoid process

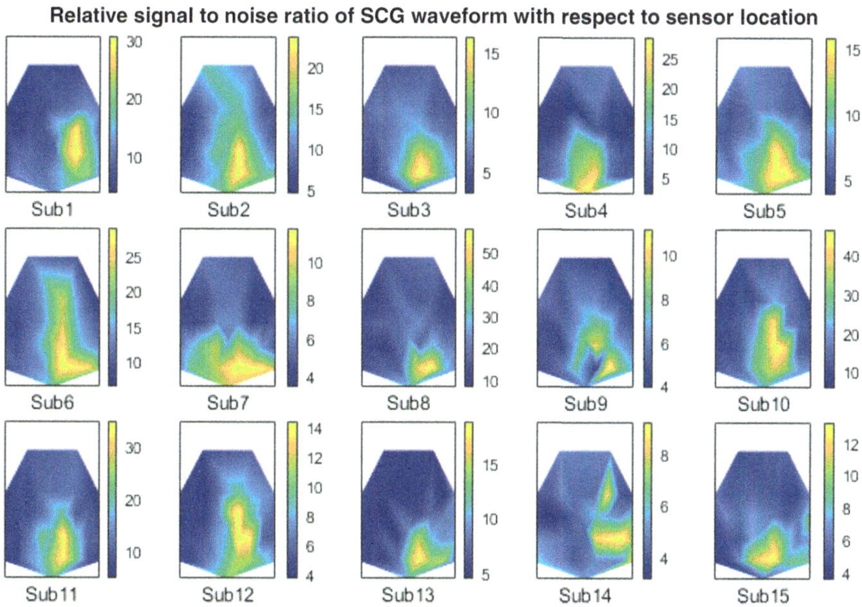

Fig. 5.17 Relative SNR of SCG signal with respect to sensor location. Figure showed that SNR values increased as the sensor moved toward left sternal border suggesting better signal quality around that region

Figure 5.17 suggests that relative SNR values are higher along the left sternal border from 3rd to 5th ICS, and it varied significantly at the right lateral border (50~80%) relative to LSB. This is coherent with SCG peak-to-peak amplitude variations. Few subjects showed higher SNR values around xiphoid process. These results suggest that a high-energy SCG with better signal quality can be acquired by attaching the sensor on the region near the left sternal border ranging from 3rd to 5th ICS which may include xiphoid process in some subjects.

5.3.3 SCG Morphological Variability

The SCG morphological variabilities of the SCG signal as described in Sect. 5.2.5.3 (intra- and inter-cluster variabilities) can contain useful features related to respiratory variation which may help predicting cardiac health (Sandler et al. 2019). The intra- and inter-cluster variability spatial distribution maps for all subjects are presented in Figs. 5.18 and 5.19.

Figures 5.18 and 5.19 suggest that the spatial distribution of SCG variability (intra- and inter-cluster variability) was found to be subject-dependent. The SCG intra- and inter-cluster variability remained comparable (within 5%) in 3-cm-wide region along the 4th ICS left sternal border, while it varied elsewhere (10~40%) relative to 4th ICS near LSB. This variation may be caused by the differences

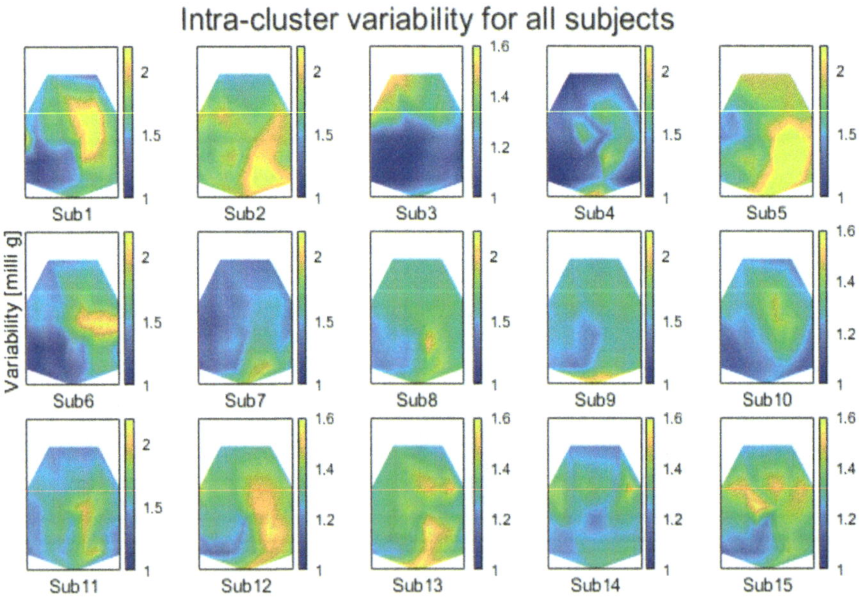

Fig. 5.18 Intra-cluster variability for all subjects. The intra-cluster variability values were comparable around the left sternal border region within 3 cm laterally spread region among most subjects

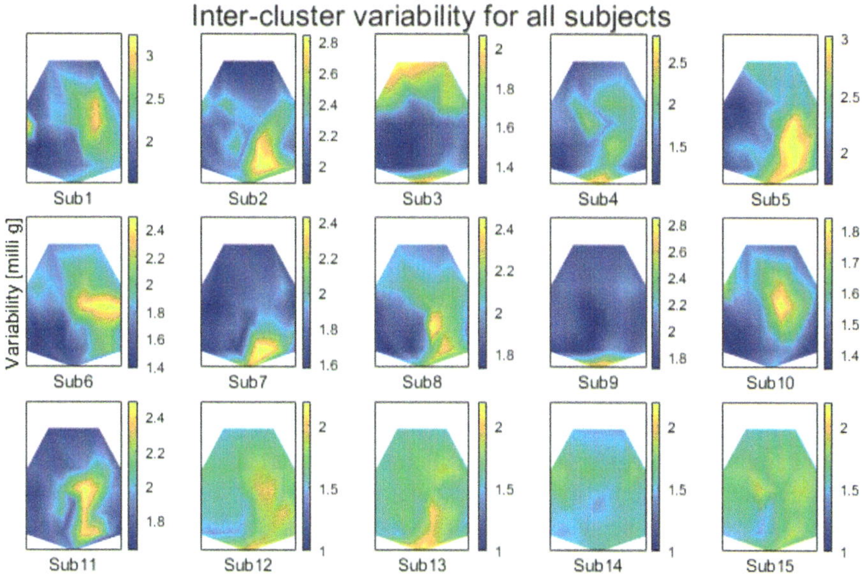

Fig. 5.19 Inter-cluster variability for all subjects. The inter-cluster variability values were consistent around the left sternal border within the 3 cm wide region for most subjects

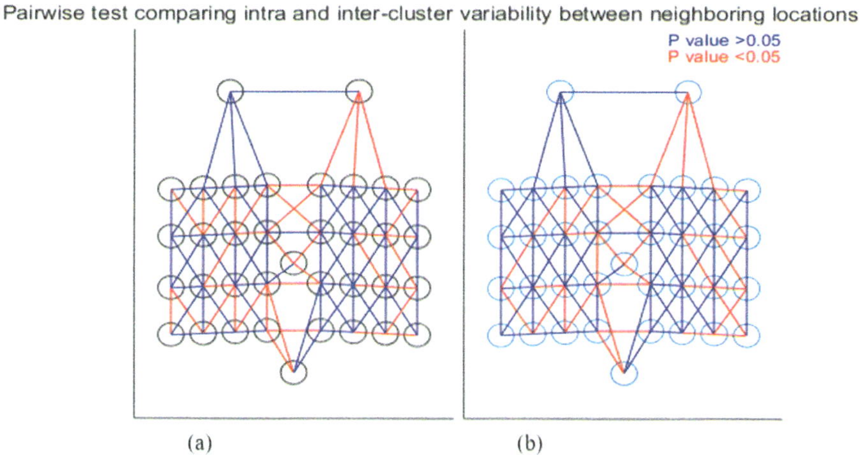

Fig. 5.20 Pairwise test p values connectivity graph comparing sensor location for (**a**) intra-cluster (**b**) inter-cluster variability between neighboring locations. The red lines link significantly different values, while blue lines link the adjacent locations with similar values. The variability values showed similarity within a 3 cm wide region lateral to left sternal border

in subject breathing patterns and variations of soft tissue concentration on the chest surface. This can also be illustrated by Fig. 5.20 which plotted the statistical significance of the differences between the SCG variability values observed at adjacent locations (using p value from pairwise t-test). In this figure, the red lines link significantly different variability values, while blue lines link the adjacent locations with similar variabilities.

5.3.4 Cardiac Timing Intervals

The spatial distribution of the CTIs, namely, pre-ejection period (PEP) and left ventricle ejection period (LVEP), is shown in Figs. 5.21 and 5.22, respectively.

The PEP values remained comparable for most of the sensor locations (0–10%) relative to 4th ICS left lower sternal border (LLSB) except the locations on right anterior axillary lines where they varied significantly (30~60%) relative to 4th ICS near LSB. For LVEP, the values are most consistent (within 2~4%) along the sternal border around 3 cm region lateral to the border. They varied around 10–20% along the right and left anterior axillary lines relative to 4th ICS. To compare PEP and LVEP values with its neighboring locations, pairwise t-test was performed, and the statistical significance between the neighboring sensor locations is represented as a connectivity chart in Fig. 5.23. The red link indicates significant difference between adjacent locations, while blue link indicates similarity.

Figure 5.23 suggests that the PEP and LVEP values were not significantly different around the left sternal border and around 3 cm wide region laterally from 4th to 5th ICS. In addition, sensor at xiphoid process showed similar values to 4th ICS near LSB for PEP and LVEP.

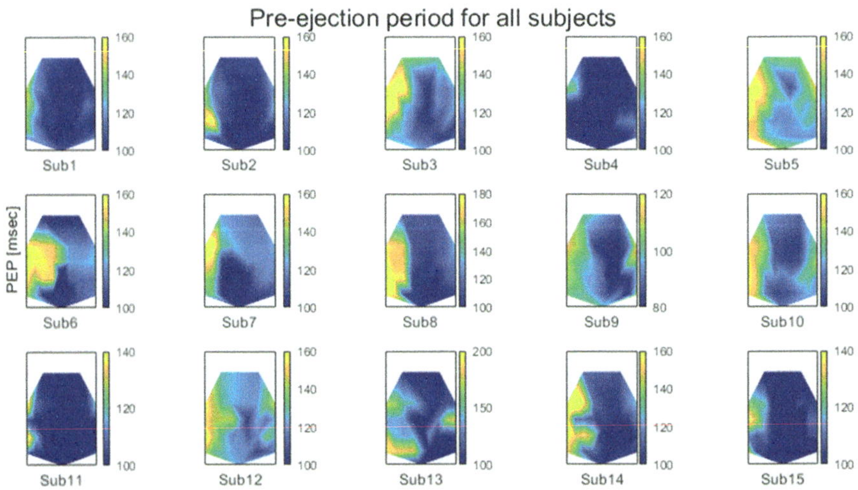

Fig. 5.21 PEP relative to sensor location for individual subjects. Figure suggests that the error in PEP is lower around the left lower sternal border region compared to right side of the sternal border

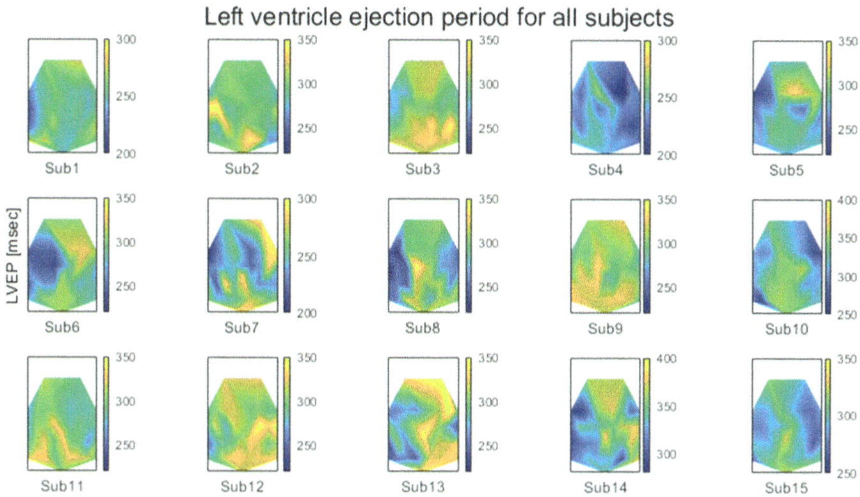

Fig. 5.22 LVEP relative to sensor location for (a) individual subjects. Figure suggests that the error in LVEP values is comparable relative to sensor locations

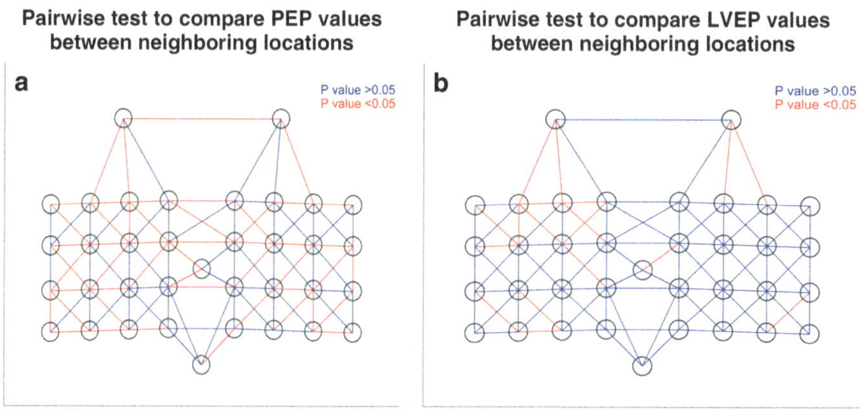

Fig. 5.23 Pairwise t-test p values connectivity graph performed for (**a**) PEP and (**b**) LVEP values between neighboring locations. The red lines link significantly different values, while blue lines link the adjacent locations with similar values. PEP and LVEP values were not significantly different at the left sternal border and at xiphoid process

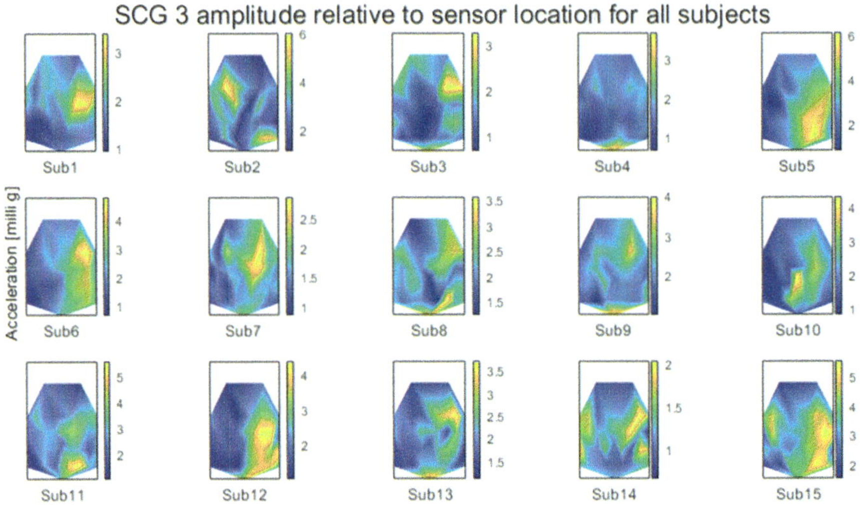

Fig. 5.24 Variation of SCG 3 amplitude relative to sensor locations

5.3.5 SCG 3 Amplitude Variation Over Sensor Location

The variation of SCG 3 amplitude relative to sensor location is plotted in Fig. 5.24.

Figure 5.24 suggests that SCG 3 amplitude values were similar (1~2 mg and were within 2–5%) around left sternal border. The SCG 3 amplitude varied (10–20%) relative to 4th ICS LLSB among most sensor locations. The pairwise test p values connectivity chart for SCG 3 amplitudes between adjacent locations is plotted in Fig. 5.25.

Fig. 5.25 suggests that SCG 3 magnitudes are not consistent as observed in previous findings in the 3-cm-wide region near the left sternal border. However, the values showed similarity just at the sternal border and xiphoid process. There may be other regions of consistent SCG 3, but these regions are away from the pericardium region and with low SCG 3 magnitude. This may be due to the inconsistent nature of the presence of SCG 3 (Correspond to S3) in healthy subjects. However, for patients with heart failure, different results may be expected with the strong likelihood of S3 presence in HF patients.

5.3.6 Maximum Instantaneous Frequency Around SCG 1 and SCG 2 Peak

The variation of maximum instantaneous frequency around SCG 1 and SCG 2 relative to sensor location is plotted in Fig. 5.26.

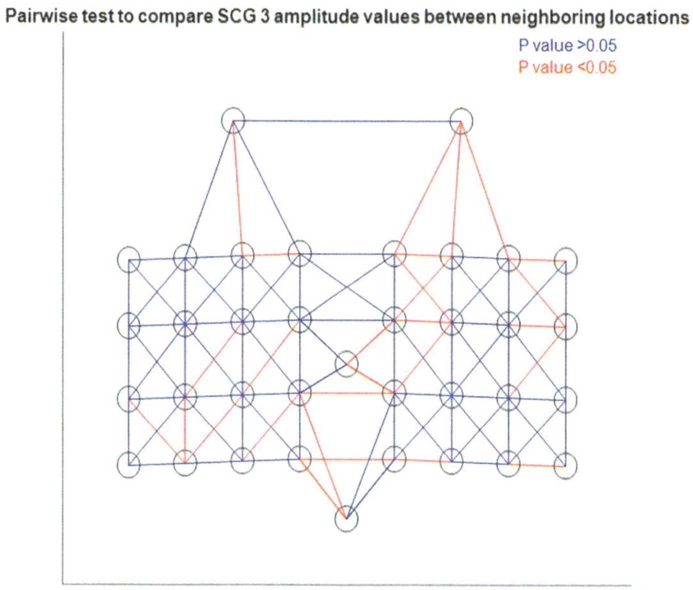

Fig. 5.25 Pairwise test of SCG 3 amplitude values between neighboring locations. The red lines link significantly different values, while blue lines link the adjacent locations with similar values. SCG 3 amplitude values were similar at left sternal border and at xiphoid process

The maximum instantaneous frequency variations around SCG 1 and 2 peak at the LSB were small (within 5%), and in other locations they varied approximately (5~10%) relative to 4th ICS near LSB. Pairwise test p value connectivity graph for Max IF around SCG 1 and SCG 2 peaks is plotted in Fig. 5.27. Pairwise test suggested that the values are not significantly different at the left sternal border locations from 3rd to 5th ICS and at xiphoid process. Other locations were also found to be consistent such as right and left lateral border in the anterior axillary lines. However, the SCG in these locations were with low signal amplitude and low feature clarity.

5.3.7 Surface Acceleration Map at Feature Points

Chest surface instant acceleration maps may help us understand the entire chest surface motion during a cardiac cycle. The surface acceleration during a cardiac cycle at important feature points relative to left sternal border near 4th ICS for a subject is shown in Fig. 5.28. Similar trend was observed for other subjects as well.

Figure 5.28 suggests that during pre-ejection period, an inward motion followed by a loud outward motion in the dorsoventral direction is observed around the left sternal border from approximately 3rd ICS to 5th ICS. During aortic closure, the surface acceleration showed a mild outward motion followed by an inward motion

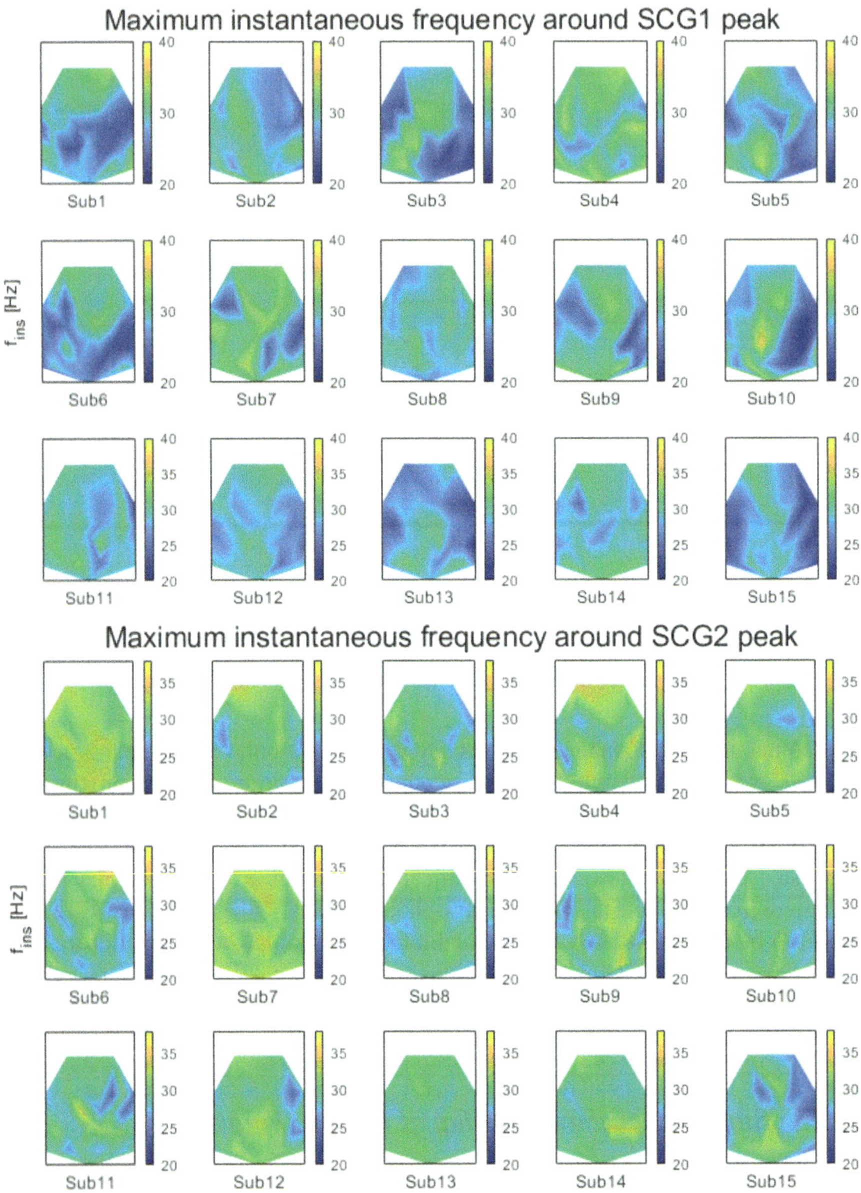

Fig. 5.26 Maximum instantaneous frequency around SCG 1 and 2 peaks. Figure suggests that the instantaneous frequency ranges from 30 to 35 Hz around the left sternal border

around the same area. A recent numerical study which modeled cardiac-related precordial vibrations (Gamage et al. 2019) suggested similar acceleration pattern at the chest surface from the finite element modeling of the cardiac motion.

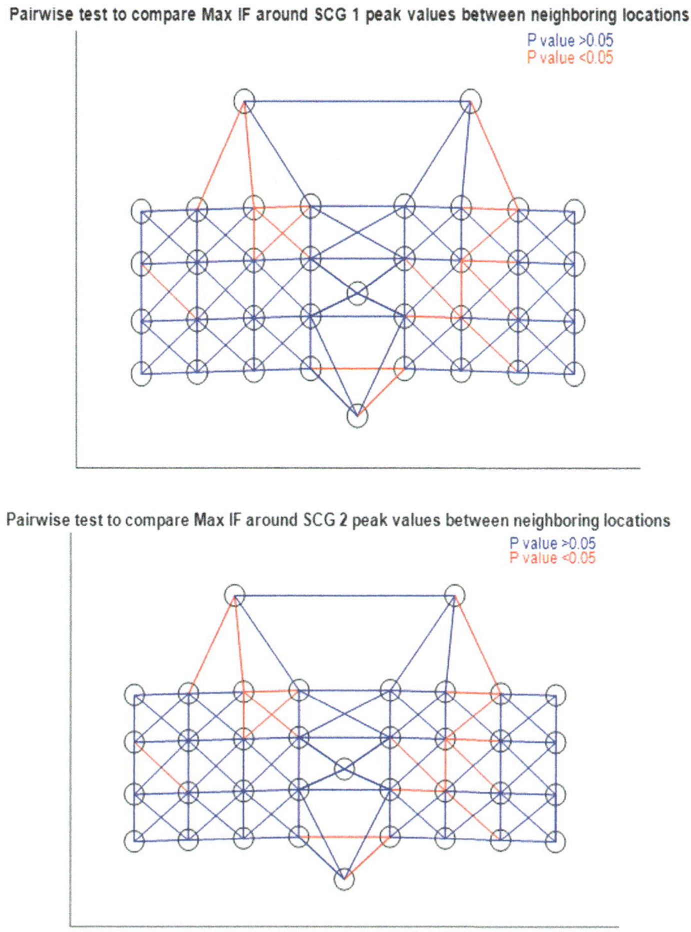

Fig. 5.27 Pairwise test p value connectivity graph for Max IF around SCG 1(top) and SCG 2 (bottom) plotted. The red link indicates significant difference between adjacent locations, while blue link indicates similar feature values. Max IF around SCG 1 and 2 peaks tend to be similar at left sternal border

5.4 Discussion

The results of the current study are consistent with previous studies (Kawamura et al. 2007; Nogata et al. 2010, 2014; Pandia et al. 2012). The current study expands the analysis by investigating more SCG features that may help increase SCG clinical utility.

The current manuscript compared SCG features between neighboring sensor locations (e.g., Figs. 5.20, 5.23, 5.25, and 5.27) to quantify the variation in features with relatively small sensor placement changes. For example, Fig. 5.20 compares

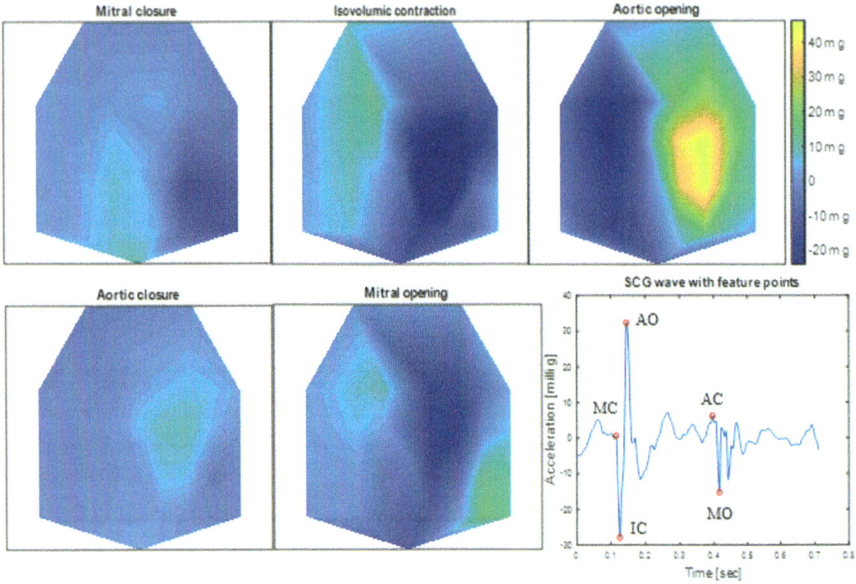

Fig. 5.28 Instantaneous chest surface acceleration during mitral closure (MC), isovolumic contraction (IC), aortic opening (AO), aortic closure (AC), and mitral opening (MO). The positive (i.e., outward) acceleration tended to be loudest around left sternal border between 3rd and 5th ICS during aortic opening and closure. During isovolumic moment, a negative (i.e., inward) acceleration was observed around the same surface region

the intra- and inter-cluster waveform variability at adjacent locations. Results suggested that although the waveform remained similar at the left side of the sternal border, they were significantly different from those at right sternal border. However, some cardiac timing intervals (PEP and LVEP) were similar for the left and right sternal borders. This increased similarity may be expected since waveform timing depends on travel distance (of cardiac vibration waves), and this distance is relatively small between left and right borders. For SCG 3 amplitudes and maximum IF (Figs. 5.25 and 5.27, respectively), SCG 3 amplitude varied significantly between left and right sternal margin (possibly due to tissue damping), while IF variation was smaller since it is independent of damping.

One limitation of the study is that it was done in young healthy male non-obese adults. To generalize findings, further investigation is needed over a wider population including females and those with cardiovascular disease.

The study used a large number of sensors to map the surface distribution of SCG to help guide sensor position choices and estimate potential sensor positioning errors. In a clinical setting, likely only one or perhaps two sensors would be used at locations where SNR and signal strength are highest. The study suggested that certain locations would be optimal based on these criteria.

5.5 Conclusion

In this study, SCG spatial variability was investigated using 36 accelerometers attached on the chest surface in 15 healthy subjects. The spatial variations of several features were studied to identify optimum location for SCG sensor placement. The magnitude of acceleration and relative signal-to-noise ratio was found higher around the left lower sternal border around a 3 cm wide laterally spread region ranging from 3rd to 5th ICS and may include the xiphoid process. In this region, SCG signal variability (i.e., intra- and inter-cluster variability) tend to be around 4–5% of SCG signal peak-to-peak amplitude. The SCG features in a 3–6 cm laterally spread region from the left sternal border found to be inconsistent and significantly different than its adjacent locations outside this region. Several potentially important SCG features (including the PEP and LVEP values) were found to be similar ($p > 0.05$) at 3-cm-wide region near the left lower sternal border. Other features including SCG 3 magnitude, maximum instantaneous frequency around SCG 1 and SCG 2 showed consistent values only along the left sternal border (ranging from 3rd ICS to 5th ICS) and xiphoid process. These results suggest that those sensor locations are optimal and should help provide guidance for accurate SCG sensor positioning. Sensor positioning optimization in turn should help advance the utility of SCG analysis for improved cardiovascular health. Further investigation is needed over a wider population including those with cardiovascular disease.

Acknowledgments This study was supported by NIH R44HL099053. Hansen A Mansy and Richard H Sandler are part owners of Biomedical Acoustics Research Company, which is the primary recipient of the above grant, as such they may benefit financially as a result of the outcomes of the research work reported in this publication.

References

J. Abrams, Current concepts of the genesis of heart sounds: I. first and second sounds. JAMA **239**(26), 2787–2789 (1978)

M.K. Azad, P.T. Gamage, R.H. Sandler, N. Raval, H.A. Mansy, Seismocardiographic signal variability during regular breathing and breath hold in healthy adults. *2019 IEEE Signal Proc. Med. Biol. Symp.***27**, 3–6 (2019)

J.M. Bland, D.G. Altman, Measuring agreement in method comparison studies. Stat. Methods Med. Res. **8**(2), 135–160 (1999)

M. Cozic, L.-G. Durand, R. Guardo, Development of a cardiac acoustic mapping system. Med. Biol. Eng. Comput. **36**(4), 431–437 (1998)

R.S. Crow, P. Hannan, D. Jacobs, L. Hedquist, D.M. Salerno, Relationship between seismocardiogram and echocardiogram for events in the cardiac cycle. Am. J. noninvasive Cardiol. **8**, 39–46 (1994)

E.W. Dijkstra, A note on two problems in connexion with graphs. Numer. Math. **1**(1), 269–271 (1959)

P.T. Gamage, M. Khurshidul Azad. A. Taebi, R.H. Sandler, H.A. Mansy, Clustering Seismocardiographic Events using Unsupervised Machine Learning, in *2018 IEEE Signal Processing in Medicine and Biology Symposium (SPMB)* (2018), pp. 1–5. https://doi.org/10.1109/SPMB.2018.8615615

P.T. Gamage, M.K. Azad, R.H. Sandler, H.A. Mansy, Modeling Seismocardiographic signal using finite element Modeling and medical image processing, in *2019 IEEE Signal Processing in Medicine and Biology Symposium (SPMB)*, (2019), pp. 1–4

P.T. Gamage, M.K. Azad, A. Taebi, R.H. Sandler, H.A. Mansy, Clustering of SCG events using unsupervised machine learning, in *Signal Processing in Medicine and Biology: Emerging Trends in Research and Applications*, ed. by I. Obeid, I. Selesnick, J. Picone, (Springer, Cham, 2020), pp. 205–233

D.D. Glower, R.L. Murrah, C.O. Olsen, J.W. Davis, J.S. Rankin, Mechanical correlates of the third heart sound. J. Am. Coll. Cardiol. **19**(2), 450–457 (1992)

J.D. Hosenpud, B.H. Greenberg, *Congestive Heart Failure* (Lippincott Williams & Wilkins, 2007)

Y. Kawamura, Y. Yokota, F. Nogata, Propagation route estimation of heart sound through simultaneous multi-site recording on the chest wall, in *2007 29th Annual International Conference of the IEEE Engineering in Medicine and Biology Society* (2007), pp. 2875–2878

M. Kompis, H. Pasterkamp, Y. Motai, G. R. Wodicka, Spatial representation of thoracic sounds, in *Proceedings of the 20th Annual International Conference of the IEEE Engineering in Medicine and Biology Society. Vol. 20 Biomedical Engineering Towards the Year* 2000 *and Beyond (Cat. No. 98CH36286)*, vol. 3 (1998), pp. 1661–1664

M. Kompis, H. Pasterkamp, G.R. Wodicka, Acoustic imaging of the human chest. Chest **120**(4), 1309–1321 (2001)

L. Luu, A. Dinh, Artifact noise removal techniques on seismocardiogram using two tri-axial accelerometers. Sensors **18**(4), 1067 (2018)

F. Nogata, Y. Yokota, Y. Kawamura, H. Morita, Y. Uno, Visualization of heart motion by analysis of chest vibration. Anal. Biomed. Signals Images **20**, 11–16 (2010)

F. Nogata, Y. Yokota, Y. Kawamura, Distribution of vibration of chest surface with heart movement. Front. Sensors **2**, 26–31 (2014)

M. Okada, Chest wall maps of heart sounds and murmurs. Comput. Biomed. Res. **15**(3), 281–294 (1982)

J. Pan, W.J. Tompkins, A real-time QRS detection algorithm. I.E.E.E. Trans. Biomed. Eng. **32**(3), 230–236 (1985)

K. Pandia, O.T. Inan, G.T.A. Kovacs, L. Giovangrandi, Extracting respiratory information from seismocardiogram signals acquired on the chest using a miniature accelerometer. Physiol. Meas. **33**(10), 1643 (2012)

J. Paparrizos, L. Gravano, Fast and accurate time-series clustering. *ACM Trans. Database Syst.***42**(2), 8 (2017)

H. Sakoe, S. Chiba, Dynamic programming algorithm optimization for spoken word recognition. IEEE Trans. Acoust. **26**(1), 43–49 (1978)

R.H. Sandler et al., Minimizing Seismocardiography variability by accounting for respiratory effects. J. Card. Fail. **25**(8), S172 (2019)

C. Sapsanis et al., StethoVest: A simultaneous multichannel wearable system for cardiac acoustic mapping, in *2018 IEEE Biomedical Circuits and Systems Conference (BioCAS)*, (2018), pp. 1–4

G. Shafiq, S. Tatinati, W.T. Ang, K.C. Veluvolu, Automatic identification of systolic time intervals in seismocardiogram. Sci. Rep. **6**, 37524 (2016)

K.Z. Siejko, P.H. Thakur, K. Maile, A. Patangay, M. Olivari, Feasibility of heart sounds measurements from an accelerometer within an ICD pulse generator. Pacing Clin. Electrophysiol. **36**(3), 334–346 (2013)

D.F. Silva, G.E. Batista, Speeding up all-pairwise dynamic time warping matrix calculation, in *Proceedings of the 2016 SIAM International Conference on Data Mining* (2016), pp. 837–845

A. Taebi, H.A. Mansy, Time-frequency distribution of Seismocardiographic signals: A comparative study. Bioengineering **4**(2), 32 (2017). https://doi.org/10.3390/bioengineering4020032.

A. Taebi, B.E. Solar, A.J. Bomar, R.H. Sandler, H.A. Mansy, Recent advances in seismocardiography. Vibration **2**(1), 64–86 (2019)
K. Tavakolian, Characterization and analysis of seismocardiogram for estimation of hemodynamic parameters, in *Applied Science: School of Engineering Science* 2010
K. Tavakolian, Systolic time intervals and new measurement methods. Cardiovasc. Eng. Technol. **7**(2), 118–125 (2016)
S.S. Virani et al., Heart disease and stroke Statistics-2020 update: A report from the American Heart Association. *Circulation*, (2020), p. CIR0000000000000757

Chapter 6
Determination of Vascular Access Stenosis Location and Severity by Multi-domain Analysis of Blood Sounds

Steve J. A. Majerus, Rohan Sinha, Binit Panda, and Hossein Miri Lavasani

6.1 Introduction and Background

Hemodialysis is a renal replacement therapy which replaces the lost function of the kidneys for individuals with acute or chronic kidney disease. For those with end-stage renal disease (ESRD), hemodialysis is essential for survival unless a kidney transplant is available. Despite the mortality risk of ESRD, successful hemodialysis can greatly prolong patient lifespans and increase the chance of receiving a donor transplant (Leypoldt 2005). During hemodialysis, arterial blood is filtered through a dialyzer to remove waste products and excess fluid before being returned to the venous system. For individuals with ESRD, hemodialysis is required typically three times per week, which requires a high-flow vascular access so core blood can be filtered efficiently. To improve hemodialysis, permanent vascular access is usually obtained using arteriovenous fistulas or grafts or central venous catheters (Fig. 6.1).

S. J. A. Majerus (✉)
Advanced Platform Technology Center, Louis Stokes Cleveland Veterans Affairs Medical Center, Cleveland, OH, USA
e-mail: steve.majerus@case.edu

R. Sinha
Advanced Platform Technology Center, Louis Stokes Cleveland Veterans Affairs Medical Center, Cleveland, OH, USA

Department of Electrical Engineering and Computer Science, Case Western Reserve University, Cleveland, OH, USA

B. Panda
Department of Biomedical Engineering, Case Western Reserve University, Cleveland, OH, USA

H. M. Lavasani
Department of Electrical Engineering and Computer Science, Case Western Reserve University, Cleveland, OH, USA

I. Obeid et al. (eds.), *Biomedical Signal Processing*,
https://doi.org/10.1007/978-3-030-67494-6_6

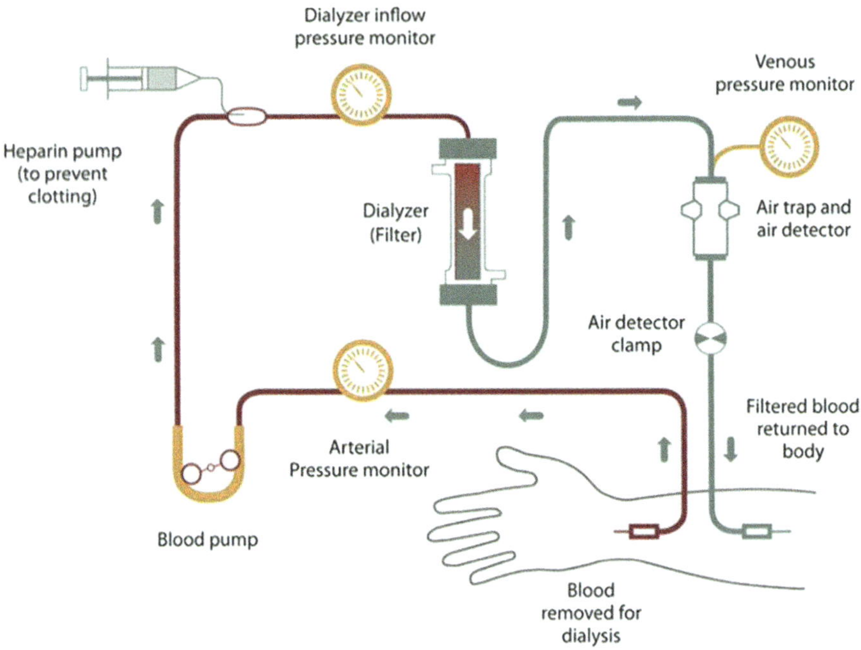

Fig. 6.1 The hemodialysis circuit removes arterial blood, filters it externally, and returns it to the body through the vascular access

Patency of a hemodialysis vascular access is the "Achilles Heel" of hemodialysis treatment (Pisoni et al. 2015). Access dysfunction accounts for two hospital visits/year (Cayco et al. 1998; Sehgal et al. 2001) for dialysis patients, and the loss of access patency greatly increases mortality risk (Lacson et al. 2010). Maintenance of vascular access is therefore a key objective in clinical guidelines for dialysis care and is often handled by dedicated vascular clinics to deal with the high volumes of individuals needing emergency interventions (Feldman et al. 1996). The predominant causes of access dysfunction are stenosis (vascular narrowing) and thrombosis (vascular occlusion), which occur in 66–73% of arteriovenous fistulas (AVFs) and 85% of arteriovenous grafts (AVGs) (Al-Jaishi et al. 2017; Huijbregts et al. 2007; Bosman et al. 1998). Venous stenosis near the artery-vein anastomosis occurs in 50–71% of grafts and fistulas, but stenoses can occur anywhere along the vascular access or central veins (Duque et al. 2017; Roy-Chaudhury et al. 2006). Clinical monitoring is essential to identify at-risk accesses for diagnostic imaging and treatment planning and to avoid emergencies, missed treatments, or loss of the access (H. Inc for OSORA CMS n.d.; Hemodialysis | NIDDK n.d.). Doppler ultrasonic imaging, for example, is a noninvasive method for characterizing vascular access function but requires a visit to a healthcare center and evaluation by specifically trained personnel (Sequeira et al. 2017). The promise of efficient, point-of-care monitoring is to proactively identify which patients might need this specialized examination to minimize vascular access dysfunction or loss.

Monitoring for vascular access dysfunction relies on data efficiently gathered in the dialysis center, most regularly through physical exam. When blood flows through a constricted vessel, the resulting high-speed flow jet induces turbulence and pressure fluctuations in the vessel wall (Seo n.d.). This produces distinct bruits which can be heard with a stethoscope during physical examination. Access surveillance, occasionally performed monthly using flow-measuring equipment, cannot detect fast-growing lesions or restenosis after angioplasty and is often a late indicator of access risk (Krivitski 2014) which reduces utility (Krivitski 2014; White et al. 2006; Moist and Lok 2019). Higher-frequency monitoring for access dysfunction would be ideal for early detection of stenosis but must be balanced against the labor and time required. Existing monitoring techniques have variable sensitivities (35–80%), in part due to the expertise dependence of bruit interpretation and physical exam techniques (Tessitore et al. 2014a). Since listening to bruits is an important aspect of physical exams, clinicians have sought to identify auditory features of bruits for quantitative analysis since the 1970s (Duncan et al. 1975).

Recording and mathematical analysis of bruits—sometimes referred to as phonoangiograms (PAGs)—is called phonoangiography because it has the same objectives of characterizing vascular stenosis as angiographic images (Seo n.d.; Kan et al. 2015; Majerus et al. 2018; Doyle et al. n.d.). The primary motivation behind phonoangiography is efficiency and objectivity, because sounds can be recorded easily from the skin surface without particular need for expertise. Signal analysis of PAGs can then be used to objectively describe the underlying turbulent flow and degree of stenosis. Recent advances in spectral and multiresolution analysis, autoregressive models, and machine learning make real-time PAG analysis feasible at the point of care for rapid patient screening. PAG monitoring has the potential to provide widespread, objective screening of hemodialysis vascular access function for early detection of accesses at-risk for thrombosis. This chapter covers relevant signal processing in the analog and digital domains and strategies for extracting classification features from an array of microphone recording sites (Figs. 6.2 and 6.3).

The chapter is organized beginning with a brief summary of prior work using PAGs to locate and classify vascular stenotic lesions. Next, an analysis of recorded bruits is presented to determine the minimum signal bandwidth and dynamic range for analog signal processing prior to digitization. Digital signal processing methods for feature extraction is reviewed, demonstrating feature extraction in spectral, temporospectral, and spatial domains based on recording site location. Finally, three digital analysis strategies are presented to locate, classify, and estimate the actual degree of stenosis using machine-learning methods. While estimation of degree of stenosis provides clinically actionable data, classification enables simpler user notification, for example, with at-home monitoring. Therefore, we highlight these differing approaches to using machine learning for stenosis characterization from acoustic analysis.

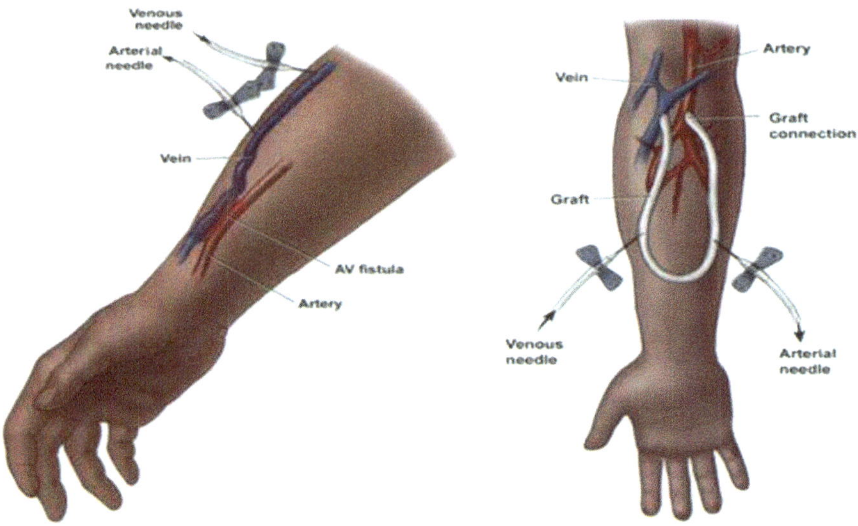

Fig. 6.2 Chronic hemodialysis is best achieved using an arteriovenous fistula vascular access, or an arteriovenous graft for individuals with compromised vascular structure. The vascular access is surgically created and monitored clinically to detect the symptoms of dysfunction such as stenosis. Note: for simplicity this image shows the venous and arterial needles at differing angles and positions; in practice, hemodialysis needles are generally placed in the venous segment of the access with the arterial needle antegrade to flow

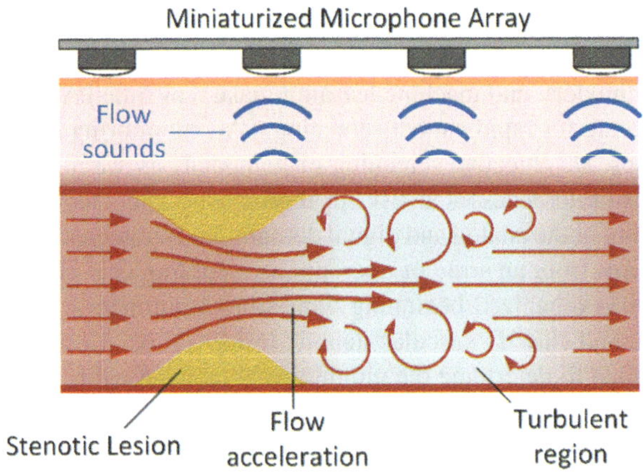

Fig. 6.3 Vascular access stenosis may be detected and quantified using flexible microphone arrays capable of detecting regions of turbulent blood flow produced in the region distal to stenosis

6.2 Prior Work in Phonoangiograhic Detection of Stenosis

PAGs have been analyzed for decades, but there is still wide variance in the descriptions of relevant spectral properties in functional and dysfunctional vascular accesses. However, there is a clear relationship between changing acoustic spectra relative to the dimensions of the stenosis. Further, there is relative agreement that PAGs recorded close to the location of stenosis have the distinctive shift in acoustic timber introduced by turbulent flow. Previous studies have analyzed PAGs from humans, from vascular bench phantoms, and from computer simulations of blood flow. Here, we describe two topics which have been studied previously: the spectral properties of PAGs in normal and stenosed cases and the impact of recording location on PAG spectra.

6.2.1 Classification of Degree of Stenosis from Phonoangiograms

Because the degree of stenosis (DOS) in a blood vessel influences the level of turbulent flow, PAG properties are related to DOS. DOS is defined as the ratio of the stenosed cross-sectional area of the blood vessel to the proximal (non-stenosed) luminal area but is also clinically calculated as the ratio in minimum diameter of the stenosed vessel section to the non-stenosed lumen diameter. When angiography is used to determine DOS, linear vessel and stenosis diameter measurements are generally used to estimate DOS within 10% (Allon and Robbin 2009). In our work, because we used computerized tomography (CT) scans of vascular stenosis phantoms (described below), we calculated DOS as the ratio in luminal area in the stenosed and non-stenosed vessel segments, because this accounted for stenosis phantoms that were not circular.

Much early work in PAG analysis represented the combined frequencies generated during systolic and diastolic phases of turbulent blood flow. Because clinical interpretation of pathologic bruits relies on detecting a high-pitched whistling character, it was hypothesized that stenosis would shift spectral power within a certain frequency band (Sung et al. 2015). Although all studies agree that the frequency range of interest is in the 20–1000 Hz band, and that DOS enhanced high-frequency spectral power, identification of specific frequency bands varied widely (Sung et al. 2015; Du et al. 2015; Du et al. 2014; Wu et al. 2015; Mansy et al. 2005; Shinzato et al. 1993; Hsien-Yi Wang et al. 2014; Chen et al. 2013; Akay et al. 1993; Obando and Mandersson 2012; Wang et al. 2011; Clausen et al. 2011; Sato et al. 2006; Gram et al. 2011; Milsom et al. 2014; Rousselot 2014; Gaupp et al. 1999; Gårdhagen n.d.).

Despite the disagreement in the precise effect of stenosis on bruit spectra, these prior studies confirmed that stenosis definitively changes PAG amplitude and pitch. The change, however, could be an enhancement or a suppression of certain frequencies depending on the impact of stenosis on blood flow. Other patient-dependent variables such as PAG amplitude and the recording location relative to stenosis must also be accounted for and are described below.

6.2.2 *Localization of Vascular Stenosis from Phonoangiograms*

Bruits are only detectable close to where they are created due to the low acoustic amplitude and acoustic attenuation of human tissue. Fluid dynamic simulations have established to a high degree of precision that stenosis induces turbulent flow at physiologic blood pressures, flow rates, and nominal lumen diameters of vascular accesses (Gaupp et al. 1999; Gårdhagen n.d.). These simulations have been confirmed by Doppler ultrasound measurements, which agree that turbulent flow occurs within 2–5 times the diameter of the unoccluded vessel distal to stenosis. Therefore, the presence of a bruit indicates stenosis or some other vascular malformation is nearby.

An important effect is that turbulence and decreased pressure occurs on the downstream side of the stenosis—for an arteriovenous vascular access, this is closer to the venous outflow tract. Therefore, bruits recorded proximally and distally to stenosis have different frequency spectra due to stenosis turbulence (Du et al. 2015). However, the acoustical influence of biomechanical properties and thickness of tissue over the vascular access varies between patients. Because tissue acts as a low-pass filter at auditory frequencies, it is presumed that the most accurate bruit recordings would be obtained in the 1–3 cm region distal to stenosis (assuming unoccluded tube diameter to be 6 mm), where turbulent flow is maximal (Gaupp et al. 1999; Gårdhagen n.d.).

6.3 In Vitro Reproduction of Vascular Bruits

The spectral content of bruits produced by human blood flow is affected by a wide range of uncontrollable factors such as vascular anatomy, blood pressure, blood concentration (hematocrit), and flow rate. We developed an in vitro vascular phantom to reproduce bruits so that relevant acoustic features and classifiers could be matched with known degree of stenosis. Acoustic recordings from the phantom system were used to validate the stenosis classification strategies described below. The reproduction performance of the phantom was validated against 3283 unique 10-s recordings obtained from 24 hemodialysis patients over 18 months (Majerus et al. 2000). Human and phantom bruits were recorded using the same digital stethoscope (Littman 3200) and compared based on aggregate power spectral density. Peak arterial pressure in the phantom was controlled using an adjustable pressure dampening system. Cardiac stroke volume was varied by changing the duty factor of a pulsatile pump. The acoustic power spectra of phantom bruits were validated against reference recordings taken from humans, as previously described (Chin et al. 2019).

Specific construction details of the vascular phantom were previously described (Chin et al. 2019; Panda et al. 2020) and are briefly introduced here (Fig. 6.4). The

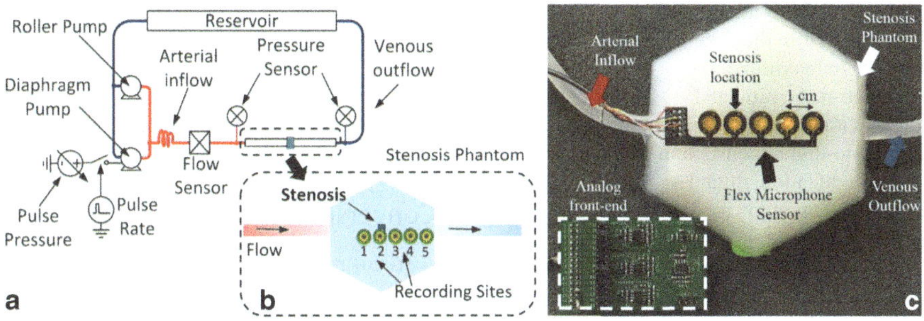

Fig. 6.4 (**a**) Vascular stenosis phantom flow diagram. Two pumping systems produced pulsatile flows in a vascular access phantom within physiological ranges of flow and pressure. The recording sites are shown in the stenosis phantom diagram (**b**). 10–85% stenosis is simulated in the center of phantom by tying a band around 6-mm silicone tubing (**c**)

phantom consisted of a 6 mm silicone tube banded by a silk suture at one location to simulate an abrupt vascular narrowing. Phantoms were produced with DOS from 10% to 85%. The banded tube was then encased below 6 mm of tissue-mimicking silicone rubber (Ecoflex 00-10). The tissue-mimicking portion also extended at least 10 cm in all directions from the stenosis. The final DOS for each phantom was then calculated from images slices taken by CT scan.

Each phantom was connected to a pulsatile flow pumping system (Cole Parmer MasterFlex L/S, Shurflo 4008). Pulsatile pressures and aggregate flow rate were measured with a pressure sensor (PendoTech N-038 PressureMAT) and flow sensor (Omega FMG91-PVDF), respectively. Pulsatile waveforms were delivered to one of the pumps at a rate of 60 beats per minute using a solid-state relay to produce flows from 600 to 1200 mL/min at peripheral peak blood pressures of 110–200 mmHg.

6.4 Signal Processing: Considerations in the Transduction of Bruits

While the main focus of this chapter is signal processing of bruits to produce phonoangiograms for classification, system-level consideration of the signal processing requirements can help optimize performance and avoid over-design. Therefore, this section will review the design considerations for a transducer and front-end interface amplifier to best capture the relevant acoustic signals to the accuracy needed for classification (Fig. 6.5).

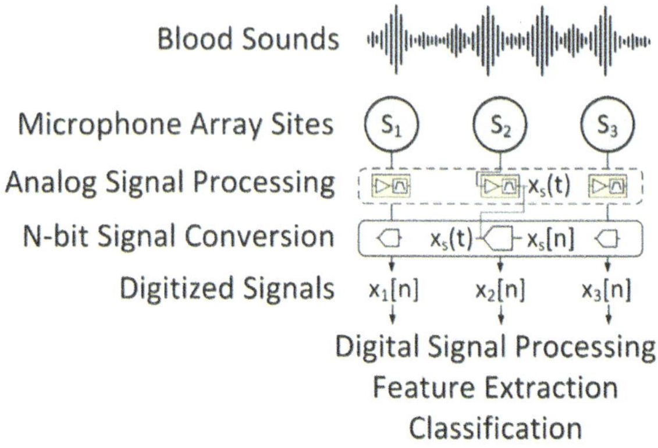

Fig. 6.5 Signal processing is required first in the analog domain to maximize signal-to-noise ratio and prevent aliasing in analog-to-digital conversion. After digitization, digital signal processing is used to extract features for classification

6.4.1 Skin-Coupled Recording Microphone Array

Fabrication details for recording arrays were detailed previously (Panda et al. 2019a), so this section will introduce new data on the bandwidth considerations for these sensors. The true spectral bandwidth and dynamic range of vascular sounds may still be unknown since only stethoscopes have been used to record these signals previously. Published analyses of PAGs report higher-pitched sounds associated with vascular stenosis (Sung et al. 2015; Du et al. 2015; Du et al. 2014; Wu et al. 2015; Mansy et al. 2005; Shinzato et al. 1993; Hsien-Yi Wang et al. 2014; Chen et al. 2013; Akay et al. 1993; Obando and Mandersson 2012; Wang et al. 2011; Clausen et al. 2011; Sato et al. 2006; Gram et al. 2011; Milsom et al. 2014; Rousselot 2014; Gaupp et al. 1999; Gårdhagen n.d.), which suggests that the reduced frequency range of stethoscopes might be insufficient for blood sounds. Therefore, acoustic recordings from the in vitro phantom were made with a reference transducer (Tyco Electronics CM-01B) with a flat frequency response to at least 2 kHz. For each recording, the 95% power bandwidth was calculated by integrating the power spectral density. To compute the power bandwidth, the power spectral density was computed using fast Fourier transform and then cumulatively integrated by frequency bin until the integration met 95% of the total power in all bins. Because electronic circuits suffer from increased flicker noise at low frequencies, and because all prior reports of PAGs indicate increased power above 100 Hz associated with vascular stenosis (Sung et al. 2015; Du et al. 2015; Du et al. 2014; Wu et al. 2015; Mansy et al. 2005; Shinzato et al. 1993; Hsien-Yi Wang et al. 2014; Chen et al. 2013; Akay et al. 1993; Obando and Mandersson 2012; Wang et al. 2011; Clausen et al. 2011; Sato et al. 2006; Gram et al. 2011; Milsom et al. 2014; Rousselot 2014; Gaupp et al. 1999; Gårdhagen n.d.), we adopted a lower integration bound of 25 Hz. This had a further benefit of enabling shorter-duration recordings (e.g., 10 s), which otherwise do not accurately capture extremely low-frequency signal components. For this analysis 10-s recordings were taken 1 cm before the simulated stenosis, at the stenosis, and 1 and 2 cm after the stenosis relative to the direction of blood flow.

Signal bandwidth was related to the degree of stenosis, as expected, but also to recording location (Figs. 6.6 and 6.7). Both effects were expected based on prior measurements and simulations indicating turbulent flow existing up to 1–2 cm from a typical stenotic lesion (Gaupp et al. 1999; Gårdhagen n.d.). These results suggest the need to record from multiple locations to accurately detect the presence and severity of a stenotic lesion. In an analysis of 156 recordings, the maximum interquartile range for 95% bandwidth was 25 Hz–1.2 kHz; the lower-frequency bound correlated with phantoms with low DOS producing little turbulent flow (Fig. 6.8). These data suggest that a signal bandwidth of at least 1.5 kHz is appropriate for measuring vascular bruits. With a safety factor, we adopted a bandwidth of 25–2.25 kHz.

The required bandwidth was achieved with a signal-to-noise ratio of 24 dB using a polyvinylidene fluoride (PVDF) film as a 2-mm diameter circular transducer. This transducer was developed to be coupled directly to the skin to measure blood sounds through direct piezoelectric transduction (Panda et al. 2019b). The small size of the transducer allowed it to be fabricated in recording arrays (M and Panda 2019). In this work we describe testing from arrays arranged as 1×5 channels spaced by 1 cm laterally (Fig. 6.4).

6.4.2 Transducer Front-End Interface Amplifier Design

Each PVDF microphone in the recording array must be coupled to an interface amplifier to amplify the signal amplitude before digital conversion. The analog performance of the interface amplifier is driven by three constraints: the electrical impedance of the PVDF transducer, the required signal bandwidth, and the required dynamic range. In this case, the dynamic range constraint is driven by the minimum signal accuracy needed for the digital signal processing and classification strategy. In a retrospective analysis of blood sounds measured from hemodialysis patients and an in vitro phantom, we determined that a minimum dynamic range of 60.2 dB was needed for accurate classification of stenosis severity (Panda et al. 2019a), which is roughly equivalent to 10-bit accuracy after digital conversion. As described in the previous section, a bandwidth of 2.25 kHz is needed to capture most of the energy in the PAG signals.

The amplifier input impedance constraint is based on the electrical model for each 2-mm transducer which was extracted using an impedance analyzer (Hioki IM3570). The PVDF transducer was modeled electrically as a resistor and capacitor in parallel (Fig. 6.9). Measured values of the sensor resistance, capacitance, and the equivalent sensor output current when recording PAGs are shown in Table 6.1.

Because the PVDF transducer has a large impedance with a small signal current, a transimpedance amplifier (TIA) was designed to convert the piezoelectric sensor current to a voltage that can be digitized. Each microphone within the array feeds

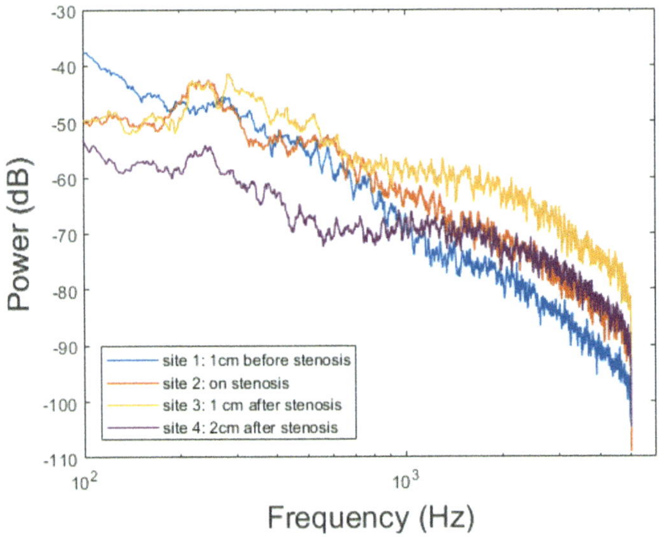

Fig. 6.6 Power spectral density recorded at different locations relative to a 75% stenosis show a site-specific signal bandwidth. In general, sites after stenosis have wider signal bandwidths because of the local presence of turbulent blood flow

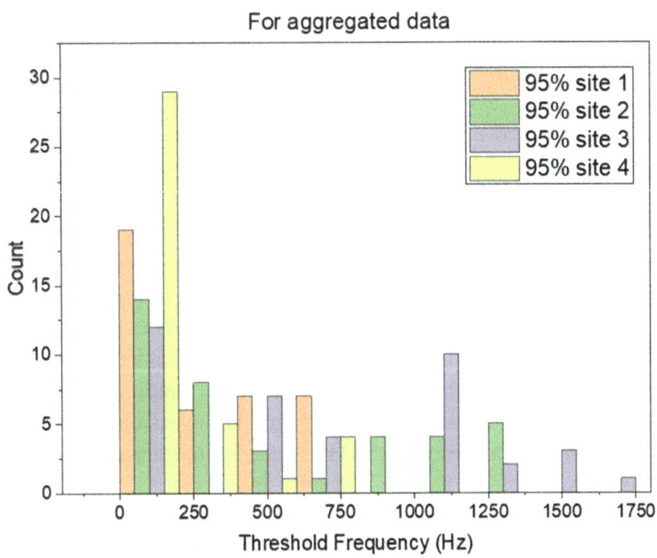

Fig. 6.7 The 95% power bandwidth for 156 PAG recordings for DOS 10-90% were aggregated based on recording site. Recordings at sites 2 and 3 indicate wider bandwidth independent of degree of stenosis or flow rate. This forms the basis of the classifier methodology, as there is a distinct correlation between elevated power and frequency content in the presence of stenosis

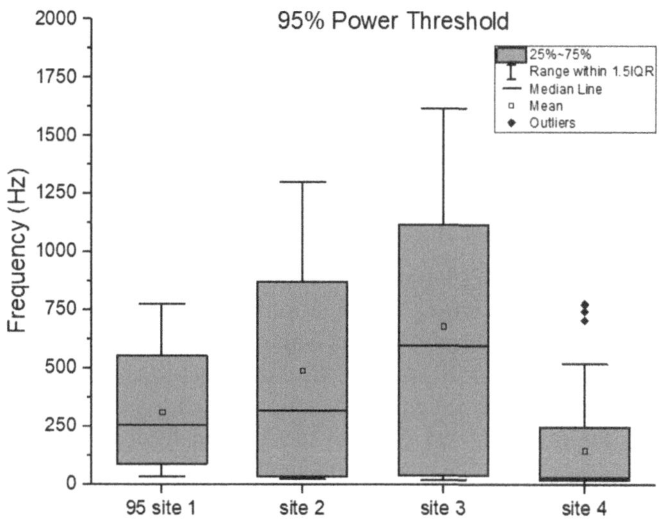

Fig. 6.8 Analysis of interquartile range for PAGs recorded with DOS 10–90% showed a required bandwidth of at least 1600 Hz to accurately capture signal dynamics in the analog signal processing section. Including a safety factor, the interface amplifier was designed for 2.25 kHz bandwidth to limit noise

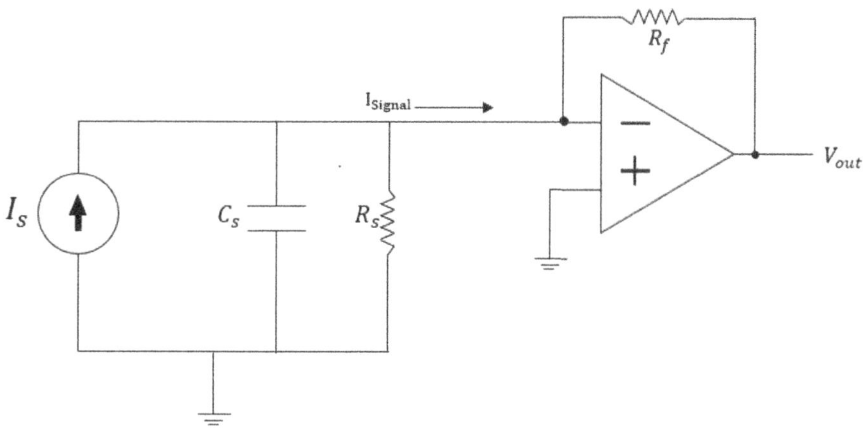

Fig. 6.9 The PVDF transducer is modeled simply as a resistor (R_S) and capacitor (C_s) in parallel with output current I_{signal} based on measured impedance at 100 Hz

Table 6.1 Measured transducer parameters for an electrical model for the PVDF sensor

Parameter	Nominal value
Current source amplitude ($\mathbf{I_{Signal}}$)	0.63 μA
Current source frequency	100 Hz
Sensor resistance ($\mathbf{R_S}$)	12.4 MΩ
Sensor capacitance ($\mathbf{C_s}$)	100 pF

Table 6.2 Design specifications for transimpedance interface amplifier

Parameter	Nominal value
Nominal input current	0.63 μA (from PVDF transducer)
Required dynamic range	60.2 dB minimum
Nominal output voltage level	30 mV peak
Low-pass signal bandwidth	2.25 kHz

a dedicated TIA. The TIA converts the current produced by the transducer to an output voltage while minimizing the input referred noise power. The TIA is an ideal interface to high impedance, current output devices, but certain critical design considerations must be made to optimize the total signal-to-noise ratio of the output signal. The most important design consideration, which has a direct impact on the sensitivity, is the input-referred noise of the TIA. In feedback TIAs built using general voltage amplifiers such as an op-amp with a shunt-shunt feedback, the input referred noise is a function of the input-referred voltage and current noise of the op-Amp (Binkley 2008). Therefore, op-amps with high input-referred voltage ($nV/\sqrt{Hz}$) and/or current noise ($nA/\sqrt{Hz}$) should be avoided.

The design specifications for the TIA were chosen assuming it would be followed by a 2nd-stage programmable gain amplifier and a 10-bit analog-to-digital converter. Therefore, a small-signal output level was chosen to limit harmonic distortion which can occur with large signal swing. The performance of the TIA dominates the analog noise floor and linearity, so these later stages are not described here. Design requirements for the TIA are summarized in Table 6.2 based on measured properties from PAGs in humans and the vascular phantom (Panda et al. 2019a).

In addition to the inherent noise of the op-amp, the feedback resistor plays a key role in the overall input-referred noise power of the TIA. Increasing the feedback resistance not only reduces the noise current associated with the resistance but also results in higher TIA gain which helps lower the overall input-referred noise of the TIA. Nevertheless, the requirement imposed on the frequency response of the TIA when interfacing with the transducer limits the amount of resistance that can be used in the feedback path. Still, optimizing the feedback resistance will lead to lower input-referred noise within the required gain bandwidth (GBW) of the TIA (Fig. 6.10).

The critical performance metrics are important in completing the design process. Major small-signal TIA performance metrics are the transimpedance gain, the 3-dB bandwidth, and input-referred noise power. Considering the transimpedance gain and the bandwidth, the feedback network is the first physical parameter that must be determined. The feedback network generally consists of a resistor and capacitor that are connected in parallel. The resistive part helps set the transimpedance gain of the TIA, while the capacitive component helps with setting the frequency response, particularly the bandwidth and the stability. The frequency response affects the TIA noise transfer function, and consequently, the input referred noise of the TIA, too. Eqs. 5, 6 demonstrate how to optimize feedback capacitor ranges, e.g.,

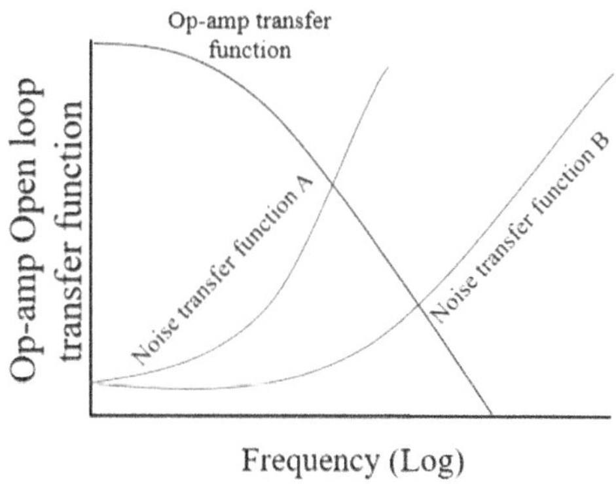

Fig. 6.10 Example of op-amp open loop transfer function and noise transfer functions versus frequency. Ideally, the noise transfer function will be flatter until the op-amp gain begins to roll off (e.g., "B")

$$\text{If } \left(\frac{R_f}{R_s}+1\right) \geq 2\sqrt{R_f * C_s * GBW} \qquad C_f = \frac{C_s}{2\left(\frac{R_f}{R_{in}}+1\right)}$$

$$\text{If } \left(\frac{R_f}{R_s}+1\right) \leq 2\sqrt{R_f * C_s * GBW} \qquad C_f = \sqrt{\frac{C_s}{R_f * GBW}}$$

Another critical consideration for feedback capacitor value is the desired cutoff frequency. This cutoff frequency determines the TIA's -3db bandwidth, f_{-3dB}, expressed as

$$f_{-3dB} = \frac{1}{2\pi * R_f * C_f}$$

Input referred power is defined by the ratio of the output noise power, divided by the TIA transfer function. This can be calculated using the SNR of the circuit (Fig. 6.11):

$$SNR = \frac{Power_{signal}}{Power_{noise}} = \frac{{I_s}^2 * R_f}{i_n^2 * R_f} = \frac{{I_s}^2}{i_n^2}$$

The TIA design process is to maximize SNR given constraints on required bandwidth, available supply voltage/current, and necessary dynamic range. The transfer function of output voltage level (V_{out}) and input current (I_{signal}) is dependent on the feedback resistance:

$$V_{out} = -\left[I_{signal} * R_f\right] + V_{ref}.$$

In this example, V_{ref} is generated by a voltage divider of R_1 and R_2. Both were selected to be $10k\Omega$ to set the reference at half of the supply voltage, i.e.,

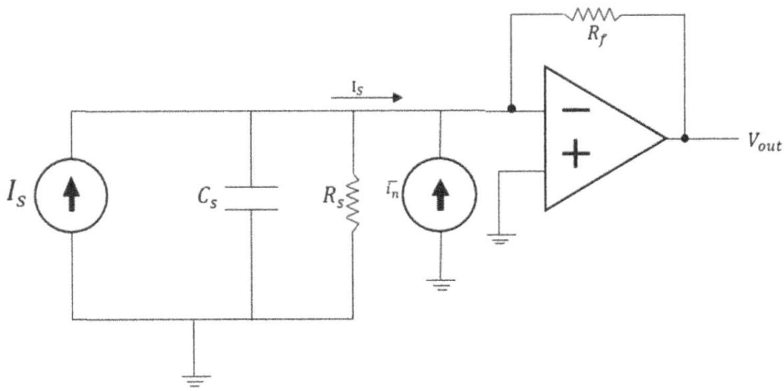

Fig. 6.11 Equivalent transducer and transimpedance amplifier circuit model for input-referred noise calculations with parallel current source, $\overline{i_n}$, functioning as input noise source

$$V_{ref} = V_{supply} * \frac{R_2}{R_1 + R_2} \text{ (where } R_2 = R_1)$$

The DC value of the output for this stage of amplification was selected to be 2.1 V. From this parameter, the feedback resistance was calculated as:

$$R_f = \frac{V_{out} - V_{ref}}{I_{signal}} = \frac{2.1V - 1.65V}{0.63\mu A} = 715k\Omega$$

The value of the feedback capacitance was determined from the required signal bandwidth. Rearranging Eq. 7 for C_f, we arrive at:

$$C_f = \frac{1}{2\pi * R_f * f_{-3dB}} = \frac{1}{2\pi * 715k\Omega * 2.25kHz} = 100\rho F$$

The minimum op-amp bandwidth for this circuit was calculated using the feedback resistance and capacitance, R_f and C_f, as well as the capacitance of the input pin of the selected op-amp (Texas Instruments OPA2378). The IN-pin capacitance is the sum of the sensor capacitance (C_s), common-mode input capacitance (C_{CM}), and differential mode capacitance (C_{Diff}) as:

$$C_{IN} = C_s + C_{CM} + C_{Diff} = 1000\rho F + 5\rho F + 4pF \cong 1000\rho F$$

$$f_{GBW} \geq \frac{C_f + C_{in}}{2\pi * R_f * C_f^2} \geq 24.7\ kHz$$

Therefore, the op-amp must have a minimum bandwidth of roughly 25 kHz. The OPA2378's 900 kHz bandwidth satisfies this requirement and is a viable component for this application. The OPA2378 has an input voltage noise density of $\frac{20nV}{Hz^{1/2}}$. The input referred voltage noise was calculated as $\frac{183nV}{Hz^{1/2}}$ which meets the 60 dB dynamic range requirement over the signal bandwidth of 2.25 kHz.

6.5 Signal Processing and Feature Classification Strategies for Acoustic Detection of Vascular Stenosis

The preceding sections described how phonoangiograms can be efficiently transduced through arrays of flexible microphones and the bandwidth and dynamic range needed for interface and data conversion electronics. After a bruit is recorded, a wide range of digital signal processing strategies can be used to extract meaningful features. Prior examples have reported that autoregressive spectral envelope estimation, wavelet sub-band power ratios, and wavelet-derived acoustic features correlate to degree of stenosis (Sung et al. 2015; Du et al. 2015; Du et al. 2014; Wu et al. 2015; Mansy et al. 2005; Shinzato et al. 1993; Hsien-Yi Wang et al. 2014; Chen et al. 2013; Akay et al. 1993; Obando and Mandersson 2012; Wang et al. 2011; Clausen et al. 2011; Sato et al. 2006; Gram et al. 2011; Milsom et al. 2014; Rousselot 2014; Gaupp et al. 1999; Gårdhagen n.d.). Features can be extracted from multiple signal processing branches and compared using machine-learning techniques, e.g., radial basis functions or random forests. However, feature extraction and model training must be constrained to prevent over-fitting on limited datasets and to improve generalized use. In this section we provide an overview of how two derived time domain signals—acoustic spectral centroid (ASC) and acoustic spectral flux (ASF)—have unique properties for bruit classification. Importantly, ASC and ASF are derived directly from the discrete wavelet transform coefficients, which reduce feature dimensionality and aid scalar feature extraction.

A specific physical system implementation provides constraints on computational complexity, accuracy, and ease of implementation which can guide the selection of features. In this section, we review the fundamental approach for extracting spectral features from a single acoustic recording site. We will then expand this signal processing into other domains, specifically into time and space, by leveraging time-synchronized recordings from an array of microphones.

6.5.1 Multi-domain Phonoangiogram Feature Calculation

Because PAGs are time domain waveforms, they can be analyzed in both the temporal or spectral domains, i.e., as one-dimensional signals in either domain. Spectral transforms such as discrete cosine transform and continuous wavelet transform combine these domains to form a two-dimensional waveform along time and frequency (or scale) axes. However, when PAGs are acquired at multiple sites along a vascular access, the spatial distribution of PAG properties provides an additional analysis domain. If PAGs are also sampled simultaneously, time domain differences between signals are correlated and can be analyzed. When features are extracted from different domains, they can be compared to each other using clustering and classifier techniques as long as they are reduced to scalar form.

In this section we review how features can be extracted from each domain with dimensional reduction to scalar values. The spectral domain provides scalar features such as average pitch. The temporospectral (combined time-spectral) domain allows segmentation of blood sounds in cardiac cycles to provide sample indices for systole onset. After temporospectral segmentation, spectral features can be separately calculated in systolic and diastolic phases. Finally, the spatial domain provides features describing the time delay between PAGs at different recording sites. Spatial analysis also enables detection of spectral changes between sites to predict where turbulent blood flow is occurring.

6.5.1.1 Spectral Domain Feature Extraction

Spectral domain feature extraction is likely the most common approach in PAG signal processing. This is intuitive because humans perceive frequency content with great sensitivity, and PAG processing seeks to replicate traditional auscultation by ear. In this section we review spectral domain feature extraction using continuous wavelet transform (CWT) to describe the spectral variance over time.

CWT over k scales $\boldsymbol{W}[k, n]$ is computed as:

$$\boldsymbol{W}[k, n] = x_{PAG}[n] * \psi[n/k],$$

where $\psi[t/k]$ is the analyzing wavelet at scale k. We used the complex Morlet wavelet because it has good mapping from scale to frequency, defined as:

$$\psi[n] = e^{-(n/2f_c)^2} e^{j2\pi f_c n},$$

where f_c is the wavelet center frequency. In the limit $f_c \to \infty$, the CWT with Morlet wavelet becomes a Fourier transform. Because of the construction of the Morlet wavelet as the wavelet $\psi[n]$ is scaled to $\psi[n/k]$, and k is a factor of 2, the wavelet center frequency will be shifted by one octave. Therefore, CWT analysis with the Morlet wavelet can be described by the number of octaves (N_O) being analyzed (frequency span) and the number of voices per octave N_V (divisions within each octave, i.e., frequency scales). Mathematically the set of scale factors k can be expressed as:

$$k[i_O, i_V] = 2^{(i_O + i_V/N_V)}.$$

$$i_O = k_0, k_0 + 1, k_0 + 2 \ldots N_O$$

$$i_V = k_0, k_0 + 1, k_0 + 2 \ldots N_V$$

Where k_O is the starting scale and defines the smallest scale value and the total number of scales $K = N_O N_V$. For PAG analysis, we compute CWT with $N_O = 6$ octaves and $N_V = 12$ voices/octave, starting at $k_O = 3$. After computing the CWT, pseudofrequencies $F[k]$ across all K scales are calculated as:

$$F[k] = f_c / k.$$

Because the CWT involves time domain convolution, each discrete sample n has a paired sequence of k CWT coefficients, i.e., it is a 2-dimensional sequence. In the context of phonoangiogram classification, features must be extracted from $\mathbf{W}[k, n]$ that are of singular dimension. Dimension reduction of $\mathbf{W}[k, n]$ can operate over all or part of the k scales at each discrete sample n, over a single k scale for all n samples, over all points of $\mathbf{W}[k, n]$, or through a more complex combination of summation over k and n.

The systolic and diastolic portions of pulsatile blood flow contain differing spectral information on turbulent flow, so we have chosen to first reduce the CWT dimensionality to n to produce time domain waveforms. This preserves the spectral differences between different times in the cardiac flow cycle. Two n-point waveforms are calculated from $\mathbf{W}[k, n]$: auditory spectral flux (ASF) and auditory spectral centroid (ASC). From these waveforms, we can compute time-independent features such as RMS spectral centroid, or we can extract time domain spectral features as explained in the next section.

ASF describes the rate at which the magnitude of the auditory spectrum changes and approximates a spectral first-order derivative. It is calculated as the spectral variation between two adjacent samples, i.e.,

$$ASF[n] = \frac{1}{K} \sqrt{\sum_{k=1}^{K} \left(|\mathbf{W}[k, n]| - |\mathbf{W}[k, n-1]| \right)^2}$$

where $\mathbf{W}[k, n]$ is the continuous wavelet transform obtained over k total scales.

To intuitively demonstrate how ASF describes a signal, Fig. 6.12 shows ASF calculated from a stepped single tone test waveform. The tone changes over [100, 200, 400, 800, 1000] stepping every 2 s. At every tonal change, the spike in the ASF waveform corresponds to the time of the spectral shift and the magnitude. The ASF waveform, therefore, describes how when, and how quickly, spectral power is shifting between bands. This is useful in mapping large variations in a PAG signal, such as the systole and diastole phases. Segmentation of these phases, therefore, uses the ASF waveform (described below).

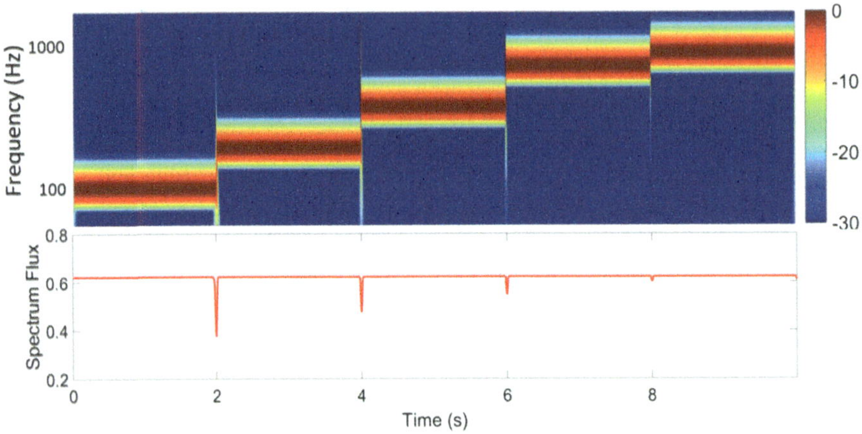

Fig. 6.12 Spectrogram of artificially generated test waveform with 6 single-tone frequencies from 100-1500 Hz. The ASF curve (lower) shows a spike at every change of frequency, approximating the spectral first derivative

ASC describes the spectral "center of mass" at each n sample in time. For Gaussian-distributed white noise, ASC will be constant at pseudofrequency *F[K/2]*. ASC is commonly used to estimate the average pitch of audio recordings, where a higher value corresponds to "brighter" acoustics with more high frequency content (Tzanetakis and Cook 2002). ASC is calculated as:

$$ASC\,[n] = \frac{\sum_{k=1}^{K} (|\boldsymbol{W}\,[k,n]|\,.fc\,[k])}{\sum_{k=1}^{K} |\boldsymbol{W}\,[k,n]|}$$

where $\boldsymbol{W}[k,n]$ is the continuous wavelet transform obtained over K total scales of the PAG and f_C[k] is the center frequency.

ASC for the same test waveform is plotted to intuitively describe how this waveform describes the time domain spectral energy of a signal (Fig. 6.13). Because only a single tone is used at each time point, ASC consistently describes the frequency of the sine wave until it changes. Because *F[k]* represents pseudofrequencies, there is not a perfect mapping between ASC pseudofrequency and real auditory frequency. The use of the Morlet waveform in the CWT improves the pseudofrequency accuracy, but for PAG classification, absolute frequency accuracy is not needed (discussed below).

Example computations of ASC and ASF waveforms, compared to the time domain and spectral domain PAG recording, demonstrate feature calculation (Fig. 6.14). After the three-dimensional $\boldsymbol{W}[k,n]$ is computed, time domain ASC and ASF waveforms are calculated. From these waveforms simple, time-invariant scalar values such as RMS or peak amplitude are calculated and used for stenosis classification.

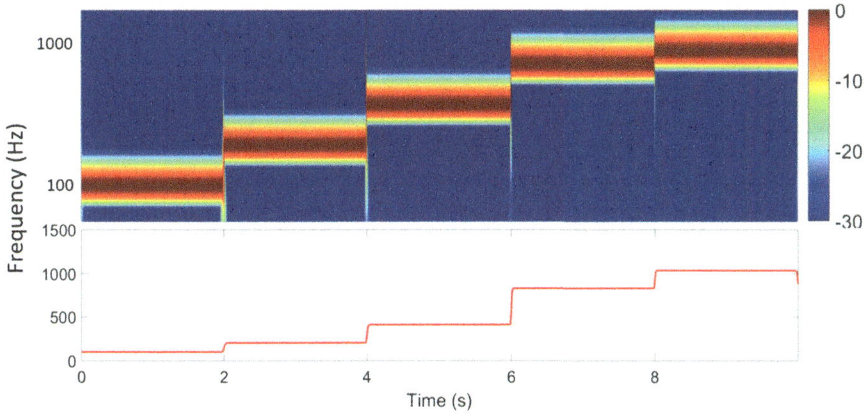

Fig. 6.13 Spectrogram of artificially generated test waveform with 6 single-tone frequencies from 100-1500 Hz. The ASC curve describes the frequency of the sine wave at each time point

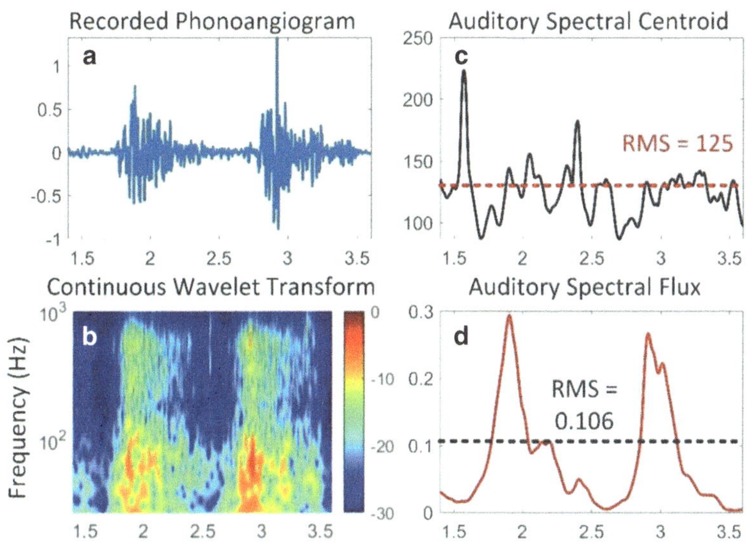

Fig. 6.14 Time-domain bruit (a) and continuous wavelet transform spectral domain (b). The descriptive signals auditory spectral centroid and flux were extracted from CWT coefficients (c,d). The RMS value of the descriptive signals is one example of a scalar feature derived from the time-domain waveform

6.5.1.2 Temporospectral Domain Feature Extraction

For PAG analysis we are primarily interested in identifying the time onset of systolic and diastolic phases. This allows separate spectral feature extraction in each phase, ratioed features by comparing spectral changes between phases, and time domain comparisons such as lengths of cardiac phases, or time shifts between recording

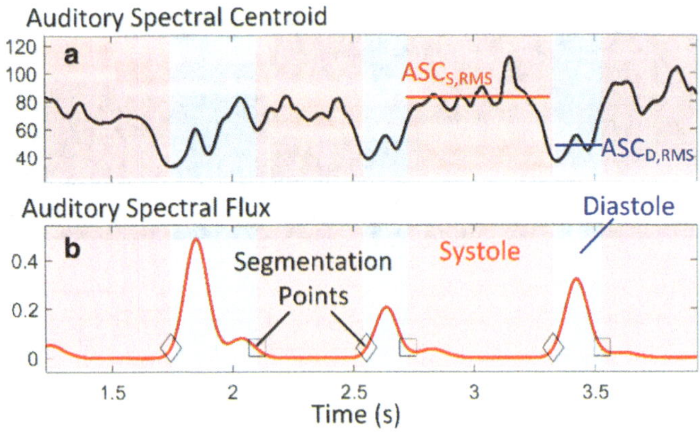

Fig. 6.15 Auditory spectral centroid (ASC) varies with degree of stenosis but also between systolic and diastolic phases (a). The auditory spectral flux (ASF) waveform enables segmentation between pulsatile phases so that the RMS value of ASC (ASC_{RMS}) can be separately calculated (b)

sites. This analysis is useful because blood flow acceleration occurs in the high-pressure systolic pulse, which gives rise to turbulence producing high spectral power. As a spectral derivative, the ASF waveform is well suited to describe the onset of systolic turbulence and is used for temporospectral segmentation.

Segmentation simply used a thresholding procedure; systolic ASF onset is defined as the time when the ASF waveform exceeds a threshold in each pulse cycle (Fig. 6.15). A suitable threshold of 25% of the ASF_{RMS} value was determined empirically using data recorded from human patients and the vascular phantom (Panda et al. 2019b). Pulse width is also used to reduce false threshold crossings. The times between threshold crossings are calculated, and any crossings which produce pulse widths less than 40% of the mean are discarded (Lázaro et al. 2013).

Temporospectral segmentation produces a set of i indices ($\boldsymbol{n}_{ASF,i}$) describing systolic and diastolic pulse widths, which themselves can be used as features. However, the indices can also be used to segment spectral waveforms such as ASF and ASC to split them into systolic ASF_S and ASC_S, and diastolic ASF_D and ASC_D. Features for each phase can be calculated by combining all segments or by averaging the feature for each segment. As an example, consider an ASC waveform segmented into P systolic segments each with length n. The RMS value of ASC in the systolic phase only is then:

$$ASC_{S,RMS} = \frac{1}{P}\sum_{i=1}^{P}\sqrt{\frac{1}{n}\sum ASC_{S,P,n}^{2}}$$

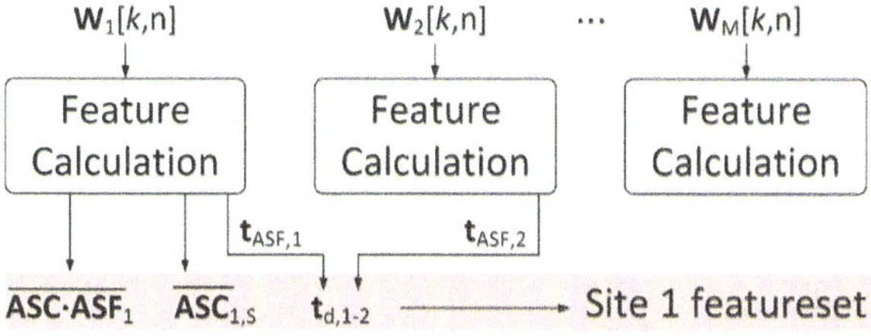

Fig. 6.16 Features can be derived for each recording site, or based on differences between sites. Since all features are scalar, they can be combined into the same featureset and used for classification

In practice, because systolic segments do not all have the same length n, any derived features are calculated for each segment independently and averaged over P segments.

Ratiometric features can also be calculated as ratios or differences between successive systolic/diastolic pairs. This reduces the effect of interference caused by recording which is correlated between adjacent segments or can be a less individual-specific feature because the diameter of the blood vessel and absolute flow rate contribute to ASC and differ between people. For example, ASC and ASF waveforms show significant differences in systolic and diastolic phases (Fig. 6.15), especially as DOS increases.

6.5.1.3 Spatial Domain Feature Extraction

The final domain analyzed in this model of PAG signal processing is the spatial domain. Features are not extracted directly from the spatial domain; rather, new features are derived as the difference in features between sites (Fig. 6.16). This is a powerful technique because not only does it accentuate regions of turbulent flow, but also the proportional feature changes between recording locations are themselves related to degree of stenosis. Therefore, spatial domain features are useful for both physical localization of stenosis and classification of degree of stenosis. Furthermore, ratiometric site-to-site feature comparisons remove some of the individual variation in features attributed to differences in anatomy. For example, the dimensionless change in systolic ASC (ASC_S) between sites 1 and 2 can be calculated as ${ASC_{2,S}}/{ASC_{1,S}}$. To obtain a similar comparison in approximate units of Hertz, a difference is used, i.e., $ASC_{2,\,S} - ASC_{1,\,S}$.

This spatial domain technique can be generalized to produce composite features for any multi-site measurement with little complications as long as the compared features are independent scalars. However, any site-to-site calculations relying on time require synchronization in sample rates between sites, or alignment of waveforms based on a reference symbol so that relative time differences can be calculated. For example, composite temporospectral features require time invariance

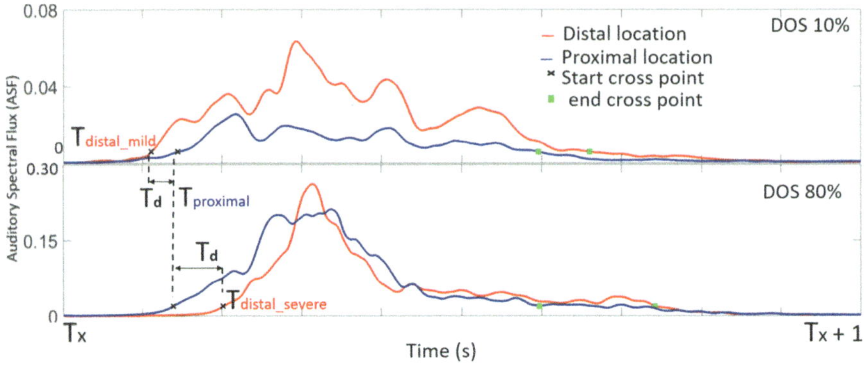

Fig. 6.17 ASF calculated at proximal and distal locations showed an inversion in T_d. At moderate and severe DOS, T_d became negative, suggesting flow velocity increase

in the calculation. Once this condition is met, composite spatial domain features based on time shifts are simple to calculate. For example, the time delay in ASF systolic onset ($\boldsymbol{n}_{ASF}$) between sites 1 and 2 can be calculated as:

$$t_{d,1-2} = {}^{1}\!/_{F_s} \left(\boldsymbol{n}_{ASF,1} - \boldsymbol{n}_{ASF,2}\right).$$

This calculation is easily performed from feature calculations for each recording site (Fig. 6.17) and is transformed to a continuous time difference in units of seconds by dividing by the sample rate F_S. Scalar features from multiple domains can be combined to form a single feature set (Fig. 6.16), especially if a machine-learning classifier will be used because the scalar features can be analyzed as if they are unitless.

6.6 Classification of Vascular Access Stenosis Location and Severity In Vitro

The clinical goal for multi-site recordings of PAGs is to both locate and describe the severity of stenosis. In our previous work, we showed that binary or ternary classification using single features was sufficient to classify DOS as mild, moderate, or severe. Analysis of this method using receiver operating characteristic (ROC) revealed detection sensitivities as high as 88–92% and specificities as high as 96–100% (Panda et al. 2020), but classification was only accurate at certain recording locations. Therefore, feature selection for an array of recording sites is important to detect differences between recording sites. This section demonstrates comparing features between sites using hyperdimensional classifiers to greatly improve the stenosis classification accuracy from PAG recordings.

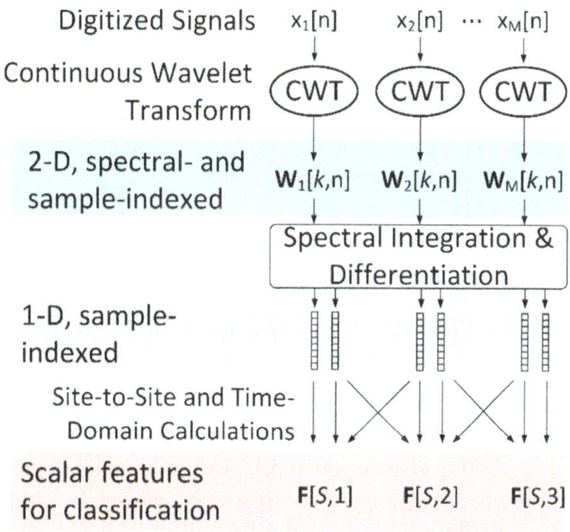

Fig. 6.18 As features are extracted, the dimensionality of the dataset is reduced to yield a final set of features. Since each site has features extracted from site-specific features and intra-site feature differences, a total featureset of F[S,M] is produced with S features over M sites

6.6.1 Multi-domain Feature Selection

The previous sections described how phonoangiograms are transduced and processed as analog signals, prior to being digitized for digital signal processing. Features are then extracted from multiple dimensions to yield a final set of M features $\mathbf{F}[S.M]$, which are site-specific to each of S recording sites (Fig. 6.18). In previous work we and others have described more than 15 features that are correlated with degree of stenosis in humans and in bench phantoms of vascular stenosis (Sung et al. 2015; Du et al. 2015; Du et al. 2014; Wu et al. 2015; Mansy et al. 2005; Shinzato et al. 1993; Hsien-Yi Wang et al. 2014; Chen et al. 2013; Akay et al. 1993; Obando and Mandersson 2012; Wang et al. 2011; Clausen et al. 2011; Sato et al. 2006; Gram et al. 2011; Milsom et al. 2014; Rousselot 2014; Gaupp et al. 1999; Gårdhagen n.d.; Chin et al. 2019; Panda et al. 2020; Panda et al. 2019a).

Machine-learning classifiers require optimized feature selection through numerous methods. Feature selection improves the performance of classifier algorithms and reduces the likelihood of over-fitting to a data set of limited size. Numerical methods such as principal component analysis are powerful tools, as is supervised feature selection which relies on trained experts to select the features describing most of the variance in the observed effect. In this work we used both automated and supervised feature selection to select the most appropriate features. In the following classification examples, we explain the rationale behind feature selection for the given classification task.

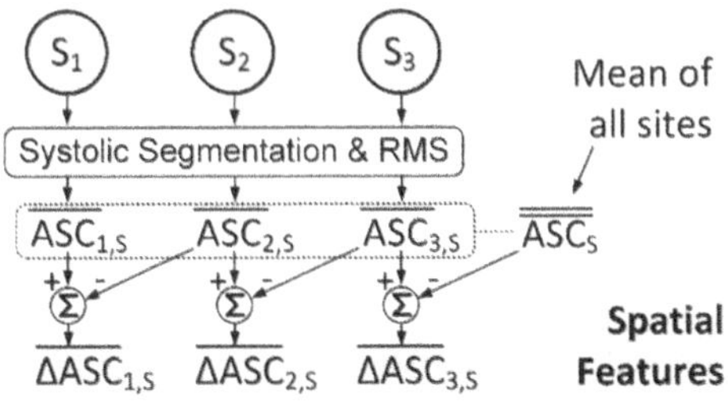

Fig. 6.19 Stenosis localization uses spatial features derived from feature differences between adjacent sites. In this example, the shift in $\overline{ASCS}$ between sites is used to detect the presence of stenosis beneath a specific recording site

6.6.2 Stenosis Spatial Localization Using Acoustic Features

Because the presence of stenosis produces turbulent flow in blood, a characteristic high-frequency sound is produced locally within 1–2 cm of the lesion (Gaupp et al. 1999; Gårdhagen n.d.). Spatial domain feature analysis is ideal to detect differences between recording sites caused by dramatic changes in blood flow patterns. To demonstrate the feasibility of detecting the location of stenosis using acoustic features alone, we tested eight stenosis phantoms on the vascular phantom previously described over variable blood flow rates of 700–1200 mL/min. This range of flows was tested at each degree of stenosis to simulate the nominal levels of human blood flow rates in arteriovenous vascular accesses. DOS for the phantoms ranged from 10% to 85%.

A vascular access is typically a uniform segment of blood vessel with few collateral veins, so we simply tested a one-dimensional recording array with five locations along the path of blood flow (Fig. 6.4). Recording sites were spaced by 1 cm and used skin-coupled microphones as previously described. While we analyzed over 15 features for stenosis localization, we found many features were correlated (Chin et al. 2019) and therefore adopted the site-to-site change in mean systolic ASC ($\overline{\Delta ASC_S}$) as the sole feature for localization (Fig. 6.19). This feature was intuitively selected because it is well documented that the presence of stenosis causes high-pitched blood sounds. Therefore, we expect that an abrupt stenosis in an otherwise smooth vessel will produce higher pitch at sites within several centimeters. Five site-to-site features for each flow rate and DOS were calculated, and including replications this yielded 370 total samples for statistical analysis.

In this experiment, the actual stenosis was located directly under location 2; location 1 was recorded 1 cm proximal, and locations 3, 4, and 5 were 1, 2, and 3 cm distal to stenosis. The interval plot (Fig. 6.20) indicated a positive shift between $\overline{\Delta ASC_S}$, differences from proximal to distal locations ($p < 0.001$ for $30\% < DOS < 90\%$) (Panda et al. 2019a). Confidence intervals and differences in group means were calculated using ANOVA followed by Tukey's test with 95% confidence intervals ($\alpha = 0.05$). Because sample data followed a normal distribution, Tukey's test was used to adjust confidence intervals based on the number of comparisons tested. Statistical analysis was performed in Minitab software (Minitab, LLC, State College, PA, USA). In general, differences between locations 3 and 4 and 4 and 5 were positive by 50–70 Hz, while the other site

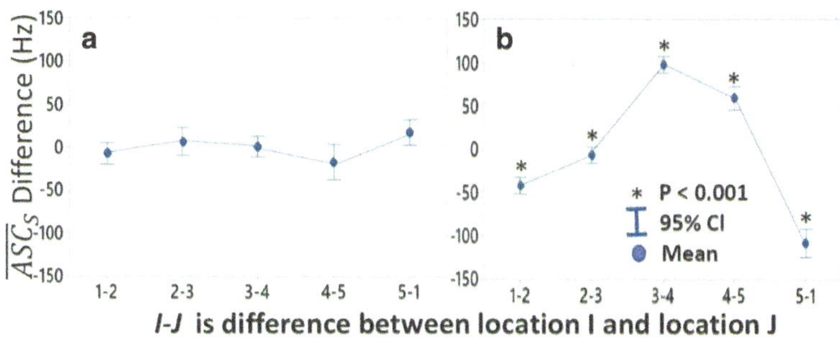

Fig. 6.20 Difference in ASC_S between adjacent locations showed no significant variation for 0% DOS (p>0.05) (**a**). A large spectral shift at locations distal to stenosis (stenosis center at location 2) (**b**). Data plotted for phantoms with 30%<DOS<90%, p<0.001 for all locations. Analysis of variance and Tukey's test were identified statistically significant differences in ASC means at significance level α=0.05

differences were negative. This suggested that a simple threshold difference of 70 Hz in $\overline{\Delta ASC_S}$, between adjacent array recording locations could identify stenosis proximally to the recording sites within 1–2 cm.

6.6.3 Stenosis Severity Classification from Acoustic Features

While the location of stenosis can be estimated by comparing feature shifts between sites to a threshold, classification of the degree of stenosis is more challenging from a single feature. This is in part because the degree of stenosis and the nonlinear properties of blood interact such that DOS nonlinearly impacts overall flow rate and turbulence pattern (Gaupp et al. 1999; Gårdhagen n.d.), introducing time-dependent changes to both acoustic spectra and intensity. Many classification strategies have been proposed and studied for a single recording site (Sung et al. 2015; Du et al. 2015; Du et al. 2014; Wu et al. 2015; Mansy et al. 2005; Shinzato et al. 1993; Hsien-Yi Wang et al. 2014; Chen et al. 2013; Akay et al. 1993; Obando and Mandersson 2012; Wang et al. 2011; Clausen et al. 2011; Sato et al. 2006; Gram et al. 2011; Milsom et al. 2014; Rousselot 2014; Gaupp et al. 1999; Gårdhagen n.d.), e.g., showing classification accuracy of about 84% using binomial Gaussian modeling (Sung et al. 2015). Here we extend classification to leverage temporospatial domain features drawn from multiple recording sites.

We chose to classify PAG data using a quadratic support vector machine (SVM) (Joachims 1998). The quadratic SVM is widely used in natural language processing tasks and is suitable for PAGs which have similar autoregressive properties as speech (Majerus et al. 2018). As a machine-learning algorithm, the SVM defines a hyperplane which is used to separate clusters of data points in a high-dimensional space. The hyperplane is used as a decision surface and is optimized to maximize the separation distance between the classes of data.

Because the data are not linearly separable, the SVM transforms the input data points into a higher dimension using a kernel function. For the quadratic SVM, the kernel K is a polynomial of order 2, i.e.,

$$K(x_1, x_2) = \left(x_1{}^{\mathrm{T}} x_2 + 1\right)^2.$$

Expanding this kernel reveals how data are expanded into higher dimension through interaction terms:

$$\begin{aligned} K(x_1, x_2) &= \left(\sum_{i=1}^{n} x_1{}^{\mathrm{T}} x_2 + 1\right)^2 \\ &= \sum_{i=1}^{n} x_{1,i}{}^2 x_{2,i}{}^2 + \sum_{i=2}^{n} \sum_{j=1}^{i-1} \left(\sqrt{2} x_{1,i} x_{1,j}\right) \left(\sqrt{2} x_{2,i} x_{2,j}\right) \\ &\quad + \sum_{i=1}^{n} \left(\sqrt{2} x_{1,i}\right) \left(\sqrt{2} x_{2,i}\right) + 1. \end{aligned}$$

This dimensional expansion changes the distances between data points in the higher-dimensional space and allows a decision surface to be constructed. The decision surface is a hyperplane optimized to the distance between the hyperplane and the nearest data points in each class. Because this quadratic optimization problem involves significant computation, SVMs are developed using machine-learning strategies and generally tuned iteratively.

For the case of DOS classification, we trained the SVM in MATLAB using the same dataset of 370 recordings described above. For each of S recording sites, a set of M features was calculated giving a total feature array **F**[*S,M*]. However, after detecting the location of stenosis, only recordings from the nearest site need to be classified, i.e., the SVM was only trained on a single feature vector **F**[*M*]. In our example with 5 recording sites, this reduced the total number of observations (recordings) to 50.

Training of the SVM was performed in MATLAB in three phases. First, PAG features were transformed to a high-dimensional space using the polynomial kernel. Then feature selection was performed to reduce the total number of features (and hence the dimensionality) of the SVM. This reduced the overall model complexity, reduced the numerical instability risk inherent to SVMs, and reduced the risk of over-fitting. Principal component analysis was used to define the three features which described variance between the data classes: $\overline{ASC \cdot ASF}$ (mean ASC multiplied by mean ASF), $\overline{ASC_S}$ (mean value of ASC in systole), and t_d (time shift in ASF onset compared to first recording site). The computation of these features is illustrated in Fig. 6.21. Then, quadratic optimization was performed to fit an optimal hyperplane between the classes of data. Model validation was performed

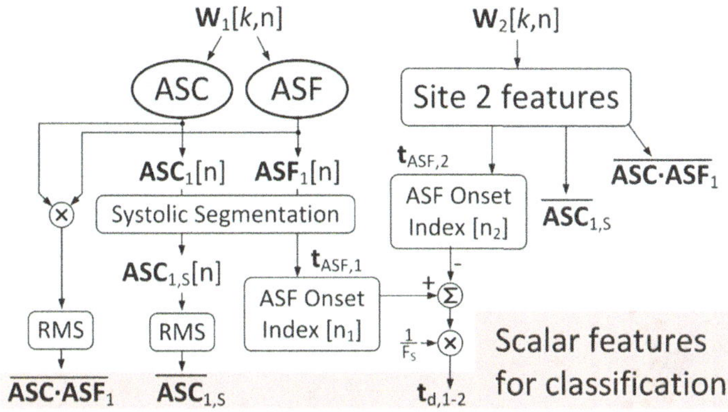

Fig. 6.21 Scalar features are derived from the time-domain ASC and ASF descriptive waveforms, including interaction features such as $\overline{ASC \cdot ASF}$. Temporo-spectral features such as systolic width can be derived, or compared to adjacent sites to compute spatial features such as t_d which describes the time shift at ASF onset in systole between time-synchronous recordings

using fivefold cross-validation such that the model was trained on ten observations and tested by classifying the remaining 40.

The quadratic SVM was designed to classify PAGs into three output classes for DOS: mild, moderate, and severe. Because these classes were ordinal (monotonic) and known a priori, quadratic SVM was selected (versus, e.g., clustering methods). Further, while DOS is a continuous variable, we chose to bin it into classification ranges because clinical monitoring does not require precise quantification of DOS; imaging is then used after a lesion is identified to more precisely determine treatment options (Sequeira et al. 2017). However, acoustic features can also be used to continuously estimate the DOS using regression, as described in the following section. Thresholding after regression can be used to similarly classify estimated DOS into ranges for clinical action.

Class definitions were chosen to be consistent with our prior work (Panda et al. 2020; Panda et al. 2019a): DOS < 30% (mild), 30% $\leq$ DOS $\leq$ 70% (moderate), and DOS > 70% (severe). Validation accuracy of the quadrative SVM on this data was 100% even though the features were not linearly separable (Fig. 6.22). Importantly, most of the classification accuracy came from the ASC and ASF features; however, adding the temporospatial measure t_d helped prevent misclassifications at high DOS which occur when the stenosis greatly reduces vascular flow rate (Table 6.3).

However, while t_d boosts classification accuracy only slightly, multiple recording locations for stenosis localization are still essential to accurate classification. For example, Table 6.4 indicates how classification accuracy drops significantly when applied to PAGs recorded more than 2 cm from the actual site of stenosis and dropping the spatial feature t_d. This suggests that accurate PAG classification requires either a priori knowledge of stenosis location or multi-site recordings to detect locations for analysis.

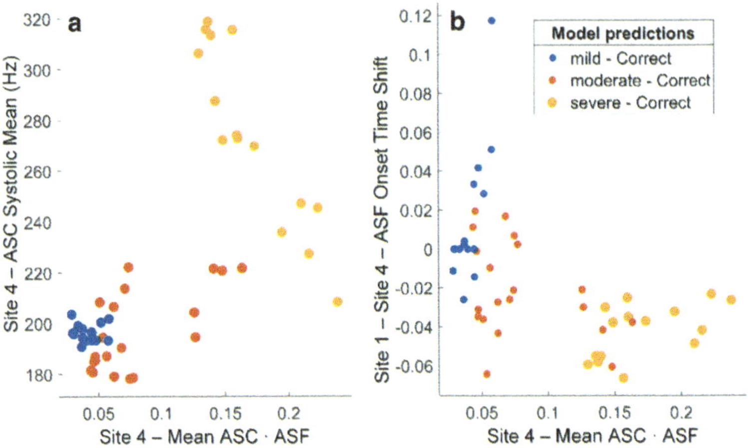

Fig. 6.22 The quadratic SVM classified DOS as mild (< 30%), moderate (30%<DOS<60%), and severe (DOS>60%) with 100% accuracy. This demonstrates the advantage of SVM as the included features are not fully separable linearly in the feature space (**a**, **b**)

Table 6.3 Performance of Quadratic SVM versus included features

Number of features	Included features	Average validation accuracy
3	$\overline{ASC \cdot ASF}, \overline{ASC_S}, t_d$	100%
2	$\overline{ASC \cdot ASF}, \overline{ASC_S}$	96%
	$\overline{ASC_S}, t_d$	84%
	$\overline{ASC \cdot ASF}, t_d$	88%
1	$\overline{ASC \cdot ASF}$	84%
	$\overline{ASC_S}$	82%
	t_d	48%

Table 6.4 Classifier accuracy of quadratic SVM versus single recording sites

Recording site	$\overline{ASC \cdot ASF}$	$\overline{ASC_S}$	$\overline{ASC \cdot ASF}, \overline{ASC_S}$
1	70%	68%	66%
2	70%	68%	78%
3	60%	54%	86%
4	84%	84%	96%

While this analysis suggested that machine-learning can be used for accurate classification of PAGs, it must be noted that cross-validation alone is only sufficient to optimize the hyperplane on the training data. The model was trained using data from a set of vascular phantoms with variable rates of blood flow, but this does not account for the wide anatomical variance seen in humans. Therefore, it is still unclear how accurately this model will function on unseen data. This remains an opportunity for future work.

6.6.4 Degree of Stenosis Estimation from Acoustic Features

The previous section discussed using acoustic features from PAGs to classify stenosis into clinically actionable ranges, but features can also be used to predict the actual degree of stenosis. Previous work in this area demonstrated that DOS could be estimated within 6% given a priori knowledge of the stenosis location (Du et al. 2015). Here, we demonstrate how features from multiple domains can be used to further improve DOS estimation using Gaussian process regression (GPR).

GPR is a regression modeling method, but unlike linear or nonlinear regression—which seeks to fit a least-squares model to minimize prediction error to a dataset *f(x)*—GPR is a Bayesian process which models *f(x)*as a Gaussian process (Rasmussen and Williams 2006). Thus, the value *f(x)* at each point x is represented as a random variable with a Gaussian distribution (Applebaum et al. 2002). The actual values used to train the model are therefore considered simply as independent observations drawn from the underlying normal probability distribution at each point. For example, observation-response pairs (x_1, y_1) and (x_2, y_2) are represented by normal distributions $P(y_1 | x_1)$ and $P(y_2 | x_2)$. Regression of a new response y_3 based on a new observation x_3 is then calculated as the conditional probability $P(y_3 | (y_1, y_2), (x_1, x_2, x_3))$

Assuming the mean of the joint distribution of all input features $\mathbf{F}[M]$ is zero (accomplished through normalization without losing information between each recording), training the GPR involves solving for the unknown covariance matrix using a radial basis function kernel $K(x_m, x_n)$, i.e.,

$$Cov\left(f\left(x_m\right), f\left(x_n\right)\right) = K\left(x_m, x_n\right) = \alpha^2 e^{-\frac{1}{2l^2}\left(x_m - x_n\right)^2}.$$

In this example the parameter α^2 is the output variance of the data, while l^2 represents the length scale of the data variance. Generally, α^2 indicates the average distance of the function from its mean, while l determines the memory length of the modeled GPR. For a GPR trained on time-invariant features, e.g., PAG features, $l = 1$. Similarly to the quadratic SVM, training data are transformed by the basis function to a higher-dimensional space. Optimization of the basis function is then performed iteratively to minimize the RMS predicted error to the input data. Model training was performed in MATLAB on the same 50 recordings used to train the quadratic SVM classifier. The RMS error of the optimized GPR was calculated using fivefold cross-validation.

While the SVM classifier was demonstrated in the previous section, SVM regression was not used for stenosis estimation. GPR was selected after feature distribution analysis, which indicated that due to the chaotic nature of turbulent fluid flow, and the dependency on variable blood flow rate, features measured at each degree of stenosis spanned a range of observations around a defined central value. Generally, for DOS > 50% extracted features followed a normal distribution when pooled across all recording sites and all flow rates. Although GPR would suffer from finite bounds on confidence intervals because DOS is bounded on the

Table 6.5 RMS error from exponential GPR model versus features and recording sites included

	Features included in model			
Sites included in model	$\overline{ASC \cdot ASF}$	$\overline{ASC_S}$	$\overline{ASC \cdot ASF}, \overline{ASC_S}$	$\overline{ASC \cdot ASF}, \overline{ASC_S}, t_d$
Site 1 only	20.0%	16.6%	10.1%	9.4%
Site 2 only	20.0%	19.0%	12.9%	9.2%
Site 3 only	21.3%	22.0%	8.6%	7.5%
Site 4 only	13.8%	16.9%	12.2%	8.0%
All sites included	8.9%	7.9%	5.2%	**4.3%**

range of 0–100%, because the model was only validated on the range of DOS from 10% to 90%, GPR out-performed other regressions, perhaps due to estimation of the underlying variance for each feature. For example, using the same features as in Table 6.5, quadratic SVM regression only achieved a best-case 8.3% RMS error.

As in the quadratic SVM classifier, the addition of more features reduced the RMS error of the regression. However, unlike the SVM, the regression required data from sites around the stenosis to improve accuracy. In this example, the actual stenosis lesion was located under Site 2 with turbulent flow occurring beneath Site 3 and Site 4 based on established models (Gaupp et al. 1999; Gårdhagen n.d.). Including features from recordings proximal and distal to the lesion greatly improved the estimation accuracy. For all tested DOS, error was in the range [−11% 14%], and for DOS>50% error was [−11% 3%] (Fig. 6.23). From this outcome we conclude two things. First, this **in vitro** experiment clearly demonstrates the need for multiple recording sites for accurate phonoangiographic estimation of degree of stenosis. In humans with more variable vascular anatomy, the need for the multiple recording sites is likely greater because the location or presence of stenosis is not known **a priori**. Second, the achieved accuracy is sufficient for clinical monitoring, which generally only needs to detect when stenosis exceeds 50% or is rapidly progressing (Sequeira et al. 2017; Valliant and McComb 2015; Tessitore et al. 2014b). Clinical imaging would still be used, so the objective for phonoangiographic monitoring is simply to identify which patients to select for imaging.

6.7 Conclusion

This chapter discussed a new technique for point-of-care clinical monitoring of a vascular access using an array of microphones. Turbulent blood flow produces bruits that are recorded by each microphone and analyzed as phonoangiograms to detect the location and severity of stenosis. Signal processing spans several domains, beginning with the analog signal processing needed to amplify and filter the PVDF microphone signals before digital conversion. In the digital domain, continuous wavelet transform was used to produce acoustic spectral centroid and acoustic spectral flux analytic signals, from which acoustic features were derived. Systolic-diastolic segmentation provided additional features or the calculation of

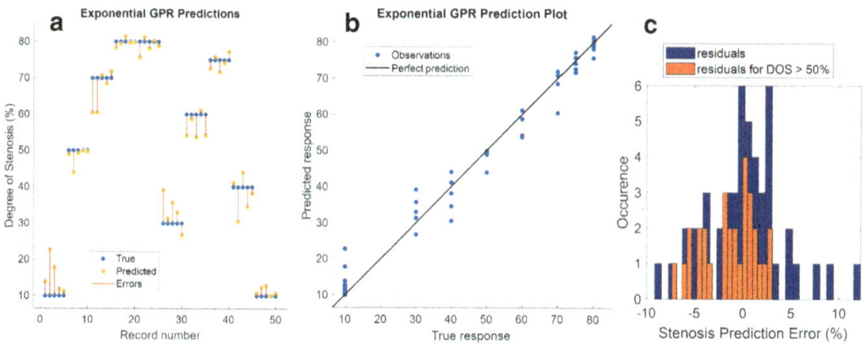

Fig. 6.23 Exponential Gaussian process regression estimated degree of stenosis for each in vitro vascular stenosis phantom (**a**). The trained model estimated degree of stenosis with RMS error of 4.3% (**b**) and error range of [−11% 14%] and [−11% 3%] for all tested stenoses and for stenoses > 50%, respectively (**c**)

ratiometric features. Techniques to calculate features from multiple domains—spectral, temporospectral, and spatial—were feasible because of time-synchronous recordings from the microphone array.

A 1×5 microphone array was used to record bruits from a vascular phantom using stenosis models of 10–90% and blood-mimicking fluid at physiologic flow rates and pressures. This produced a dataset of recordings from which features were calculated. Stenosis localization was demonstrated using a simple binary classifier against a pitch-shift threshold to detect which recording site was nearest the stenotic lesion. A quadratic support vector machine classifier was trained using multi-domain features from a single recording site and achieved 100% accuracy when classifying the degree of stenosis as mild, moderate, or severe. Finally, estimation of the actual degree of stenosis was demonstrated using an exponential Gaussian process regression. The regression model combined features recorded from four sites to estimate degree of stenosis with 4.3% RMS error. Because the clinical threshold for elective surgery for vascular stenosis is 50% (Sequeira et al. 2017; Valliant and McComb 2015; Tessitore et al. 2014b) (and clinical monitoring for stenosis does not need to be as accurate as angiographic imaging), this suggests that phonoangiographic analysis is feasible for point-of-care monitoring.

Acknowledgements This work was supported in part by RX001968-01 from US Dept. of Veterans Affairs Rehabilitation Research and Development Service, the Advanced Platform Technology Center of the Louis Stokes Cleveland Veterans Affairs Medical Center, and Case Western Reserve University. The contents do not represent the views of the US Government.

References

Y.M. Akay, M. Akay, W. Welkowitz, J.L. Semmlow, J.B. Kostis, Noninvasive acoustical detection of coronary artery disease: A comparative study of signal processing methods. I.E.E.E. Trans. Biomed. Eng. **40**(6), 571–578 (1993)

A.A. Al-Jaishi, A.R. Liu, C.E. Lok, J.C. Zhang, L.M. Moist, Complications of the arteriovenous fistula: A systematic review. J. Am. Soc. Nephrol. **28**(6), 1839–1850 (2017)

M. Allon, M.L. Robbin, Hemodialysis vascular access monitoring: Current concepts. Hemodial. Int. **13**(2), 153–162 (2009)

D. Applebaum, G. Grimmett, D. Stirzaker, M. Capiński, T. Zastawniak, M. Capinski, Probability and random processes. Math. Gaz. **86**, 185 (2002)

D. M. Binkley, Tradeoffs and Optimization in Analog CMOS Design. 2008

P.J. Bosman, P.J. Blankestijn, Y. Van der Graaf, R.J. Heintjes, H.A. Koomans, B.C. Eikelboom, Comparison between PTFE and denatured homologous vein grafts for haemodialysis access: A prospective randomised multicentre trial. Eur. J. Vasc. Endovasc. Surg. **16**, 126 (1998)

A. V Cayco, A. K. Abu-Alfa, R. L. Mahnensmith, and M. A. Perazella, "Reduction in Arteriovenous Graft Impairment: Results of a Vascular Access Surveillance Protocol," 1998

W.-L.L. Chen, C.-H.H. Lin, T. Chen, P.-J.J. Chen, C.D. Kan, C.-D. Kan, Stenosis detection using burg method with autoregressive model for hemodialysis patients. J. Med. Biol. Eng. **33**(4), 356–362 (2013)

S. Chin, B. Panda, M.S. Damaser, S.J.A. Majerus, Stenosis characterization and identification for Dialysis vascular access, in *2018 IEEE Signal Processing in Medicine and Biology Symposium, SPMB 2018 – Proceedings*, (2019)

I. Clausen, S.T. Moe, L.G.W. Tvedt, A. Vogl, D.T. Wang, A miniaturized pressure sensor with inherent biofouling protection designed for in vivo applications. Proc. Annu. Int. Conf. IEEE Eng. Med. Biol. Soc. EMBS, 1880–1883 (2011)

D.J. Doyle, D.M. Mandell, R.M. Richardson, Monitoring hemodialysis vascular access by digital phonoangiography. Ann. Biomed. Eng. **30**(7), 982

Y.-C.C. Du, C.-D.D. Kan, W.-L.L. Chen, C.-H.H. Lin, Estimating residual stenosis for an arteriovenous shunt using a flexible fuzzy classifier. Comput. Sci. Eng. **16**(6), 80–91 (2014)

Y.-C.C. Du, W.-L.L. Chen, C.-H.H. Lin, C.-D.D. Kan, M.-J.J. Wu, Residual stenosis estimation of arteriovenous grafts using a dual-channel phonoangiography with fractional-order features. IEEE J. Biomed. Heal. Inform. **19**(2), 590–600 (2015)

G.W. Duncan, J.O. Gruber, C.F. Dewey, G.S. Myers, R.S. Lees, Evaluation of carotid stenosis by phonoangiography. N. Engl. J. Med. **293**(22), 1124–1128 (1975)

J.C. Duque, M. Tabbara, L. Martinez, J. Cardona, R.I. Vazquez-Padron, L.H. Salman, Dialysis arteriovenous fistula failure and angioplasty: Intimal hyperplasia and other causes of access failure. Am. J. Kidney Dis. **69**(1), 147–151 (2017)

H.I. Feldman, S. Kobrin, A. Wasserstein, Hemodialysis vascular access morbidity. J. Am. Soc. Nephrol. **7**(4), 523–535 (1996)

R. Gårdhagen. Turbulent Flow in Constricted Blood Vessels Quantification of Wall Shear Stress Using Large Eddy Simulation.

S. Gaupp, Y. Wang, T. V How, and P. J. Fish, "Characterisation of vortex shedding in vascular anstomosis models using pulsed doppler ultrasound," 1999

M. Gram et al., *Stenosis Detection Algorithm for Screening of Arteriovenous Fistulae* (2011), pp. 241–244

H. Inc for OSORA CMS. Medicare Claims Processing Manual Chapter 8-Outpatient ESRD Hospital, Independent Facility, and Physician/Supplier Claims Transmittals

"Hemodialysis | NIDDK"

H.-Y. Hsien-Yi Wang, C.-H. Cho-Han Wu, C.-Y. Chien-Yue Chen, B.-S. Bor-Shyh Lin, Novel noninvasive approach for detecting arteriovenous fistula stenosis. I.E.E.E. Trans. Biomed. Eng. **61**(6), 1851–1857 (Jun. 2014)

H.J.T.A.M. Huijbregts, M.L. Bots, F.L. Moll, P.J. Blankestijn, Hospital specific aspects predominantly determine primary failure of hemodialysis arteriovenous fistulas. J. Vasc. Surg. **45**(5), 962–967 (2007)

T. Joachims, Advances in kernel methods: Support vector. Learning (1998)

C.-D. Kan, W.-L. Chen, J.-F. Wang, P.-H. Sung, and L.-S. Jang, "Phonographic Signal with a Fractional-Order Chaotic System: A Novel and Simple Algorithm for Analyzing Residual Arteriovenous Access Stenosis View Project Stenosis Detection Using Burg Method with Autoregressive Model for Hemodialysis Patients View Project," 2015

N. Krivitski, Why vascular access trials on flow surveillance failed. J. Vasc. Access **15**(7_suppl), 15–19 (2014)

E. Lacson, W. Wang, J.M. Lazarus, R.M. Hakim, R.M. Hakim, Change in vascular access and hospitalization risk in long-term hemodialysis patients. Clin. J. Am. Soc. Nephrol. **5**(11), 1996–2003 (2010)

J. Lázaro, E. Gil, R. Bailón, A. Mincholé, P. Laguna, Deriving respiration from photoplethysmographic pulse width. Med. Biol. Eng. Comput. **51**(1–2), 233–242 (2013)

J.K. Leypoldt, Hemodialysis adequacy. Chronic Kidney Dis. Dial. Transplant., 405–428 (2005)

S. M, S.M.B. Panda, Vascular stenosis detection using temporal-spectral differences in correlated acoustic measurements. IEEE Signal Process. Med. Biol. (2019)

S.J.A. Majerus et al., *Bruit-enhancing phonoangiogram filter using sub-band autoregressive linear predictive coding* (2000), pp. 4–7

S.J.A.A. Majerus et al., Bruit-enhancing phonoangiogram filter using sub-band autoregressive linear predictive coding, in *Proceedings of the Annual International Conference of the IEEE Engineering in Medicine and Biology Society, EMBS*, vol. 2018, (2018), pp. 1416–1419

H.A. Mansy, S.J. Hoxie, N.H. Patel, R.H. Sandler, Computerised analysis of auscultatory sounds associated with vascular patency of haemodialysis access. Med. Biol. Eng. Comput. **43**(1), 56–62 (2005)

I. Milsom, K.S. Coyne, S. Nicholson, M. Kvasz, C.I. Chen, A.J. Wein, Global prevalence and economic burden of urgency urinary incontinence: A systematic review. Eur. Urol. **65**(1), 79–95 (2014)

L. Moist, C.E. Lok, Con: Vascular access surveillance in mature fistulas: Is it worthwhile? Nephrol. Dial. Transplant. **34**(7), 1106–1111 (2019)

P.V. Obando, B. Mandersson, Frequency tracking of resonant-like sounds from audio recordings of arterio-venous fistula stenosis, in *2012 IEEE International Conference on Bioinformatics and Biomedicine Workshops*, (2012), pp. 771–773

B. Panda, S. Mandal, S. Member, S.J.A. Majerus, S. Member, S.J.A. Majerus, Flexible, skin coupled microphone Array for point of care vascular access monitoring. IEEE Trans. Biomed. Circuits Syst. **13**(6), 1494–1505 (2019a)

B. Panda, S. Chin, S. Mandal, S. Majerus, Skin-coupled PVDF microphones for noninvasive vascular blood sound monitoring, in *2018 IEEE Signal Processing in Medicine and Biology Symposium, SPMB 2018 – Proceedings*, (2019b)

S.M.B. Panda, S. Chin, S. Mandal, Noninvasive vascular blood sound monitoring through flexible PVDF microphone. Emerg. Trends Signal Process. Med. Biol. (2020)

R.L. Pisoni, L. Zepel, F.K. Port, B.M. Robinson, Trends in US vascular access use, patient preferences, and related practices: An update from the US DOPPS practice monitor with international comparisons. Am. J. Kidney Dis. **65**(6), 905–915 (2015)

C. E. Rasmussen and C. K. I. Williams, Gaussian processes for machine learning. 2006

L. Rousselot. Acoustical monitoring of model system for vascular access in haemodialysis. September, 2014

P. Roy-Chaudhury, V.P. Sukhatme, A.K. Cheung, Hemodialysis vascular access dysfunction: A cellular and molecular viewpoint. J. Am. Soc. Nephrol. **17**(4), 1112–1127 (2006)

T. Sato, K. Tsuji, N. Kawashima, T. Agishi, H. Toma, Evaluation of blood access dysfunction based on a wavelet transform analysis of shunt murmurs. J. Artif. Organs **9**(2), 97–104 (2006)

A.R. Sehgal, A. Dor, A.C. Tsai, Morbidity and cost implications of inadequate hemodialysis. Am. J. Kidney Dis. **37**(6), 1223–1231 (2001)

J. H. Seo. A coupled flow-acoustic computational study of bruits from a modeled stenosed artery
A. Sequeira, M. Naljayan, T.J. Vachharajani, Vascular access guidelines: Summary, rationale, and controversies. Tech. Vasc. Interv. Radiol. **20**(1), 2–8 (2017)
T. Shinzato, S. Nakai, I. Takai, T. Kato, I. Inoue, K. Maeda, A new wearable system for continuous monitoring of arteriovenous fistulae. ASAIO J **39**(2), 137–140 (1993)
P.H. Sung, C.D. Kan, W.L. Chen, L.S. Jang, J.F. Wang, Hemodialysis vascular access stenosis detection using auditory spectro-temporal features of phonoangiography. Med. Biol. Eng. Comput. **53**(5), 393–403 (2015)
N. Tessitore, V. Bedogna, G. Verlato, A. Poli, The rise and fall of access blood flow surveillance in arteriovenous fistulas. Semin. Dial. **27**(2), 108–118 (2014a)
N. Tessitore et al., Should current criteria for detecting and repairing arteriovenous fistula stenosis be reconsidered? Interim analysis of a randomized controlled trial. Nephrol. Dial. Transplant. **29**(1), 179–187 (2014b)
G. Tzanetakis, P. Cook, Musical genre classification of audio signals. IEEE Trans. Speech Audio Process. **10**(5), 293 (2002)
A. Valliant, K. McComb, Vascular access monitoring and surveillance: An update. Adv. Chronic Kidney Dis. **22**(6), 446–452 (2015)
Y.-N. Wang, C.-Y. Chan, and S.-J. Chou, "The Detection of Arteriovenous Fistula Stenosis for Hemodialysis Based on Wavelet Transform," 2011
J.J. White, S.J. Ram, S.A. Jones, S.J. Schwab, W.D. Paulson, Influence of luminal diameters on flow surveillance of hemodialysis grafts: Insights from a mathematical model. Clin. J. Am. Soc. Nephrol. **1**(5), 972–978 (2006)
M.-J. Wu et al., Dysfunction screening in experimental arteriovenous grafts for hemodialysis using fractional-order extractor and color relation analysis. Cardiovasc. Eng. Technol. **6**(4), 463–473 (2015)

Chapter 7
Fast Automatic Artifact Annotator for EEG Signals Using Deep Learning

Dong Kyu Kim and Sam Keene

7.1 Introduction

The study of the brain, neuroscience, to understand about ourselves better has been a great research area that combines the efforts of scientists and engineers across various disciplines. Due to the brain's complexity, the understanding of the basis of learning, perception, and consciousness is sometimes described as the "ultimate challenge" of biological sciences (Aminoff 2001). Currently, many advances in neuroscience come from analyzing recordings of the brain. However, due to the overwhelming amount of electrochemical activities in the brain, the collection of reliable data is still one of the biggest challenges in neuroscience (Louis et al. 2016).

There are two main branches of brain signal acquisition methods: invasive and non-invasive methods. Invasive methods involve placements of electrodes inside the brain or insertion of needles through the subject's head to collect precise and highly local data. On the other hand, non-invasive methods such as electroencephalogram (EEG) and magnetic resonance imaging (MRI) suffer from noise and various artifacts (Louis et al. 2016). Due to the high interest and potential in this area of research, in addition to relatively cheap and accessible EEG recording machines (DellaBadia et al. 2002), there are a lot of interesting data available for analysis. However, a lot of EEG data suffer from artifacts which are unwanted signals present in the recordings as a result of the procedure of measurements. Artifacts in EEGs are both physiological and technical, and they require well-trained observers to be identified well (Louis et al. 2016). If there is a system that can distinguish

D. K. Kim (✉) · S. Keene
Electrical Engineering Department, The Cooper Union, New York, NY, USA
e-mail: dongkyuk@usc.edu

I. Obeid et al. (eds.), *Biomedical Signal Processing*,
https://doi.org/10.1007/978-3-030-67494-6_7

between artifacts, and cerebral data automatically, neuroscience can advance further as reducing the effect of artifacts will increase the signal-to-noise ratio so that brain activity can be detected more precisely.

To achieve this goal, Temple University has constructed a large dataset of EEG signals from various subjects that are specifically labeled for artifacts (Obeid and Picone 2016) to aid engineers and scientists to build models that detect and remove the artifacts. Previously, Golmohammadi and colleagues developed a model that automatically analyzes EEG signals to help physicians diagnose brain-related disorders such as seizures using hybrid deep learning architectures. This model integrates hidden Markov models, deep learning models, and statistical language models to deliver a composite model that has a true positive rate of 90% while having a false alarm rate of below 5% on events of clinical interests: spike and sharp waves, periodic lateralized epileptiform discharges, and generalized periodic epileptiform discharges (Golmohammadi et al. 2019). This model proves the viability of big data and deep learning methods in detecting events in EEG signals.

The work in Golmohammadi et al. (2019) attempts to classify artifacts as well as the mentioned events of clinical interest, but the model developed was only able to distinguish 14.04% of the artifacts correctly from the data. As the goal of that model was to detect seizures and epilepsy, no further analysis of artifacts was done, but it was noted that transient pulse-like artifacts such as eye movements and muscle movements can significantly degrade the performance. In this chapter, a method that can quickly identify the presence of artifacts and the type of the artifacts during the data acquisition is proposed so that a clinician can resolve the problem immediately and ensure the collected data is cleaner. To achieve this goal, multiple deep learning models with varying model size, inference time, and accuracies were developed and optimized to compare and contrast between advantages and disadvantages of different approaches. The key feature of the models is that all the inferences are done directly on the signals with a minimal preprocessing such as normalizing and aggregating enough samples to be used for predictions by the model. The system aims to be memory efficient, and computationally light, while being fast enough to be implemented on portable systems such as Raspberry Pi. Such portable systems would be able to detect and classify artifacts in real-time, potentially in a clinical setting.

7.2 Related Works

There have been numerous efforts to combat the artifact problems in EEG signals. A lot of research has been done to reduce the effects of artifacts by utilizing prior knowledge such as how some artifacts behave in the signal. Artifact removal and detection tools of this nature tend to examine the statistical characteristics of the signals.

Nolan, Whelan, and Reilly (Nolan et al. 2010) proposed FASTER, Fully Automated Statistical Thresholding for EEG artifact Rejection, which uses independent component analysis (ICA) to separate EEG signals into neural activity and artifacts. ICA works by separating multivariate signals into additive subcomponents by assuming that different subcomponents are statistically independent of each other. The advantage of using ICA is that ICA reduces the statistical dependencies of different components of the signal, by separating the components (Lee et al. 1999). After the separation, the model uses a statistical comparison charts to check for features such as correlation with signal components, mean, variance, spatial, etc. This model was tested on simulated EEGs and real EEGs and had a true positive rate of over 90% in detecting artifacts when the model was given data with more than 64 channels. However, the true positive rate drops to 5.88% when the number of channels provided decreases to 32. Besides, the algorithm takes an hour per 400 s to yield the results using a machine with a 64-bit dual-core machine. Nevertheless, the model not only detects the signal quite accurately but also can remove the artifact, as any separated component of the signal can be extracted. This model can detect eye movements, EMG artifacts, linear trends, and white noise.

Similarly, Singh and Wagatsuma (2017) used Morphological Component Analysis (MCA), which uses a dictionary of multiple bases to guarantee the reconstruction of original signals. MCA is applied to the EEG signal so that the signal is deconstructed into a combination of bases in the dictionary. Singh and Wagatsuma hypothesized that three dictionaries of bases are dominant, and they are undecimated wavelet transform (UDWT), discrete sine transform (DST), and DIRAC (standard unit vector basis). The decomposition was able to show that EEG signals and their artifacts are represented by different dictionaries of bases, indicating that given the decomposition result, artifacts can be distinguished from the signals of interest. Singh and Wagatsuma successfully categorized which dictionary corresponds well with the signal or the artifact. This research demonstrates that an ensemble of different signal processing techniques could work well for artifact classification. The drawback of this method is similar to that of Nolan's. MCA takes about 6 s on 1024 samples of data that are sampled at 173.61 Hz. This corresponds to spending around 1.01 s of computation time per 1 s of a signal. As a result, this computational time is not suitable for fast EEG artifact detection. There are numerous other additional statistical approaches to separate the real EEG signal from the artifacts, such as canonical correlation analysis, which Clercq used to remove muscle artifacts from the EEG signals (Clercq et al. 2006).

All of the statistical approaches of the problem require a deconstruction of EEG signals into multiple components and analyzing each component to determine which components are responsible for artifacts and which are responsible for the real signal. Though they are highly interpretive, the separation procedure takes a lot of computation, and correct prior knowledge, such as the number of artifacts, a set of orthogonal bases that work well with the time-series data, or the general behavior of artifacts, is required. Due to the complex nature of the EEG signals, deep learning with its ability to learn hidden features from the raw data has shown great promises (Goodfellow et al. 2016).

According to the review paper by Roy et al. (2019), among the 156 papers about applying deep learning to EEG signals that the authors reviewed from January 2010 to July 2018, some papers applied data preprocessing techniques and artifact rejection techniques such as the ICA mentioned above to combat the artifacts, while some papers just used the raw EEG signals. Given that the majority of the papers did not use any artifact removal schemes, Roy et al. suggest that using deep learning on EEG signals directly might avoid the artifact removal step without any performance degradation. However, all the papers mentioned in Roy's review paper specifically target certain applications such as detecting epilepsy, monitoring sleep, and making a brain-computer interface, and none of the papers mentioned targets the detection of artifacts specifically. The review paper suggests that convolutional neural networks (CNNs) and recurrent neural networks (RNNs) are the most used networks in this field; 40% of the studies use CNNS and 14% use RNNs.

Other works relating to deep learning and EEG signals or EEG like signals not mentioned in the review paper above include Krishnaveni's work on ocular artifact removal in EEG signals (Krishnaveni et al. 2007) and Hasasneh's work on automatic classification of ocular and cardiac artifacts in magnetoencephalography (MEG) (Hasasneh et al. 2018). Both of these works include some data preprocessing. Hasasneh's work utilizes ICA, and Krishnaveni's work utilizes the Joint Approximation Diagonalisation of Eigen-matrices (JADE) algorithm to separate the real signals from the artifact signals before using neural networks. The detection rates for the test data for both of these works are 94.4% and 92%, respectively. However, both of them only address one or two types of artifacts at the same time, while the model proposed will include four different artifacts to be classified separately with no preprocessing such that the model can be applied directly to the raw data.

There have been many attempts and there have been successful attempts in detecting artifacts and classifying them using statistical machine learning and inferences, but there are not much done using deep learning. Deep learning approaches are particularly adept at optimizing an arbitrary large model and recognizing complex patterns (Goodfellow et al. 2016). The previous methods require mathematical models for artifact events or seizure events to classify the signals accurately; hence the performance of the models depends highly on the accuracy of the proposed mathematical models. However, the usage of deep learning models can alleviate the incorrect modeling error as no accurate mathematical model is needed to classify different events. In addition, the statistical analysis of large temporal data is computationally heavy and takes a long time. While training a deep learning model to optimize the parameters may take a long time, the inference time for the completed model is relatively short compared to that of statistical models. To use these advantages, many works have attempted to classify different aspects of the EEG signals for monitoring purposes for seizure and sleep disorders using deep learning. However, not a lot of works have been done in detecting and classifying artifacts using deep learning, especially classifying multiple artifacts instead of detecting a small number of artifacts.

7.3 Method

7.3.1 Resources

The dataset used to develop our model is the Temple University Hospital's EEG Artifact Corpus. This dataset was developed to help researchers build models to reduce the harmful effects of artifacts for EEG event classification algorithms such as seizure detection algorithms. The version of the dataset is v1.0.0, and the dataset is derived from the v1.1.0 of the TUH EEG Corpus (Obeid and Picone 2016). The TUH EEG Corpus is the largest publicly available database of clinical EEG data that contains over 30,000 EEGs spanning from 2002 to present, and the Artifact Corpus is a subset of the original corpus that has been specifically labeled to enhance artifact related research. There are 310 observations with 213 subjects with varying durations and sampling rates.

The experiments to build our model were done using Python. Specifically, the version of the python that was used is 3.6.8. Additional libraries used are matplotlib v3.0.2, numpy v1.16.0, tqdm v4.31.1, scipy v1.2.0, tensorflow v1.12.0, and keras v2.2.4. matplotlib and tqdm library were used for making plots and monitoring progress, and numpy, scipy, tensorflow, keras libraries were used to build a deep learning model and test. All the experiments were done using a machine equipped with 16GB memory, AMD FX(tm)-6300 Six-Core Processor 3.5GHz, and a Geforce GTX 1070 8GB graphics card. The data drive in which the corpus was in was a standard hard drive with 7200RPM. Finally, the environment was a Windows 10 operating system with a virtual environment with all the above libraries created using conda for the Anaconda Python distribution.

7.3.2 Data Preprocessing

The data corpus contains three different configurations of EEG. The first is the AR (averaged reference) where the average of a finite number of electrodes is used as a reference. This means that the average is subtracted from the signals of each electrode for every time point to account for the common noise. The second configuration is the LE (linked ears reference) which is based on the assumption that ears do not have any electrical activity so that ears can be used as reference points (Lopez et al. 2016). The third configuration is the AR_A which is a modified version of the AR configuration, where A1_REF and A2_REF are not used. All the data contain standard measurements that one could expect from the 10–20 International System. For the AR, and the LE configurations, 22 channels can be derived from the available channel information, while for the AR_A configuration, only 20 channels can be derived. This is because the AR_A configuration lacks the EEG A1_REF and the EEG A2_REF channels. The computations necessary to derive the channels

Table 7.1 List of channels with appropriate computation

Channel number	Computation
1	FP1-F7
2	F7-T3
3	T3-T5
4	T5-01
5	FP2-F8
6	F8-T4
7	T4-T6
8	T6-02
9	A1-T3
10	T3-C3
11	C3-CZ
12	CZ-C4
13	C4-T4
14	T4-A2
15	FP1-F3
16	F3-C3
17	C3-P3
18	P3-01
19	FP2-F4
20	F4-C4
21	C4-P4
22	P4-02

are tabulated in Table 7.1. The AR_A configuration lacks channel number 9 and 14 from Table 7.1.

There are only seven occurrences of the AR_A configuration with four subjects, and as this configuration lacks similarity to other configurations, this configuration was discarded for the experiments. Too few examples of different data would hinder the model from learning the important aspects of the artifacts, and for deep learning models, consistent data size is important. The tradeoff is either to give up 2 channels across all 303 observations or to give up 7 observations, and we have decided to give up these 7 observations. Hence, for the experiment, there are 303 observations with 209 subjects available.

Another way to alleviate this problem is to fill in the missing channels. Nolan's work describes a method to fill in any missing channels using adjacent channels (Nolan et al. 2010). However, since the missing A1 and A2 electrodes in the AR_A configuration are reference points that are placed on ears, they cannot be interpolated from other electrodes, as all the other electrodes are on the head. We decided that guessing the signals on ears based on signals from the brain would not be accurate at all. As a result, we decided not to use the interpolation method and thus discard this configuration.

The original data are in the European Data Format (EDF), which is a standard file format designed for the storage of medical time series data. All the EDF

Table 7.2 Possible labels and corresponding descriptions

Label	Description
eyem	Eye movements
chew	Chewing
shiv	Shivering
elpp	Electrode related artifacts such as electrode pops, static electrodes, lead artifacts
musc	Muscle related artifacts
bckg	Background noise
null	Undefined annotation

files provided have all the electrode information so that channels defined in the instruction can be derived easily using the computations tabulated in Table 7.1. In addition, the corresponding label files contain the artifact class labels for the whole EEG session and also for each channel.

There are seven possible labels and the labels and the corresponding descriptions are tabulated in Table 7.2. The label files provide the start time and the stop time of the existing artifacts in seconds. The files have the confidence level of the label, which indicates the probability that the artifact is what the label says it is. All the labels in this data corpus have the confidence levels of 1, and the background noise label, "bckg," is not available for this dataset. This is because the corpus is still in the beginning stage of the development so it does not have a lot of data available so the "bckg" label seems to be lacking in this version. As a result, the model is developed to classify five artifacts and a "null" label. The "null" label is defined to be any undefined annotation, in this corpus; this label is given to signals that do not seem to have artifacts.

The EEG signals in the dataset have varying sampling frequencies of 250 Hz, 256 Hz, 480 Hz, and 500 Hz. As deep learning models require input features to be consistent that is input features need to be of the same size and having different sampling rates for temporal data can harm the performance of the model. For example, if we were to optimize the model to infer using 500 time points, this is equivalent to using 2 s if the sampling frequency is 250 Hz, and 1 s if the sampling frequency is 500 Hz. Then the two samples have different kinds of information available, as the former sample will have more seconds of information, while the latter sample will have more detailed information on a smaller time window.

To alleviate this problem, all the signals were resampled to 250 Hz, which is the lowest sampling rate using a Fourier method. Then the signals were separated into 1-second segments without overlaps. The separation is done so that the input signal to the model is kept small. The deep learning model size depends on the number of layer parameters, which depends on the complexity of the layer and the input size. Also, the separation allows the model to be able to infer on any instance, which means we can determine whether the segment of the signal is affected by artifacts at any time using the small accumulated data around the specific time. The 1-second segment was chosen as the lowest frequency of brain waves is around

Table 7.3 Occurrences and the percentage of original 1-second segment samples of each label

Label	Occurrences	Percentage (%)
eyem	7471	2.16
chew	2727	0.79
shiv	1338	0.39
elpp	2663	0.77
musc	4892	1.41
null	327,222	94.49
Total:	346,313	100

3 Hz, which allows the segment to have at least three occurrences of the smallest wave. In addition, all the observations end at a whole second, so that there is no loss of information when the time window for segments is 1 s.

After the resampling and the separation, 303 observations of varying lengths turn into 346,313 1-second segments. The breakdown of the number and the corresponding percentage of samples available for each label are tabulated in Table 7.3. There is a high imbalance of data due to many examples with the label "null." This is due to the nature of the signal as the artifact content in the clinical EEG waves collected should be ideally low. There are only 1338 observations of "shiv," which consists of 0.39% of all the data available. Due to the relatively small number of occurrences, this label caused problems in developing models. When a preliminary study was done to investigate possible research directions, the "shiv" label caused problems by not being able to separate into three sets required for the development of the models. Since there are too few samples of "shiv" available, and most of the samples are from the same subject, when the dataset is separated into the train, the test, and the validation sets, depending on the random state of the machine, samples with "shiv" label are only found in one or two of the three sets. To illustrate this problem, a recurrent neural network model was trained for 100 epochs on the dataset with the "shiv" label. The confusion matrix for this model is shown in Fig. 7.1. The model completely fails to classify the "shiv" label and predicts all the "shiv" events to be either a "musc" event, an "elpp" event, or a "null" event. In fact, the model does not predict anything to be the "shiv" event. The reason why the model failed to do so was because there was no "shiv" label available in the training set, which caused the model to never be exposed to the label. As a result, we decided to leave out the "shiv" label from the experiments. The updated numbers and the updated percentages of samples available for each label are tabulated in Table 7.4.

The data were divided into a train set, a validation set, and a test set. The ratio among the three was 0.75:0.10:0.15. The ratio was determined arbitrarily while making sure a good amount of data was available for each of the sets. The data division was done on the unique patient ID that was provided in the EEG corpus. The reason why the division was done on the IDs rather than the sessions is that we wanted to ensure that the training and the testing were not performed on the same patient as the goal of the models is to generalize to detect artifacts on new subjects. Out of the 209 subjects, 157 subjects were allocated to the training set, 21 subjects were allocated to the validation set, and 31 patients were allocated to the test set.

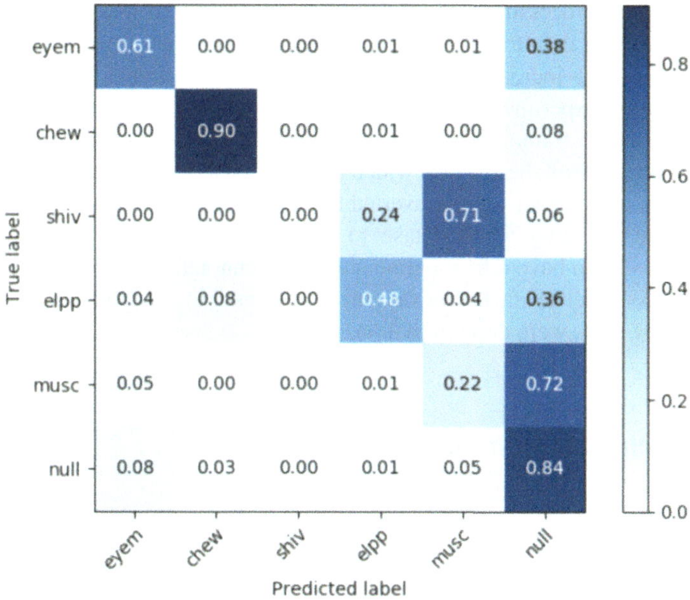

Fig. 7.1 Confusion matrix of the RNN-based model with all the labels

Table 7.4 Occurrences and the percentage of 1-second segment samples of each label after the removal of "shiv"

Label	Occurrences	Percentage (%)
eyem	7471	2.17
chew	2727	0.79
elpp	2663	0.77
musc	4892	1.42
null	327,222	94.85
Total	344,975	100

This translates to 224 sessions in the train set, 23 sessions in the validation set, and 56 sessions in the test set. The order of the patient ID has been shuffled before the division to remove any lingering pattern.

In addition to the sampling rate change, the signals are normalized. As the neural network models generally perform better when the data are in the $(-1,1)$ range, the dynamic range of the EEG signals is modified. All the signals were normalized to have a 0 mean, and a standard deviation of 1. The statistics of the whole training set were used for the normalization, and these statistics are used for all the sets as statistics of the unseen data are assumed to be not available. The mean of the training set was 1.5977595, and the standard deviation was 219.39517. In order to normalize, the mean was subtracted from all the signals and the resulting values were divided by the standard deviation.

All the EDF files are in the 16-bit floating-point format; however as the Tensorflow library does not work with the 16-bit floating-point format, all the data after the preprocessing were all converted to the 64-bit floating-point format. Converting all the data to the 64-bit floating-point format and saving the data as numpy array objects increased the size of the whole dataset from 5.39GB to 14.2GB. From our initial experiments, it was evident that the extra precision degraded the performance of the training process as the speed of the hard drive reading the data could not keep up with the speed at which the model was training. In order to combat this problem, all the data were converted to the 32-bit floating-point format, which decreased the size of the whole dataset to 7.1GB.

As the goal is to have a fast, online automatic annotator for artifacts, no further signal processing or artifact removal currently available was applied. All the data preprocessing steps were done in python.

7.3.3 Preliminary Studies

In order to examine the dataset to learn the general characteristics and the general behavior, a deep learning model with two fully connected layers was built. The input layer was flattened to reduce the dimension so that the fully connected layer that follows can access all the data. Each fully connected layer had 1024 nodes and was activated by a ReLu (Rectified Linear Unit). The ReLu was chosen as the activation function as it tends to have a good convergence and is computationally light compared to other activations such as the sigmoid function. The Adam optimizer (Kingma and Ba 2015) was used, with the default setting. The default setting is that the learning rate is 0.001, the beta-1 value is 0.9, and the beta-2 value is 0.999 with no decay. The Adam optimizer was used for all the experiments as it is computationally efficient and has a small memory requirement. This fully connected model was trained using the training set for 10 epochs with the batch size of 32. The model was validated using the validation set created, and this model was never tested with the test set. The loss function that was used is "categorical_crossentropy," which is defined as below:

$$L_i = -\sum_{n=1}^{N} \left(y_{i,n} \log \left(\hat{y}_{i,n} \right) \right). \tag{7.1}$$

i denotes the index of the observation, and n denotes the class label. y and $\hat{y}$ denote the true label and the estimated probability of the label, respectively. This is a categorical cross-entropy for N number of classes. The model minimizes this loss function by maximizing the estimated probability of the class when the true label for the class matches the estimation. The model trains completely with an accuracy of 94.4%, which is around the accuracy that one will get with a baseline classifier that guesses all the signals as "null" that yields an accuracy of around 94.9%. The relative frequencies of labels other than "null" were so insignificant as shown in Table 7.4 that the model never attempted to optimize the parameters to account for

Table 7.5 Occurrences and the percentage of 1-second segment samples of each label after the subsampling of "null"

Label	Occurrences	Percentage (%)
eyem	7471	26.20
chew	2727	9.56
elpp	2663	9.34
musc	4892	17.16
null	10,763	37.74
Total	28,516	100

artifact labels. This was evident in the behavior of the test and validation losses and accuracies which just fluctuated a bit without making a meaningful movement over the 10 epochs.

In order to combat the label-imbalance problem, another dataset was prepared. In this dataset, the "null" label is sampled such that every 30th "null" observation is included in the dataset. The number 30 was chosen with one purpose of making the "null" label to be not dominating the dataset, but still be the most frequently occurring label. This effectively reduces the number of "null" observations to around 10,000, which still lets this label to be the most dominant, but not overwhelming. After the sampling, the breakdown of the occurrences and the percentage of each label are tabulated in Table 7.5.

Using the newly created dataset, the model was retrained for 10 epochs. During the first two epochs, the validation accuracy increased to 33%, and the accuracy fluctuated around 33% for the rest of the eight epochs. This indicates that the model's complexity is not high enough for this task.

7.3.4 Version 1: Recurrent Neural Network Approach

Using the prior knowledge that EEG signals are temporal, and previous works on detecting artifacts relied on statistical significances of various signal features such as mean and standard deviation, the recurrent neural network (RNN) seems to be a logical choice for the replacement of a network of 2 fully connected layers. The rationale is that since RNNs have access to the previous outputs as well as the current inputs, they would be adept at capturing patterns spread across time. After trying out different combinations of recurrent layers, long short-term memory (LSTM) layer was found out to be the most successful.

LSTM is a specific architecture of an RNN that was proposed by Hochreiter and Schmidhuber in 1997 to combat the vanishing or exploding gradient problems that are common among RNNs (Hochreiter and Schmidhuber 1997). These problems occur as having access to all the previous outputs essentially leads to a large chain of connections between the error and the input. Hence the gradient information could be vanishing or exploding depending on the situation as the information is propagated back to update the weights.

Table 7.6 Model structure for the RNN-based classifier

Layer (type)	Output shape	Number of parameters
Input_1 (InputLayer)	(None, 22, 250)	0
LSTM_1 (LSTM)	(None, 50)	60,200
Dense_1 (Dense)	(None, 1024)	52,224
Dense_2 (Dense)	(None, 5)	5125

The success of a model was determined by predicting the behavior of the training the model from just observing the first few epochs. The different models have been compared by how much training loss was reduced in three epochs and how much validation loss was reduced as a result of those three epochs. For the cases in which the loss function for this dataset did not decrease significantly (by 0.1 or more), the losses never decreased in a reasonable time, and the model tended to overfit to the training data. The final model that was decided is organized in Table 7.6. The total number of trainable parameters is 117,549, and this translates to 225 KB of weights when the weights are saved.

The LSTM layer is to extract the temporal information embedded in the signal. The final dense layers are to do the classification tasks at the end. The parameters on each layer were chosen such that the model is as light as possible without sacrificing significant performance degradation. For the number of cells in the LSTM layer, a varying number of cells was tried such as 5, 10, 25, 50, 100, 200, and 250, and increasing the number of cells decreased the performance by overfitting. However, having too few cells resulted in degraded performance as well. Hence, the number of cells in the LSTM layer was chosen to be 50. The "None" is the placeholder for the batch size. Changing the number of the batch size does not change the number of parameters.

The model was trained on the training data using categorical cross-entropy as the loss function. The model was optimized using the Adam optimizer with the default learning rate and the beta values. The batch size was 32, and the model was trained for 100 epochs. Each epoch takes about 40 s, and the training roughly took about half an hour. The result of this model will be given in the section.

7.3.5 Version 2: Convolutional Neural Network Approach

Another approach that we investigate is using convolutional neural networks (CNNs). As all the channels are available and ordered such that the arrangement reflects the actual spatial closeness of the electrodes roughly, we hypothesize that there will be certain localities across different channels that will be visible in certain channels. As EEG measures net neural activity, if an area of the brain gets triggered, all the electrodes that are near that area will be triggered, which makes channels that are close in the ordered list to have similar activity. As CNNs are known to work well with image data by using the fact that pixels that are related are close together in images, it seems possible that convolutional layers will also work well with this task. As there is only one-dimensional information available per time frame, 1-D convolutional layers were used instead of 2-D convolutional layers.

While the convolutional layers capture the spatial information, we have added the max-pooling layers to capture the temporal information by grouping up time frames together. Extracting spatial information and temporal information is done multiple times so that any hidden information can be extracted.

Before the max-pooling layers, batch normalization layers are added so that the values of the latent space representation of the input signals are normalized and scaled. Parameter changes in layers during the training cause the layers to yield different outputs each iteration. This forces all the layers to readjust to the new distribution of the outputs every iteration, which delays the training. The batch normalization layer normalizes the activations to reduce these internal covariate shifts to make the training process to be faster, and more stable, especially for deep and large neural networks (Ioffe and Szegedy 2015). Finally, the model has a flattening layer to prepare the data shape to be usable by fully connected layers, and the model uses fully connected layers to do the classification task.

Two versions of the deep convolutional neural network models have been constructed. One version is "deeper" than the other one to see whether adding more layers helped with the classification or not. The structures of both versions are organized in Tables 7.7 and 7.8.

Both versions were optimized using the Adam optimizer with the default setting. The batch size was 32, and the model was trained for 30 and 100 epochs, respectively. The first CNN model was highly overfitting to the train set at around epochs 40, as the validation loss went up by 10 times. The source of this behavior could not be tracked, so the number of epochs that the shallow CNN model was trained for was decreased to 30 epochs. The shallow CNN model took about 20 s per epochs, and the deeper model took about 40 s per epochs.

The hyperparameters used in the model, such as the filter sizes and the output sizes, for the convolutional layers were optimized based on observations of the first few epochs during the training phase just as we did in the development of the RNN based model.

7.3.6 Ensemble Method

In addition to all the methods with different approaches, the final method that incorporates all the models was created. This model takes in the logit outputs of

Table 7.7 Model structure for the shallow CNN-based classifier

Layer (type)	Output shape	Number of parameters
Input_1 (InputLayer)	(None, 22, 250)	0
conv1d_1 (Conv1D)	(None, 16, 250)	1072
batch_normalization_1	(None, 16, 250)	1000
max_pooling1d_1	(None, 16, 125)	0
conv1d_2 (Conv1D)	(None, 32, 125)	1568
batch_normalization_2	(None, 32, 125)	500
max_pooling1d_2	(None, 32, 63)	0
conv1d_3 (Conv1D)	(None, 64, 63)	6208
batch_normalization_3	(None, 64, 63)	252
max_pooling1d_3	(None, 64, 32)	0
conv1d_4 (Conv1D)	(None, 128, 32)	24,704
batch_normalization_4	(None, 128, 32)	128
max_pooling1d_4	(None, 128, 16)	0
conv1d_5 (Conv1D)	(None, 256, 16)	98,560
batch_normalization_5	(None, 256, 16)	64
max_pooling1d_5	(None, 256, 8)	0
conv1d_6 (Conv1D)	(None, 512, 8)	393,728
batch_normalization_6	(None, 512, 8)	32
flatten_1	(None, 4096)	0
dense_1(Dense)	(None, 1024)	4,195,328
dense_2(Dense)	(None, 5)	5125

each of the three models and simply adds the logits to do the decision-making by choosing the label with the highest logit. Different methods of adding up the logits were tested such as weighing one of the three models higher than the other two or excluding one of the models, but weighing all the models equally without exclusion had the highest validation accuracy.

For all the models, binary classification versions were constructed and trained using the same settings to examine how well models detect artifacts. The binary classification task for this problem is determining whether a 1-second segment contains an artifact or not, which will be denoted as either "artifact" or "null." The only deviation for these new models from the original models is the last dense layer. Instead of returning a label of length 5, the binary classification versions return the output label of length 2 (artifact, null). This causes the parameter numbers to be multiplied by 2/5 on the last dense layer. The number of total trainable parameters for the shallow CNN classifier is 4728269, and for the deeper CNN classifier is 11,548,141. When weights are saved, the shallow CNN classifier requires 18.0 MB, while the deep CNN classifier requires 44.1 MB. The results for both versions are given in the following chapter. All the construction of the models and the pipelines for the input and the output for the EEG signals are done in python.

Table 7.8 Model structure for the deep CNN-based classifier

Layer (type)	Output shape	Number of parameters
Input_1 (InputLayer)	(None, 22, 250)	0
conv1d_1 (Conv1D)	(None, 16, 250)	1072
batch_normalization_1	(None, 16, 250)	1000
max_pooling1d_1	(None, 16, 125)	0
conv1d_2 (Conv1D)	(None, 32, 125)	1568
batch_normalization_2	(None, 32, 125)	500
max_pooling1d_2	(None, 32, 63)	0
conv1d_3 (Conv1D)	(None, 64, 63)	6208
batch_normalization_3	(None, 64, 63)	252
max_pooling1d_3	(None, 64, 32)	0
conv1d_4 (Conv1D)	(None, 128, 32)	24,704
batch_normalization_4	(None, 128, 32)	128
max_pooling1d_4	(None, 128, 16)	0
conv1d_5 (Conv1D)	(None, 256, 16)	98,560
batch_normalization_5	(None, 256, 16)	64
max_pooling1d_5	(None, 256, 8)	0
conv1d_6 (Conv1D)	(None, 512, 8)	393,728
batch_normalization_6	(None, 512, 8)	32
max_pooling1d_6	(None, 512, 4)	0
conv1d_7 (Conv1D)	(None, 1024, 4)	1,573,888
batch_normalization_7	(None, 1024, 4)	16
max_pooling1d_7	(None, 1024, 2)	0
conv1d_8 (Conv1D)	(None, 1024, 2)	3,146,752
batch_normalization_8	(None, 1024, 2)	8
conv1d_9 (Conv1D)	(None, 1024, 2)	3,146,752
batch_normalization_9	(None, 1024, 2)	8
flatten_1	(None, 2048)	0
dense_1(Dense)	(None, 1024)	2,098,176
dense_2(Dense)	(None, 1024)	1,049,600
dense_3(Dense)	(None, 5)	5125

7.4 Results and Discussion

After optimizing hyperparameters, and model structures using validation set accuracy, each model was tested using the test set. We find in all the models that there are limitations in precisely predicting labels, and we were interested in whether the models can act as indicators for artifact presence. So, in addition to being trained to do multi-class classification, the models were retrained to do binary classification with the same number of epochs and optimizer settings.

One thing to note for the binary classification is that the evaluation of the binary classification based on the accuracies depends highly on the threshold that is set for the detection. For example, when there are many examples of "null," or no artifacts, high accuracy could be achieved by intentionally raising the threshold of detection for artifacts high so that most of the examples are classified as "null." Then the system will have high accuracy while failing to act as a respectable classifier for artifacts.

To evaluate the performance of the detection systems receiver operating characteristic (ROC) curves are used, which illustrate the ability of the systems to diagnose with different thresholds. The ROC curve plots the probability of detection versus the probability of false alarm (Richards 2005). The probability of detection which is also known as the true positive rate (TPR), sensitivity, or recall denotes the proportion of actual positives that are correctly identified. Using the problem of this chapter as an example, the true positive rate is the proportion of segments that contain the artifacts that are correctly classified by the model among all the segments that contain the artifacts. The probability of false alarm, which is often referred to as the fall-out, the Type I error, or the false-positive rate (FPR), denotes the proportion of negatives that are misidentified as positives. Using this task as an example again, the false-positive rate would be the proportion of segments that do not contain artifacts that are classified as containing artifacts by the model.

A perfect classifier has a true positive rate of 1.0 and a false positive rate of 0.0, which makes the ROC curve to pass the upper left corner. Hence, a ROC curve that closely approaches the upper left corner indicates a system that discriminates well (Zweig and Campbell 1993). To numerically compare the performance of different ROC curves, the area under the curve (AUC) is computed to indicate how close the ROC curve is to the upper left corner. For example, AUC ranges from 0 to 1, and AUC value of 1 corresponds to the perfect separation case where the true positive rate is 1.0 and the false-positive rate is 0.0 (Hand and Till 2001).

For all the ROC curves provided in this chapter, the area under the curve is also computed and provided.

7.4.1 Recurrent Neural Network-Based Classifier

The recurrent neural network model was trained for 100 epochs. At the end of the training, the train set accuracy was 0.7168, and the validation accuracy was 0.4262. However surprisingly, the test set accuracy was 0.5801, and the confusion matrix is shown in Fig. 7.2.

The model does well on predicting "eyem" and predicting "null." However, the model cannot predict the electrode popping "elpp" label and the muscle movement "musc" label that well. Unfortunately, this pattern persists in all the results. Our conjecture of the behavior of the model is that eye movement and chewing labels have certain localities. For example, we expect electrodes located near the mouth to be more affected by chewing, and electrodes that are far away from mouth to be less affected. This causes specific channels to be affected while leaving other channels to be like "null." As there is a distinguishing feature to be extracted consistently across all the patients, the model does well on the "eyem" and the "chew" labels.

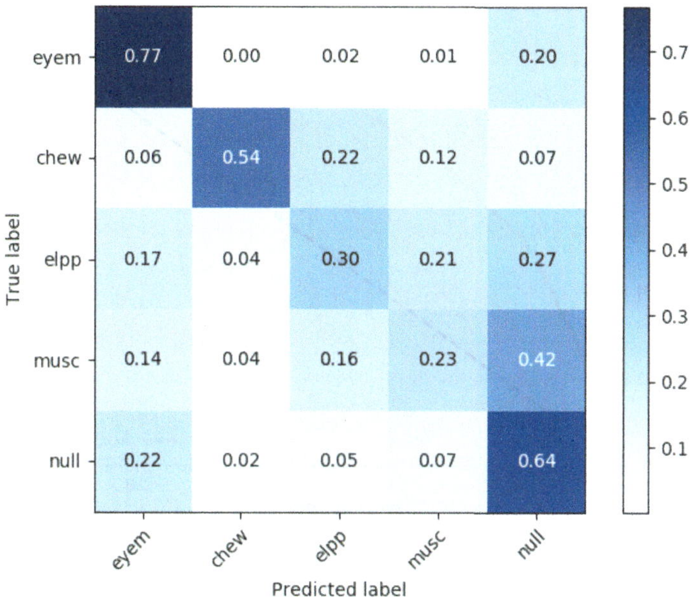

Fig. 7.2 Confusion matrix of the RNN-based model on the test

However, for the cases of "elpp," and "musc", the region of the channels, which are affected, is ambiguous. "elpp" causes similar noise pattern to occur when it occurs, but this can be anywhere, and similar observation could be made regarding "musc."

To see if the RNN-based model is at least powerful enough to indicate the presence of artifacts, the model was retrained to do the binary classification. The RNN-based model trained to the train set accuracy of 0.9885, with the validation accuracy of 0.6254. When tested on the test set, the highest accuracy was 0.7126. In Fig. 7.3, the ROC curve for the RNN based model is shown to visualize the performance of the system. The orange line is the ROC curve, and the dotted blue line is the straight line connecting the (0,0), and (1,1) points. The straight line indicates the worst possible detection system. At around the false-positive rate of 0.424, the true positive rate is 0.800. This indicates that the model would work in a system roughly but would not be recommended in any device that requires high accuracy. The area under the curve is 0.75.

7.4.2 *Convolutional Neural Network-Based Classifier*

Similar evaluations were done on the shallow CNN model and the deeper CNN model. The confusion matrices are shown in Figs. 7.4 and 7.5, and ROC curves are shown in Figs. 7.6 and 7.7.

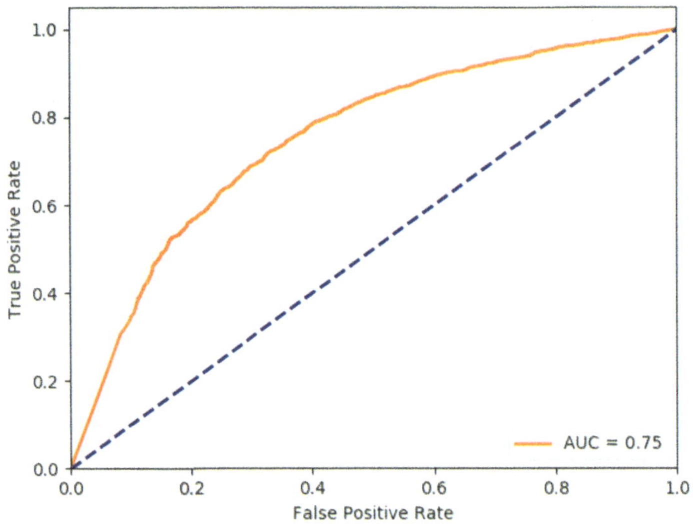

Fig. 7.3 ROC curve for the RNN-based model

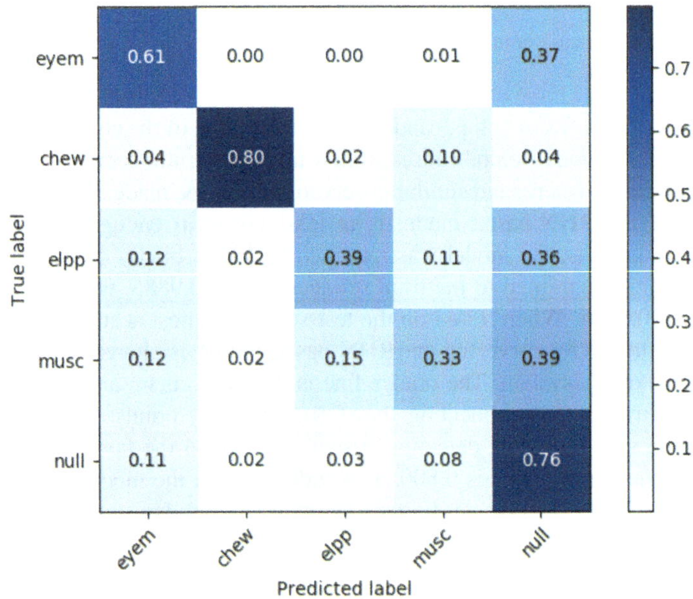

Fig. 7.4 Confusion matrix of the shallow CNN-based model

The shallow CNN-based model was trained for 30 epochs, due to its tendency to overfit when it was trained for more than 40 epochs. The model was trained until the train accuracy of 0.7409 and the validation accuracy of 0.4203. The final test accuracy was 0.6515. Given that both the RNN-based model and the CNN-based

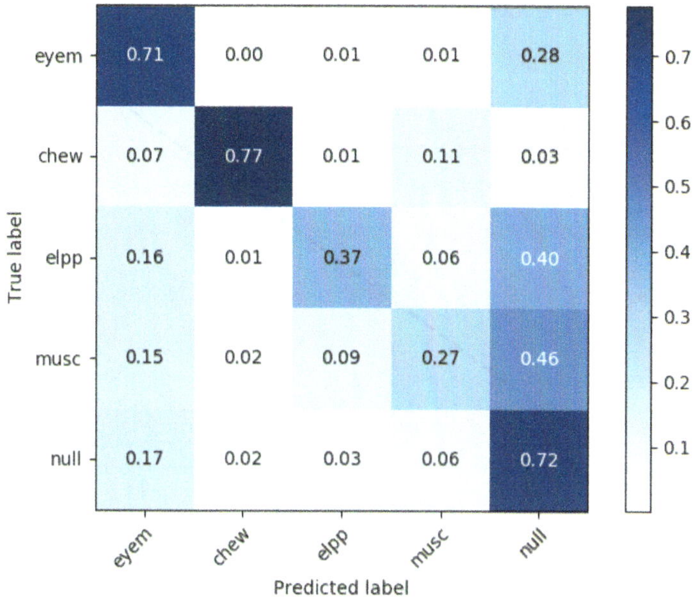

Fig. 7.5 Confusion matrix of the deep CNN-based model

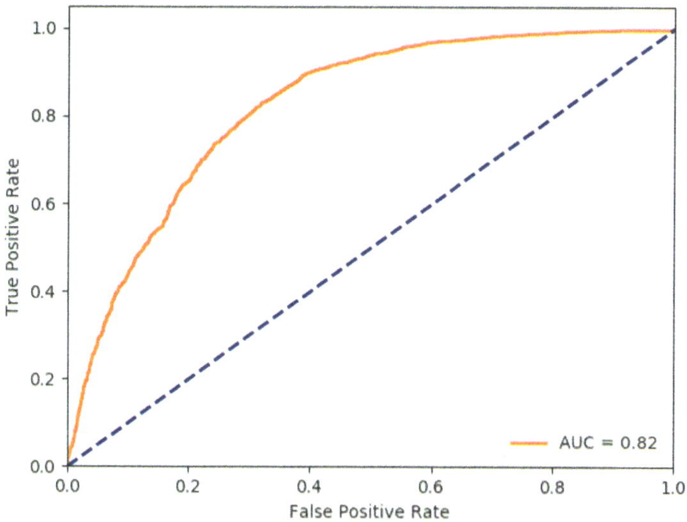

Fig. 7.6 ROC curve for the shallow CNN-based model

model trained until the validation accuracy was around 0.42, the fact that CNN-based model did about 7% better in predicting the 5-class classification problem was interesting. One possibility is that the difference in the complexities of both models causes the difference. Comparing the number of trainable parameters, the CNN-

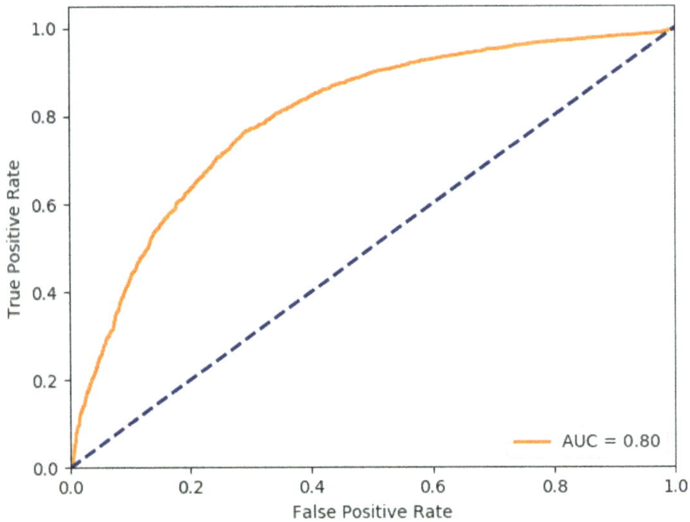

Fig. 7.7 ROC curve for the deep CNN-based model

based model is 4 times bigger, and this may have helped the model to generalize better. However, as evident in Fig. 7.4, this model does significantly better in predicting "eyem" and "chew" than "elpp," and "musc", which is similar to what we observed for the RNN-based model.

The result for the deep CNN-based model is similar. The model was trained to the 100th epochs, the train accuracy of 0.9472 was reached, and the validation accuracy at this epoch was 0.4430. This validation accuracy is slightly higher than that of the shallow CNN-based model. The final test accuracy was 0.6517, which is 0.0002 higher than that of the shallow CNN model. This is likely to be from just noise. The confusion matrix shown in Fig. 7.5 indicates a similar behavior compared to the other models. Hence, we can conclude that CNN-based models work better in multi-class models, but RNN-based model is much lighter, and simply making CNN-based models more complex does not improve the performance of the model significantly.

The more interesting findings are ROC curves. The same analytic method that converts a five-class classification task into a binary classification task was applied to both versions of the CNN-based models just as in the RNN-based model. The shallow CNN model was retrained for 30 epochs, and the deep CNN based model was retrained for 100 epochs. The train set accuracies were 0.8108 and 0.9684, the validation accuracies were 0.5227 0.6008, and the test accuracies were 0.6958 and 0.7499 for the shallow and the deep CNN-based models, respectively. Although these numbers might be misleading as the accuracy depends on the threshold of the binary classifier, for the binary classification problem, the more complex and deeper model has a performance improvement of about 0.05. The receiver operating characteristic curves of CNN-based models are shown in Figs. 7.6 and 7.7.

These ROC curves, compared to that of the RNN based model, have a significantly higher area under the curve, indicating that CNN-based models perform better. Numerically, the areas under the curve for the shallow CNN-based model and the deep CNN-based model are 0.82 and 0.80, respectively, which are larger than that of the RNN-based model which is 0.75. At the true positive rate of 0.800, the false-positive rates are 0.424, 0.295, and 0.339 for the RNN, the shallow CNN, and the deep CNN-based models, respectively. This indicates that CNN-based models can predict the presence of artifact correctly, with fewer false alarms compared to the RNN-based model.

7.4.3 Ensemble Method

Lastly, the ensemble method was examined in the same procedure. The ensemble method incorporates all the other methods by adding the logits produced at the output layers of the other methods. The confusion matrix is shown in Fig. 7.8. The ensemble method's accuracy measures are higher compared to all the other methods, except for the "musc" label. The shallow CNN-based model achieves the accuracy of 0.33 on the "musc" label, while the ensemble method achieves 0.28. Regardless, the ensemble method achieves the overall accuracy of 0.6759, which is the highest among all the methods. In addition to the confusion matrix, the ROC curve for the binary classification version of the model is produced. The ROC curve is shown in Fig. 7.9, with all the ROC curves from other models for better comparison.

Interestingly the ROC curve for the shallow CNN-based model has a similar area under the curve as the ensemble method. The shallow CNN-based model has higher true positive rates in certain regions than the ensemble method, and the ensemble method performs superior to the shallow CNN-based model in the regions of lower thresholds.

For the binary classification problem, as the main purpose is to accurately point out the artifact events, the time-lapse system was proposed to further enhance the performance. The idea comes from the fact that artifacts often come in bursts, such that the previous segment's label correlates well with the new segment that follows. This method does not change any of the models but rather works directly on the logits produced by the models. A sliding window adds all the logits in the window to produce a new logit that the classifier uses. Different methods of producing the new logit were tried such as taking the maximum or doing a weighted sum of the logits, but simply adding all the logits worked the best. Different sizes of sliding windows were tried, ranging from 1 to 10, but a 2-second window produced the best result. The ROC curves for the highest performing window setting are shown in Fig. 7.10.

The time-lapse method improves all the ROC curves, especially lifting the regions in the lower false positive rates. At the true positive rate of 0.800, the new time-lapse method yields the false-positive rates of 0.310, 0.288, 0.268, and 0.258 for the RNN-based, the shallow CNN-based, the deep CNN-based, and ensemble

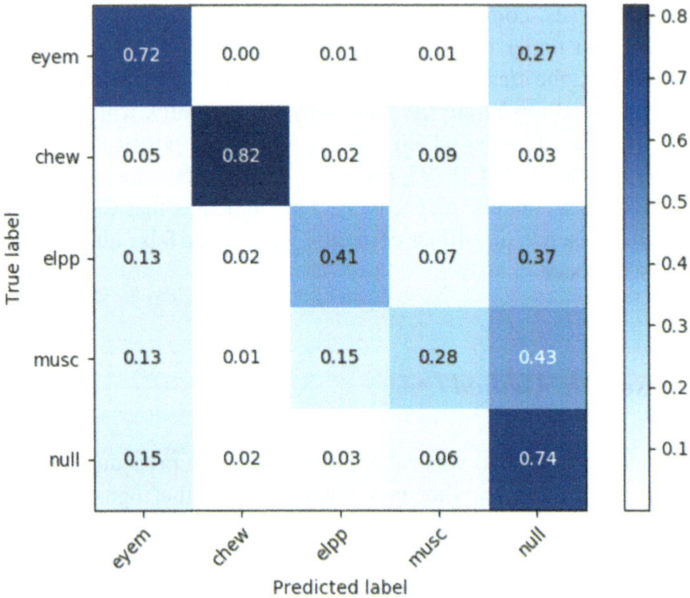

Fig. 7.8 Confusion matrix of the ensemble method

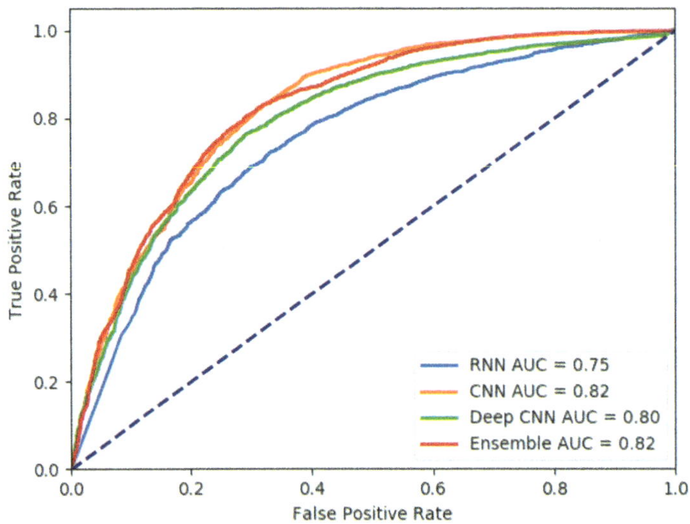

Fig. 7.9 ROC curves for all the models

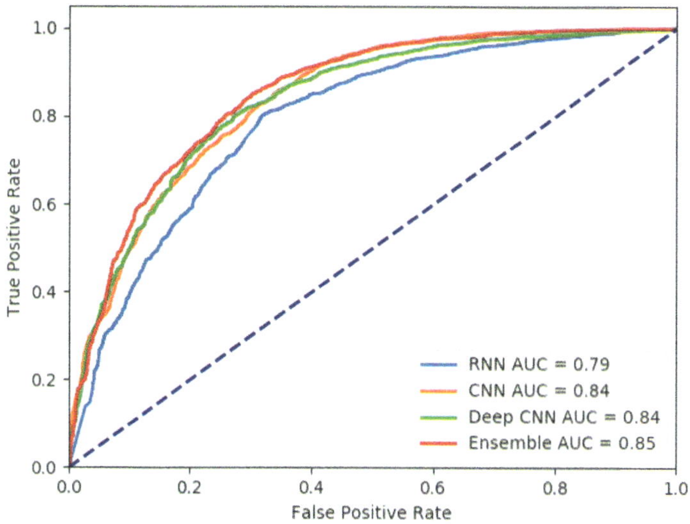

Fig. 7.10 ROC curves for all the models with the time-lapse method

methods, respectively. This is a slight improvement from the false-positive rate of 0.295 from the shallow CNN model without the sliding window. The ensemble method does the best for this method proposed.

In order to see the viability of the model in real-life settings, all the binary classification models were tested on a test set that contains all the "null" information without the sampling procedure. The five-class classification accuracies of the models are 0.7234, 0.7612, 0.7534, and 0.7808, for the RNN based, the shallow CNN-based, the deep CNN-based, and ensemble methods, respectively. Only one confusion matrix from the best result is shown as all the confusion matrices behave similarly. The resulting confusion matrix is shown in Fig. 7.11. The increase in the accuracy comes from the fact that there are more "null" labels in the dataset; hence the accuracy converges to the accuracy of predicting the "null" label which is around 0.78 for the ensemble method.

The ROC curves for the binary classification problem using all the models on the original data are shown in Figs. 7.12 and 7.13. Figure 7.12 shows the ROC curves of the models without the time-lapse method, and Fig. 7.13 shows the ROC curves of the models with the time-lapse method. The areas under the curves are significantly higher than those of the sampled data cases. These curves indicate the viability of the models in a real clinical setting.

Lastly, the average time elapsed in processing one example was computed for each model, for each classification problem to see whether the model is feasible for doing an on-line signal processing task of indicating whether the artifact exists or not. For the reference, there are 5797 observations in the test set. In addition, the time elapsed while loading the Tensorflow module and the libraries as well as loading the data was not accounted for. The results for the accuracy with default

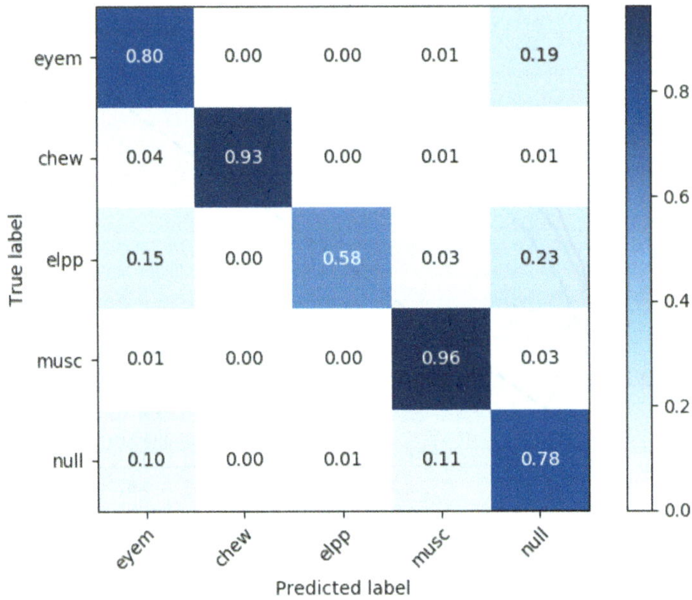

Fig. 7.11 Confusion matrix of the ensemble method on the original data

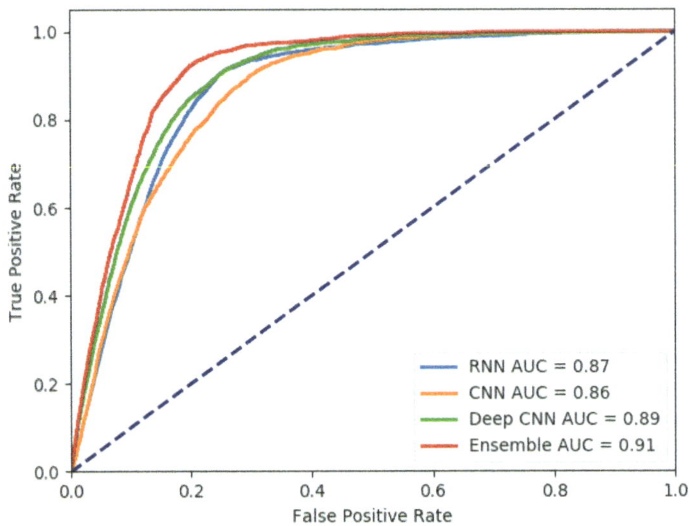

Fig. 7.12 ROC curves for all the models on the original data

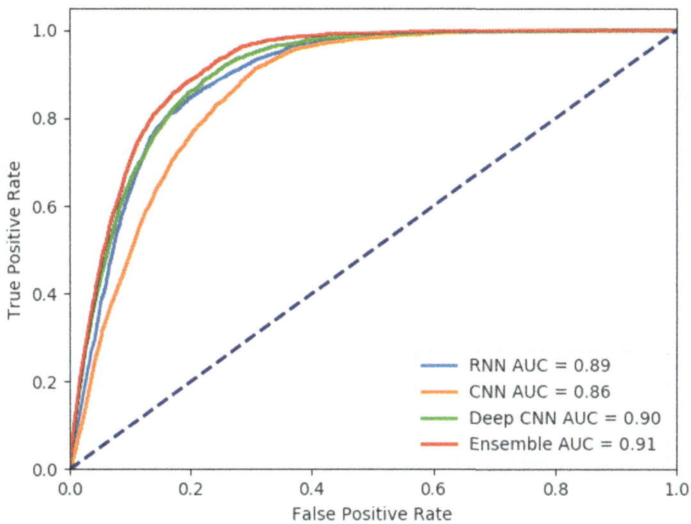

Fig. 7.13 ROC curves for all the models with the time-lapse method on the original data

Table 7.9 The Time elapsed, the accuracy, and the size of each model

Model	Average time elapsed (ms/sample)	Test set accuracy (%)	Size of the model (KB)
RNN	0.707	58.01	476
RNN-binary	0.677	71.26	464
CNN	0.483	65.15	18,526
CNN-binary	0.468	69.58	18,514
DeepCNN	0.595	65.17	45,189
DeepCNN-binary	0.568	74.99	45,177
Ensemble	N/A	67.59	64,191

thresholds, which looks at the maximum confidence level of each label, the average time elapsed, and the size of each model are tabulated in Table 7.9. All the test results on this table are from the sampled test data.

All the average time elapsed for inference for all the models is less than 1 ms, for each of the 1-second segment. This indicates that the model is able to predict the presence and the kind of artifact almost instantaneously. Also, the sizes of the models are small enough to be implemented in a Raspberry Pi, which could make this model highly portable. Since the original EEG signals were expressed in 16-bit floating-point values, the model can be further compressed if all the parameters are converted to 16-bit floating-points instead of 32-bit floating-points. This compression is approximately half the size of the model, further improving the portability. All the evaluations were done in python.

7.5 Conclusion

The chapter proposes three types of deep learning-based machine learning model that learns to distinguish artifacts from the real signal and classify artifacts. Three models, the RNN-based model and the two CNN based models of different depth, have been constructed and evaluated. In addition, the ensemble model was created that utilizes all the other methods. The ensemble model, which has the best overall performance, achieves a 67.59% five-class classification accuracy, and a true positive rate of 80% at the false positive rate of 25.82% for the binary classification problem. The models are light and fast enough to be implemented in a portable device, such as Raspberry Pi. The largest model only has 65 MB of trainable parameters, and the slowest model only takes about 0.7 ms to predict on a 1-second long EEG signal. The speed of the ensemble model has not been tested but given that the slowest component in the model occupies less than 0.1% of the segment implies we expect it to be fast enough for the goal. We expect the time elapsed to be slightly more than the three models combined. As this model can successfully detect whether artifacts are present in the collected signals quickly, and can tell what type of artifacts they are, physicians can use this device while collecting data to check whether the data that are being collected are free of artifacts or not. If the data are being affected by any artifacts, physicians can quickly check which artifact is present and act in response to that artifact. This work is significant to the research community as it adds deep learning as one of the tools that the community can use in recognizing artifacts in EEG signals and potentially removing them also.

Clinicians indicate that a sensitivity, which is the true positive rate, of 95%, and specificity, the false positive rate, of below 5% to be the minimum requirement for clinical acceptance (Golmohammadi et al. 2019). As none of the models achieve that guideline yet, there are many more investigations needed in optimizing the models. Hence for future works, an investigation into incorporating different features that can be extracted quickly, and larger and more complex models to reach the recommended guideline can be done. In addition, since the models were trained, validated, and tested on the first version of the EEG artifact corpus which only consists of observations from 310 patients, in the future when there are more data available, the model could be trained again to see whether the lack of data was part of the inadequate performance. Also, since classification within the artifacts, excluding the "null" label, seems to work at high accuracies evident from the confusion matrix, and the binary classification of artifacts can have arbitrarily high true positive rate, an investigation on a two-step system seems to be another interesting path to take on. This research envisioned to have a portable device that can be used during data acquisition. Building a portable machine that runs these models to predict the presence of artifacts and to classify the artifacts should be the next step. Finally, testing this machine in a real-life setting will be beneficial to see if the machine works and to see if there are additional adjustments and improvements to make.

Acknowledgments We would like to thank the Department of Electrical Engineering at The Cooper Union and Temple University Hospital for supporting this research by providing us the necessary resources.

References

M. Aminoff, Principles of neural science. 4th edition. Muscle Nerve **24**(6), 839–839 (2001)

W. Clercq, A. Vergult, B. Vanrumste, W. Paesschen, S. Huffel, Canonical correlation analysis applied to remove muscle artifacts from the electroencephalogram. IEEE Trans. Biomed. Eng. **53**(12), 2583–2587 (2006)

J. DellaBadia, W. Bell, J. Keyes, V. Mathews, S. Glazier, Assessment and cost comparison of sleep-deprived EEG, MRI and PET in the prediction of surgical treatment for epilepsy. Seizure-Eur. J. Epilepsy **11**(5), 303–309 (2002)

M. Golmohammadi, A. Torbati, S. Diego, I. Obeid, J. Picone, Automatic analysis of EEGs using big data and hybrid deep learning architectures. Front. Hum. Neurosci. **13** (2019)

I. Goodfellow, Y. Bengio, A. Courville, *Deep Learning* (MIT Press, 2016)

D. Hand, R. Till, A simple generalisation of the area under the ROC curve for multiple class classification problems. Mach. Learn. **45**(2), 171–186 (2001) Retrieved from https://academic.microsoft.com/paper/1912982817

A. Hasasneh, N. Kampel, P. Sripad, N. Shah, J. Dammers, Deep learning approach for automatic classification of ocular and cardiac artifacts in MEG data. J. Eng. **2018**, 1–10 (2018)

S. Hochreiter, J. Schmidhuber, Long short-term memory. Neural Comput. **9**(8), 1735–1780 (1997)

S. Ioffe, C. Szegedy, Batch normalization: Accelerating deep network training by reducing internal covariate shift. International conference on machine learning, 448–456 (2015)

D. Kingma, J. Ba, *Adam: A Method for Stochastic Optimization* (International conference on learning representations, 2015)

V. Krishnaveni, S. Jayaraman, A. Gunasekaran, K. Ramadoss, Automatic removal of ocular artifacts using JADE algorithm and neural network. *International Journal of Computer and Information*. Engineering **2**(4), 1330–1341 (2007)

T.-W. Lee, M. Girolami, T. Sejnowski, Independent component analysis using an extended infomax algorithm for mixed subgaussian and supergaussian sources. Neural Comput. **11**(2), 417–441 (1999)

S. Lopez, A. Gross, S. Yang, M. Golmohammadi, I. Obeid, J. Picone, An analysis of two common reference points for EEGS, in *2016 IEEE Signal Processing in Medicine and Biology Symposium (SPMB), 2016*, (2016), pp. 1–5. Retrieved from https://academic.microsoft.com/paper/2586273059

E. Louis, Frey, L., Britton, J., Hopp, J., Korb, P., Koubeissi, M., ... Pestana-Knight, E. Electroencephalography (EEG): An Introductory Text and Atlas of Normal and Abnormal Findings in Adults, Children, and Infants (2016)

H. Nolan, R. Whelan, R. Reilly, FASTER: Fully automated statistical thresholding for EEG artifact rejection. J. Neurosci. Methods **192**(1), 152–162 (2010)

I. Obeid, J. Picone, The Temple University Hospital EEG data corpus. Front. Neurosci. **10**, 196 (2016). https://doi.org/10.3389/fnins.2016.00196

M. Richards. Fundamentals of Radar Signal Processing (2005)

Y. Roy, H. Banville, I. Albuquerque, A. Gramfort, T. Falk, J. Faubert, Deep learning-based electroencephalography analysis: a systematic review. arXiv preprint arXiv **1901.05498** (2019)

B. Singh, H. Wagatsuma, A removal of eye movement and blink artifacts from EEG data using morphological component analysis. Comput. Math. Methods Med. **2017**, 1861645 (2017)

M. Zweig, G. Campbell, Receiver-operating characteristic (ROC) plots: A fundamental evaluation tool in clinical medicine. Clin. Chem. **39**(4), 561–577 (1993)

Chapter 8
Objective Evaluation Metrics for Automatic Classification of EEG Events

Vinit Shah, Meysam Golmohammadi, Iyad Obeid, and Joseph Picone

8.1 Introduction

Electroencephalograms (EEGs) are the primary means by which physicians diagnose and manage brain-related illnesses such as epilepsy, seizures, and sleep disorders (Yamada and Meng 2017). Automatic interpretation of EEGs by computer has been extensively studied for the past 40 years (Roy et al. 2019; Craik et al. 2019; Wilson and Emerson 2002; Gotman et al. 1997; Gotman 1982) with mixed results. Even though many published research systems report impressive levels of accuracy, widespread adoption of commercial technology has yet to happen in clinical settings primarily due to the high false alarm rates of these systems (Clifford et al. 2016; Cvach Maria 2014; Bridi et al. 2014). In this chapter, we investigate the gap in performance between research and commercial technology and discuss how these perceptions are influenced by a lack of a standardized scoring methodology.

There are in general two ways to evaluate machine learning technology: user acceptance testing (von Goethem and Hambling 2013; Banchs et al. 2006) and objective performance metrics based on annotated reference data (Picone et al. 1990; Michel et al. 2017). User acceptance testing is slow, time-consuming, and expensive. It has never been a practical way to guide technology development because algorithm developers need rapid turnaround times on evaluations. Hence evaluations using objective performance metrics, such as sensitivity and specificity,

V. Shah
The Neural Engineering Data Consortium, Temple University, Philadelphia, PA, USA

M. Golmohammadi
The Neural Engineering Data Consortium, Temple University, Philadelphia, PA, USA

Internet Brands, El Segundo, CA, USA

I. Obeid · J. Picone (✉)
ECE Department, Temple University, Philadelphia, PA, USA

I. Obeid et al. (eds.), *Biomedical Signal Processing*,
https://doi.org/10.1007/978-3-030-67494-6_8

are common in the machine learning field (Altman and Bland 1994; Wozencraft and Jacobs 1965; Martin et al. 1997). When using objective performance metrics, it is very important to have a rich evaluation dataset and a performance metric that correlates well with user and application needs. The metric must have a certain level of granularity so that small differences in algorithms can be investigated and parameter optimizations can be evaluated. For example, in speech recognition applications, word error rate has been used for many years because it correlates well with user acceptance testing and provides the necessary level of granularity to guide technology development. Despite many years of research focused on finding better performance metrics (Wang et al. 2003; Mostefa et al. 2006), word error rate remains a valid metric for technology development and assessment in speech recognition.

Sequential pattern recognition applications, such as speech recognition, keyword search, or EEG event detection, require additional considerations. Data are not simply assessed with an overall judgment (e.g., "did a seizure occur somewhere in this file?"). Instead, the locality of the hypothesis must be considered – to what extent did the start and end times of the hypothesis match the reference transcription. This is a complex issue since a hypothesis can partially overlap with the reference annotation, and a consistent mechanism for scoring such events must be adopted.

Unfortunately, there is no such standardization in the EEG literature. For example, Wilson and Emerson (2002) advocates using a term-based metric involving sensitivity and specificity. A term was defined as a connection of consecutive decisions of the same type of event. A hypothesis is counted as a true positive when it overlaps with one or more reference annotations. A false positive corresponds to an event in which a hypothesis annotation does not overlap with any of the reference annotations. Kelly et al. (2010) recommends using a metric that measures sensitivity and false alarms. A hypothesis is considered a true positive when time of detection is within 2 min of the seizure onset. Otherwise it is considered a false positive. Baldassano et al. (2016) uses an epoch-based metric that measures false positive and negative rates as well as latency. The development, evaluation, and ranking of various machine learning approaches are highly dependent on the choice of a metric.

A large class of bioengineering problems, including seizure detection, involve prediction as well as classification. In prediction problems, we are often concerned with how far in advance of an event we can predict an outcome. The accuracy of a prediction varies with latency. By convention, we refer to negative latency as prediction before the event has occurred. Positive latency means a system outputs a hypothesis after an event has occurred. It is not uncommon for machine learning systems to have significant amounts of latency – often tens of seconds for seizure detection. Similarly, prediction of a seizure before the seizure has occurred is an extremely valuable technology with far-reaching clinical implications if the onset of a seizure can be predicted long in advance (e.g., tens of minutes) of the actual event. This gives healthcare providers a chance to perform a medical intervention as well as allows the patient to make necessary preparations for a medical emergency.

Measuring performance as a function of latency adds some complexity to the process. Winterhalder et al. (2003) have studied this problem extensively and argue for scoring based on long-term considerations. In this chapter, we are not concerned with these types of prediction problems. We are focused mainly on assessing the accuracy of classification of events and assessing the proximity of these classifications to the actual event. We refer to this as time-aligned scoring.

Therefore, in this chapter, we analyze several popular scoring metrics and discuss their strengths and weaknesses on sequential decoding problems. We introduce several alternatives, such as the actual term-weighted value (ATWV) (Wegmann et al. 2013; Fiscus et al. 2007) and time-aligned event scoring (TAES), and discuss their relevance to the seizure detection problem. We present a comparison of performance for several systems using these metrics and discuss how this correlates with a proxy for overall user acceptance involving a combination of sensitivity and false alarm rate.

Comparing systems using a single operating point is, of course, not always correct. It is quite possible that the systems are simply operating at different points on what is known as their receiver operating characteristic (ROC) curve. This was a problem well-studied in the mid-1960s with the emergence of communication theory (Wozencraft and Jacobs 1965). In machine learning, we often prefer to analyze systems using a detection error trade-off (DET) curve (Fiscus et al. 2007; Mason and Graham 2002; Hajian-Tilaki 2013). These curves provide a holistic view of performance but make it difficult to tune a system at a specific operating point. We will also briefly discuss holistic measures based on DET analysis.

8.2 Basic Error Measures and Relevant Derived Measures

Researchers in biomedical fields typically report performance in terms of sensitivity and specificity (Japkowicz and Shah 2014). In a two-class classification problem such as seizure detection, it is common to characterize performance in terms of four basic error measures:

- True positives (TP): the number of "positives" detected correctly.
- True negatives (TN): the number of "negatives" detected correctly.
- False positives (FP): the number of "negatives" detected as "positives".
- False negatives (FN): the number of "positives" detected as "negatives".

False positives, also known as type I errors, play a very important role in sequential decoding applications since they tend to dominate performance considerations. Throughout this chapter, we will quantify, or normalize, false positives by using the false alarm (FA) rate, which is simply the number of false positives divided by the total amount of data measured in units of time. We typically compute FAs/24 h – the number of false alarms per day. This is a useful figure of merit for critical care applications in healthcare.

There are a large number of measures derived from these four basic quantities that appear extensively in the sequential decoding literature. These are summarized concisely in (Confusion matrix 2017). For example, in information retrieval applications, systems are often evaluated using:

$$\text{Sensitivity (Recall)} = (TP/(TP + FN)), \tag{8.1}$$

$$\text{Specificity (Selectivity)} = (TN/(TN + FP)), \tag{8.2}$$

$$\text{Accuracy} = ((TP + TN)/(TP + FN + TN + FP)), \tag{8.3}$$

$$\text{Precision} = (TP/(TP + FP)) \tag{8.4}$$

More recently, integrated measures such as the F1 score and the Matthews correlation coefficient (MCC) (Chicco and Jurman 2020) have become popular for tasks ranging from information retrieval to binary classification:

$$F1 = ((2 \times \text{Precision} \times \text{Recall}) / (\text{Precision} + \text{Recall})), \tag{8.5}$$

$$\begin{aligned} MCC = {} & ((TP \times TN) - (FP \times FN)) \\ & /\sqrt{((TP + FP)(TP + FN)(TN + FP)(TN + FN))} \end{aligned} \tag{8.6}$$

In the field of machine translation, the bilingual evaluation understudy (BLEU) metric, which measures the similarity between two strings of text, was one of the first objective evaluation metrics to claim a high correlation with human judgments of quality (Papineni et al. 2002).

However, none of these measures address the time scale over which the scoring must occur, which is critical in the interpretation of these measures for many real-time bioengineering applications. When the time alignment of the reference event and the hypothesized event is important, and spurious hypotheses play a critical role in overall system performance, evaluation metrics must take into account the accuracy of the start time and end time of these detected events. We refer to this as the temporal localization problem. Accurate temporal localization is critical if sequential decoding technology is to be successfully applied in clinical settings.

In some applications, it is preferable to score every unit of time. With multichannel signals, such as EEGs, scoring for each channel for each unit of time is appropriate since significant events such as seizures occur on a subset of the channels present in the signal. However, it is more common in the literature to simply score a summary decision per unit of time that is based on an aggregation of the per-channel inputs (e.g., a majority vote). We refer to this type of scoring as *epoch-based* (Liu et al. 1992; Navakatikyan et al. 2006).

An alternative, that is more common in speech and image recognition applications, is *term-based* (Fiscus et al. 2007; Xiong et al. 2017), in which we consider the start and stop time of the event, and each event identified in the reference annotation is counted once. There are fundamental differences between the two conventions.

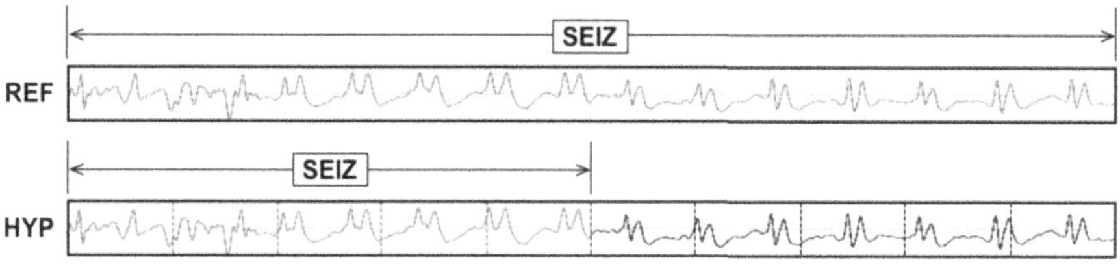

Fig. 8.1 A hypothesis (HYP) has a 50% overlap with the reference (REF)

For example, one event containing many epochs will count more heavily in an epoch-based scoring scenario. Epoch-based scoring generally weights the duration of an event more heavily since each unit of time is assessed independently.

Time-aligned scoring is essential to the evaluation of sequential decoding systems. But to implement such scoring in a meaningful way, there needs to be universal agreement on how to assess overlap between the reference and the hypothesis. For example, Fig. 8.1 demonstrates a typical issue in scoring. The machine learning system correctly detected 5 s of an event 10 s in duration. Essentially 50% of the event is correctly detected, but how that is reflected in the scoring depends on the specific metric. Epoch-based scoring with an epoch duration of 1 *sec* would count 5 FN errors and 5 TP detections. Term-based scoring would potentially count this as a correct recognition depending on the way overlaps are scored.

Term-based metrics score on an event basis and do not count individual frames. A typical approach for calculating errors in term-based scoring is the any-overlap method (OVLP) (Gotman et al. 1997; Wilson et al. 2003). TPs are counted when the hypothesis overlaps with the corresponding event in the reference annotation. FPs correspond to situations in which a hypothesis does not overlap with the corresponding event in the reference. The metric ignores the duration of the term in the reference annotation. In Fig. 8.2, we demonstrate two extreme cases for which the OVLP metric fails. In each case, 90% of the event is incorrectly scored. In Example 1, the system does not detect approximately 9 s of a seizure event, while in Example 2, the system incorrectly labels an additional 9 s of time as seizure. OVLP is considered a very permissive way of scoring, resulting in artificially high sensitivities. In Fig. 8.2, the OVLP metric will score both examples as 100% TP. These kinds of significant differences in scoring, and in the interpretation of the results, necessitate a deeper look at the characteristics of several popular evaluation metrics and motivate the need for industry-wide standardized scoring. That is the focus of this book chapter.

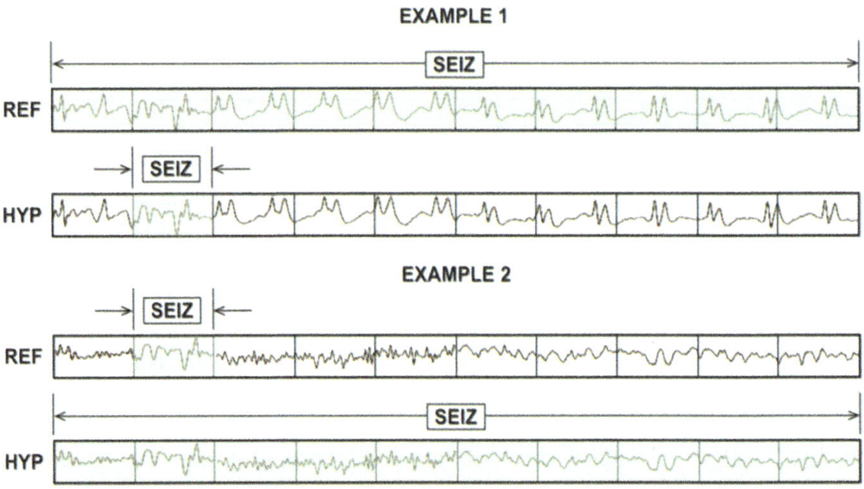

Fig. 8.2 TP scores for the Any-Overlap method are 100% even though large portions of the event are miss (Example 1) or false alarm (Example 2)

8.3 Evaluation Metrics

The proper balance between sensitivity and FA rate is often application specific and has been studied extensively in a number of research communities. For example, evaluation of voice keyword search technology was carefully studied in the Spoken Term Detection (STD) evaluations conducted by the National of Standards and Technology (NIST) (Wegmann et al. 2013; Fiscus et al. 2007; Fiscus 2013). These evaluations resulted in the introduction of a single metric, ATWV, to address concerns about trade-offs for the different types of errors that occur in voice keyword search systems. Despite being popular in the voice processing community, ATWV has not been widely used outside the voice processing community.

Therefore, in this chapter, we present a detailed comparison of five important scoring metrics popular in a wide range of machine learning communities. These are briefly described below:

1. *NIST Actual Term-Weighted Value (ATWV):* based on NIST's popular scoring package (F4DE v3.3.1), this metric, originally developed for the NIST 2006 Spoken Term Detection evaluation, uses an objective function that accounts for temporal overlap between the reference and hypothesis using the detection scores assigned by the system.
2. *Dynamic Programming Alignment (DPALIGN):* similar to the NIST package known as SCLite (Fiscus 2017), this metric uses a dynamic programming algorithm to align terms. It is most often used in a mode in which the time alignments produced by the system are ignored.

3. *Epoch-Based Sampling (EPOCH):* treats the reference and hypothesis as temporal signals, samples each at a fixed epoch duration, and counts errors accordingly.
4. *Any-Overlap (OVLP):* assesses the overlap in time between a reference and hypothesis event, and counts errors using binary scores for each event.
5. *Time-Aligned Event Scoring (TAES):* similar to (4) but considers the percentage overlap between the two events and weights errors accordingly.

It is important to understand that each of these measures estimates TP, TN, FP, and FN through some sort of error analysis. From these estimated quantities, traditional measures such as sensitivity and specificity are computed, as shown in Eqs. (8.1)–(8.6). As a result, we will see that sensitivity is a function of the underlying metric, and this is why it is important there be community-wide agreement on a specific metric.

We also include two derived measures in our analysis:

6. *Interrater Agreement (IRA):* uses EPOCH scoring to estimate errors and calculates Cohen's Kappa coefficient (Navakatikyan et al. 2006) using the measured TP, TN, FP, and FN.
7. *Area Under the Curve (AUC):* reduces a ROC or DET curve to a single scalar figure of merit by measuring the area encompassed by the curve.

IRA is popular for comparing the variability in human annotations when manually annotating reference data. We consider this a derived measure because it relies on one of the first five measures to estimate errors. Similarly, AUC relies on the generation of an ROC or DET curve, which in turn depends on one of the first five measures to estimate errors.

We now briefly describe each of these approaches and provide several examples that illustrate their strengths and weaknesses. These examples are drawn on a compressed timescale for illustrative purposes and were carefully selected because they demonstrate the strengths and weaknesses of the algorithms we are evaluating.

8.3.1 NIST Actual Term-Weighted Value (ATWV)

ATWV is a measure that balances sensitivity and FA rate. ATWV essentially assigns an application-dependent reward to each correct detection and a penalty to each incorrect detection. A perfect system results in an ATWV of 1.0, while a system with no output results in an ATWV of 0.0. It is possible for ATWV to be less than zero if a system is doing very poorly (for example a high FA rate). Experiments in voice keyword search have shown that an ATWV greater than 0.5 typically indicates a promising or usable system for information retrieval by voice applications. We believe a similar range is applicable to EEG analysis.

The metric accepts as input a list of N-tuples representing the hypotheses for the system being evaluated. Each of these N-tuples consists of a start time, end time, and system detection score. These entries are matched to the reference annotations using an objective function that accounts for both temporal overlap between the reference and hypotheses and the detection scores assigned by the system being evaluated. These detection scores are often likelihoods or confidence scores (Wegmann et al. 2013). The probabilities of errors due to misses and false alarms at a detection threshold θ are computed using:

$$P_{Miss(kw,\theta)} = 1 - N_{Correct(kw,\theta)} \Big/ N_{Ref(kw)}, \tag{8.7}$$

$$P_{FA(kw,\theta)} = N_{Spurious(kw,\theta)} \Big/ N_{NT(kw)}, \tag{8.8}$$

where $N_{Correct(kw,\theta)}$ is the number of correct detections of terms with a detection score greater than or equal to θ, $N_{Spurious(kw,\theta)}$ is the number of incorrect detections of terms with a detection score greater than or equal to θ, and $N_{NT(kw)}$ is the number of non-target trials for the term *kw* in the data. The number of non-target trials for a term is related to the total duration of source signal in seconds, T_{Source}, and is computed as $N_{NT(kw)} = T_{Source} - N_{Ref(kw)}$.

A term-weighted value (TWV) is then computed that quantifies a trade-off between misses and FAs. ATWV is defined as the value of TWV at the system's chosen detection threshold. Using a predefined constant, β, that was optimized experimentally ($\beta = 999.9$) (Fiscus et al. 2007), ATWV is computed using:

$$TWV_{(kw,\theta)} = 1 - P_{Miss(kw,\theta)} - \beta \; P_{FA(kw,\theta)}. \tag{8.9}$$

A standard implementation of this approach is available from NIST via GitHub (Fiscus 2017).

This metric has been widely used throughout the human language technology community for almost 20 years. This is a very important consideration in standardizing such a metric – researchers are using a common shared software implementation that ensures there are no subtle implementation differences in scoring software implementation between sites or researchers. There are always numerous parameters associated with this type of software and the only ways to make sure algorithms are producing identical results are (1) the existence of a common (open source) software package or (2) the distribution of a detailed set of regression tests that establish the equivalency of the implementations. The former has been a standard methodology for 40 years in the human language technology community, but the bioengineering communities have not quite achieved this level of standardization yet.

To demonstrate the features of this approach, consider the case shown in Fig. 8.3. The hypothesis for this segment consists of several short seizure events, while the reference consists of one long event. The ATWV metric will assign a TP score of 100% because the midpoint of the first event in the hypothesis annotation is mapped to the long seizure event in the reference annotation. This is somewhat

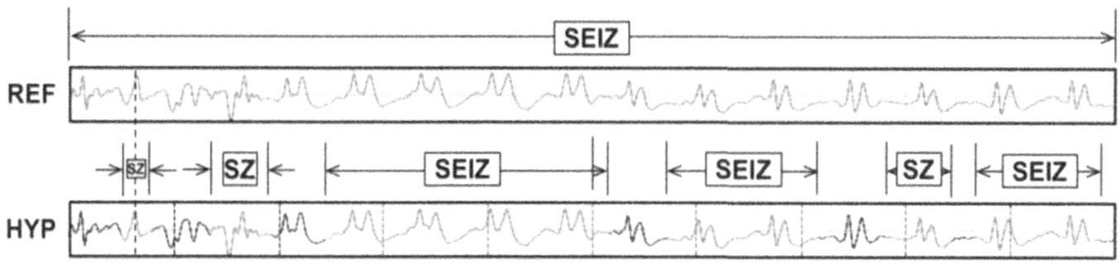

Fig. 8.3 ATWV scores this segment as 1 TP and 5 FPs

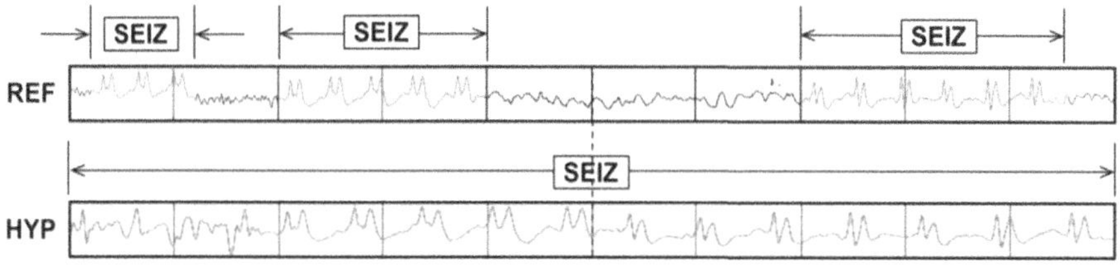

Fig. 8.4 ATWV scores this segment as 0 TP and 3 FN events

generous given that 50% of the event was not detected. The remaining 5 events in the hypothesis annotation are counted as false positives. The ATWV metric is relatively insensitive to the duration of the reference event, though the 5 false positives will lower the overall performance of the system. The important issue here is that the hypothesis correctly detected about 70% of the seizure event, and yet because of the large number of false positives, it will be penalized heavily.

In Fig. 8.4 we demonstrate a similar case in which the metric penalizes the hypothesis for missing three seizure events in the reference. Approximately 50% of the segment is correctly identified. Scoring that penalizes repeated events that are part of a larger event in the reference makes sense in an application like voice keyword search because in human language, each word hypothesis serves a unique purpose in the overall understanding of the signal. However, for a two-class event detection problem such as seizure detection, such scoring too heavily penalizes a hypothesis for splitting a long event into a series of short events.

8.3.2 Dynamic Programming Alignment (DPALIGN)

The DPALIGN metric essentially performs a minimization of an edit distance (the Levenshtein distance) (Picone et al. 1990) to map the hypothesis onto the reference. DPALIGN determines the minimum number of edits required to transform the hypothesis string into the reference string. Given two strings, the source string $X = [x_1, x_2, \ldots, x_n]$ of length n and target string $Y = [y_1, y_2, \ldots, y_m]$ of length m, we define $d_{i,j}$, which is the edit distance between the substring $x_1 : x_i$ and $y_1 : y_j$, as:

```
    Ref: bckg seiz SEIZ SEIZ bckg seiz bckg
    Hyp: bckg seiz BCKG **** bckg seiz ****
(Hits: 4 Sub: 1 Ins: 0 Del: 2 Total Errors: 3)

    Ref: bckg seiz BCKG **** bckg seiz ****
    Hyp: bckg seiz SEIZ SEIZ bckg seiz bckg
(Hits: 4 Sub: 1 Ins: 2 Del: 0 Total Errors: 3)
```

Fig. 8.5 DPALIGN aligns symbol sequences based on edit distance, ignoring the actual time alignments present in the reference annotation and the system output

$$d_{i,j} = \begin{cases} d_{i-1,j} + del \\ d_{i,j-1} + ins \\ d_{i-1,j-1} + sub \end{cases} . \tag{8.10}$$

The quantities being measured here are often referred to as substitution (sub), insertion (ins), and deletion (del) penalties. For this study, these three penalties are assigned equal weights of 1.0. A dynamic programming algorithm is used to find the optimal alignment between the reference and hypothesis based on these weights. Though there are versions of this metric that perform time-aligned scoring in which both the reference and hypothesis must include start and end times, this metric is most commonly used without time alignment information.

The metric is best demonstrated using the two examples shown in Fig. 8.5. In the first example, the reference annotation has a series of 7 events, while the hypothesis contains 5 events. The hypothesis substitutes background for the second seizure event and omits the third seizure event and the last background event. Hence, there are a total of three errors: two deletions and one substitution. In the second example, the reference annotation and hypothesis have been swapped to demonstrate the symmetry of the error calculations. The hypothesis generated two insertions and one substitution.

In practice, there are often multiple alignments that make sense based only on the labels associated with the annotations. As long as the algorithm is consistent about its choices, scoring will be fine. To accurately resolve such ambiguities, the actual endpoints of the hypotheses must be compared to the endpoints in the reference annotations. NIST distributes the ability to score this way, often referred to as time-aligned scoring, in their open-source package (Fiscus 2017). But this scoring mode is a little more complicated from a data interface point of view and has not been as popular. Though this type of scoring might at first seem highly inaccurate since it ignores time alignments of the hypotheses, it has been surprisingly effective in scoring machine learning systems in sequential data applications (e.g., speech recognition) (Picone et al. 1990; Martin et al. 1997; Fiscus et al. 2007).

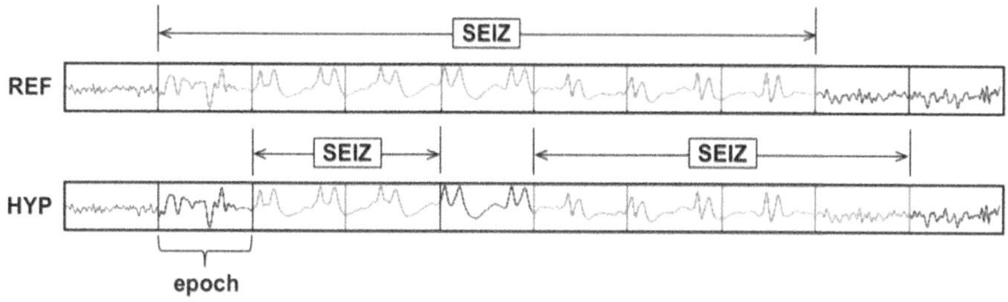

Fig. 8.6 EPOCH scoring directly measures the similarity of the time-aligned annotations. TP, FN, and FP are 5, 2, and 1, respectively

8.3.3 Epoch-Based Sampling (EPOCH)

Epoch-based scoring uses a metric that treats the reference and hypothesis as signals. These signals are sampled at a fixed frame rate, or epoch, duration. The corresponding label in the reference is compared to the hypothesis. Similar to DPALIGN, substitutions, deletions, and insertion errors are tabulated with an equal weight of 1.0 for each type of error. This process is depicted in Fig. 8.6. Epoch-based scoring requires that the entire signal be annotated (every second of the signal must be accounted for in the reference and hypothesis annotations), which is normally the case for sequential decoding evaluations. It attempts to account for the amount of time the two annotations overlap, so it directly addresses the inconsistencies demonstrated in Figs. 8.3 and 8.4.

One important parameter to be tweaked in this algorithm is the frequency with which we sample the two annotations, which we refer to as the scoring epoch duration. The scoring epoch duration is ideally set to an amount of time smaller than the unit of time used by the classification system to make decisions. For example, the hypothesis in Fig. 8.6 contains decisions made for every 1 *sec* of data. The scoring epoch duration should be set less than 1 *sec*. We set this parameter to 0.25 s for most of our work because our analysis system epoch duration is typically 1 *sec*. We find in situations like this the results are not overly sensitive to the choice of the scoring epoch duration as long as it is below the frame rate of the classification system, which is 1 *sec* in this case. This parameter simply controls the precision used to assess the accuracy of segment boundaries.

Because EPOCH scoring samples the annotations at fixed time intervals, it is inherently biased to weigh long seizure events more heavily. For example, if a signal contains one extremely long seizure event (e.g., 1000 *secs*) and two short events (e.g., each 10 *secs* in duration), the accuracy with which the first event is detected will dominate the overall scoring. Since seizure events can vary dramatically in duration, this is a cause for concern.

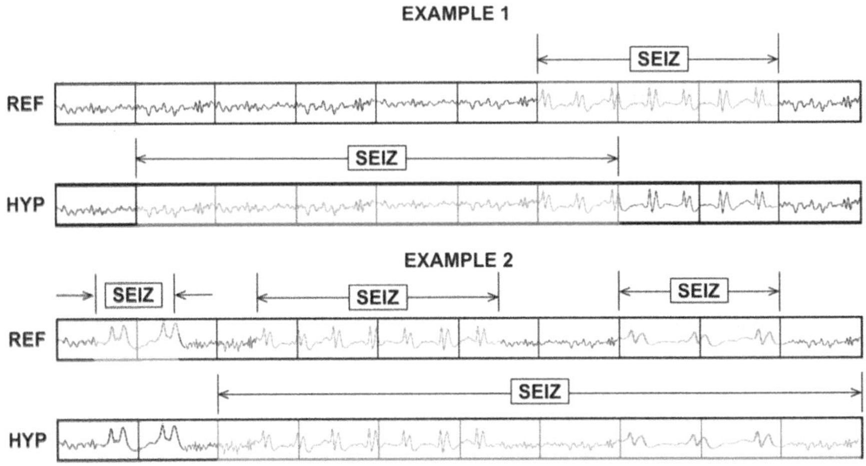

Fig. 8.7 OVLP scoring is very permissive about the degree of overlap between the reference and hypothesis. The TP score for Example 1 is 1 with no false alarms. In Example 2, the system detects 2 out of 3 seizure events, so the TP and FN scores are 2 and 1, respectively

8.3.4 Any-Overlap Method (OVLP)

In Sect. 8.2, we briefly introduced the OVLP metric and indicated; it was a popular choice in the neuroengineering community (Gotman et al. 1997; Wilson et al. 2003). OVLP is a more permissive metric that tends to produce much higher sensitivities. If an event is detected in close proximity to a reference event, the reference event is considered correctly detected. If a long event in the reference annotation is detected as multiple shorter events in the hypothesis, the reference event is also considered correctly detected. Multiple events in the hypothesis annotation corresponding to the same event in the reference annotation are not typically counted as FAs. Since the FA rate is a very important measure of performance in critical care applications, this is another cause for concern.

The OVLP scoring method is demonstrated in Fig. 8.7. It has one significant tunable parameter – a guard band that controls the degree to which a misalignment is still considered as a correct match. In this study, we use a fairly strict setting for this parameter – 1 *ms*. This has the effect of requiring some overlap between the two events in time – essentially a guard band of zero. The guard band needs to be tuned based on the needs of the application. Sensitivity generally increases as the guard band is increased.

8.3.5 Time-Aligned Event Scoring (TAES)

Though EPOCH scoring directly measures the amount of overlap between the annotations, there is a possibility that this metric also too heavily weighs single long events. Seizure events can vary in duration from a few seconds to several minutes (a seizure that lasts longer than 5 min is considered a medical emergency). In some applications, correctly detecting the number of events is as important as their duration.

In machine learning, the Jaccard index (Dodge 2008) is widely used for the analysis of such overlapping events. The Jaccard index is the ratio between the intersection and the union of two events. However, this metric lacks the ability to specify the degree of the misses and false alarms separately. Hence, since the FA rate is of great interest in bioengineering applications, the TAES metric was designed to tabulate these errors separately. The essential parameters for calculation of sensitivity and specificity such as TP, TN, and FP for the TAES scoring metric are defined as follows:

$$TP = \frac{H_{stop} - H_{start}}{Ref_{dur}}, \; where \; R_{start} \leq H \leq R_{stop}, \tag{8.11}$$

$$TN = \frac{1 - (TH_{stop} - TH_{start})}{Ref_{dur}}, \; where \; R_{start} \leq H \leq R_{stop}, \tag{8.12}$$

$$FP = \begin{cases} \frac{H_{stop} - R_{stop}}{Ref_{dur}}, & if \; H_{stop} \geq R_{stop}, H_{start} \geq R_{start} \; and \; H_{stop} - R_{stop} \leq 1, \\ \frac{R_{start} - H_{start}}{Ref_{dur}}, & if \; R_{start} \geq H_{start}, R_{stop} \geq H_{stop} \; and \; R_{start} - H_{start} \leq 1, \\ 1, & otherwise. \end{cases} \tag{8.13}$$

where H and R represent the reference and hypothesis events, respectively, and Ref_{dur} represents the duration of the reference events.

TAES gives equal weight to each event, but it calculates a partial score for each event based on the amount of overlap. The TP score is the total duration of a detected term divided by the total duration of the reference term. The FN score is the fraction of the time the reference term was missed divided by the total duration of the reference term. The FP score is the total duration of the inserted term divided by total amount of time this inserted term that was incorrect according to the reference annotation. FPs are limited to a maximum of 1 per event. Therefore, like TP and FN, a single FP event contributes only a fractional amount to the overall FP score if it correctly detects a portion of the same event in the reference annotation (partial overlap). Moreover, if multiple reference events are detected by a single long hypothesis event, all but the first detection are considered as FNs. These properties of the metric help manage the trade-off between sensitivity and FAs by balancing the contributions from short and long duration events. An example of TAES scoring is depicted in Fig. 8.8.

8.3.6 Interrater Agreement (IRA)

Interrater agreement (IRA) is a popular measure when comparing the relative similarity of two annotations. We refer to this metric as a derived metric since it is computed from error counts collected using one of the other five metrics. IRA is most often measured using Cohen's Kappa coefficient (McHugh 2012), which compares the observed accuracy with the expected accuracy. It is computed using:

$$\kappa = \frac{p_0 - p_e}{1 - p_e}, \tag{8.14}$$

where p_o is the relative observed agreement among raters and p_e is the hypothetical probability of chance agreement.

The range of the Kappa coefficient is $[-1, 1]$ where $\kappa = 1$ corresponds to complete agreement and $\kappa = -1$ which corresponds to no agreement. It has been used extensively to assess interrater agreement for experts manually annotating seizures in EEG signals. Values in the range of $0.5 \leq \kappa \leq 0.8$ are common for these types of assessments (Halford et al. 2015). The variability among experts mainly involves fine details in the annotations, such as the exact onset of a seizure. These kinds of details are extremely important for machine learning, and hence we need a metric that is sensitive to small variations in the annotations. For completeness, we use this measure as a way of evaluating the amount of agreement between two annotations.

8.3.7 A Brief Comparison of Metrics

A simple example of how these metrics compare on a specific segment of a signal is shown in Fig. 8.9. A 10 s section of an EEG signal is shown subdivided into 1 s segments. The reference has three isolated events. The system being evaluated outputs one hypothesis that starts in the middle of the first event and continues through the remaining two events.

ATWV scores the system as 1 TP and 2 FNs since it assigns the extended hypothesis event to the center reference event and leaves the other two undetected. The ATWV score is 0.33 for seizure events and 0.25 for background events, resulting in an average ATWV of 0.29. The sensitivity and FA rates for seizure events for this metric are 33% and 0 per 24 *hrs.*, respectively.

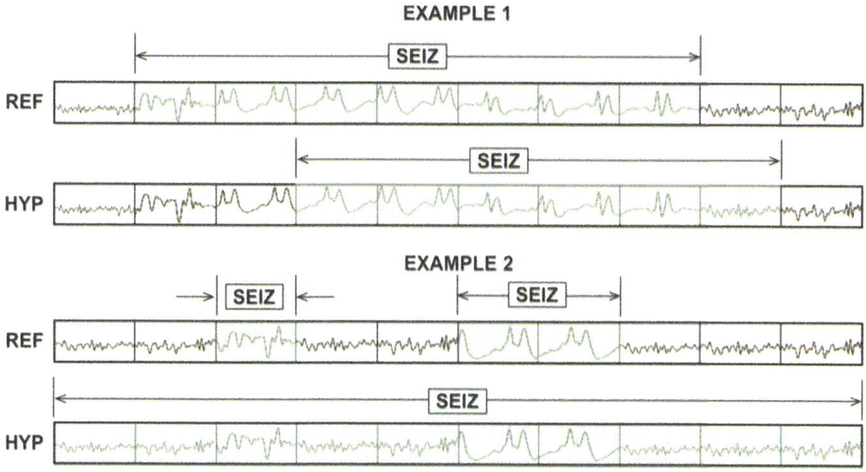

Fig. 8.8 An example that summarizes the differences between scoring metrics

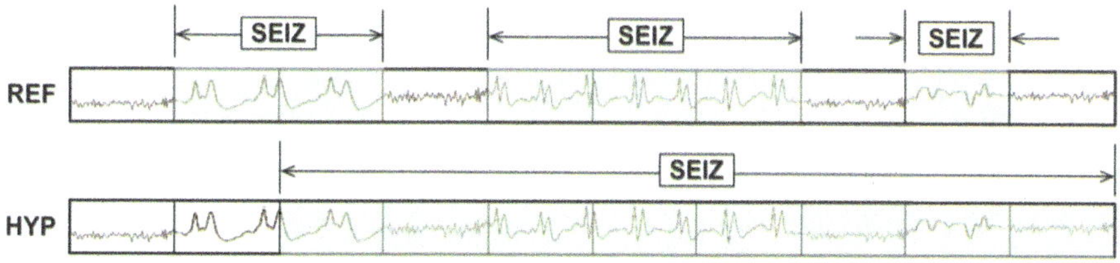

Fig. 8.9 TAES scoring accounts for the amount of overlap between the reference and hypothesis. TAES scores Example 1 as 0.71 TP, 0.29 FN, and 0.14 FP. Example 2 is scored as 1 TP, 1 FN, and 1 FP

DPALIGN scores the system the same way since time alignments are ignored and the first event in each annotation is matched together, leaving the other two events undetected.

The EPOCH method scores the alignment 5 TP, 3 FP, and 1 FN using a 1 *sec* epoch duration because there are 4 epochs for which the annotations do not agree and 5 epochs where they agree. The sensitivity is 83.33%, and the FA rate per 24 *hrs* is very high because of the 3 FPs.

The OVLP method scores the segment as 3 TP and 0 FP because the detected events have partial to full overlap with all the reference events, giving a sensitivity of 100% with an FA rate of 0. TAES scores this segment as 0.5 TP and 2.5 FN because the first event is only 50% correct and there are FN errors for the 5th to 7th and 9th epochs (an example of multiple overlapping reference events), giving a sensitivity of 16.66% and a corresponding high FA rate.

IRA for seizure events evaluated using Cohen's Kappa statistic is 0.09 for this example because there are essentially 4 errors for 4 seizure events. IRAs below 0.5 indicate a poor match between the reference and the hypothesis.

Table 8.1 The TUSZ Corpus (v1.1.1)

Description	Train	Eval
Patients	196	50
Sessions	456	230
Files	1505	984
No. seizure events	870	614
Seizure (secs)	51,140	53,930
Non-seizure (secs)	877,821	547,728
Total (secs)	928,962	601,659

It is difficult to conclude from this example which of these measures are most appropriate for EEG analysis. However, we see that ATWV and DPALIGN generally produce similar results. The EPOCH metric produces larger counts because this metric samples time rather than events. OVLP produces a high sensitivity, while TAES produces a low sensitivity but a relatively higher FA rate. In the next section, we conduct a more rigorous evaluation of these metrics using the output of several automatic seizure detection systems.

8.4 Evaluation

In order to evaluate the behavior of our scoring metrics, we analyzed the performance of several machine learning systems on a seizure detection task. We briefly introduce the TUH seizure detection corpus. Next we introduce five different hybrid machine learning architectures based on deep learning principles. We then conduct a very detailed statistical analysis of the performance of these systems using the scoring metrics introduced in Sect. 8.3.

8.4.1 The TUH EEG Seizure Corpus

To demonstrate the differences between these metrics on a realistic task, we have evaluated a range of machine learning systems on a seizure detection task based on the TUH EEG Seizure (TUSZ) Corpus (Shah et al. 2018). This is a subset of the TUH EEG Corpus developed at Temple University (Obeid and Picone 2016) that has been manually annotated. An overview of the corpus is given in Table 8.1. This is the largest open-source corpus of its type. It consists of clinical data collected at Temple University Hospital. TUSZ represents a very challenging machine learning task because it contains a rich variety of common real-world problems (e.g., patient movements and artifacts) found in clinical data as well as various types of seizures (e.g., absence, tonic-clonic). It is worth noting that seizure data represents an extremely unbalanced dataset – only about 8% of the data are annotated as seizure events.

The version of the seizure database used for this study was v1.1.1 which contains 196 patients in the training set and 50 patients in the evaluation set, making it adequate to accurately assess fine differences in algorithm performance for machine learning algorithms. Although this database provides event-based as well as term-based annotations, for our study we only used the term-based annotations: a single decision is made at each point in time based on examination of all channels. Though annotations are channel-based (each channel is annotated independently), these annotations are aggregated to produce a single decision at each point in time. More information about the annotation process is available in Ochal et al. (Ochal et al. 2020).

8.4.2 Machine Learning Architectures

For EEG signals, it is appropriate to use algorithms which can learn spatial as well as temporal context efficiently. Sequential algorithms such as hidden Markov models (HMMs), recurrent neural networks (RNNs), and convolutional neural networks (CNNs) are perfect candidates as the building blocks of the recognition system. We developed five different hybrid networks which use these algorithms in their system design so that we had a variety of classification algorithms represented in our study. A general architecture for the five machine learning systems evaluated is shown in Fig. 8.10.

The first step in this architecture is to convert an EEG signal, typically stored in a European Data Format (EDF) file (Kemp 2013), to a sequence of feature vectors. Linear frequency cepstral coefficients features (Harati et al. 2015) are created using a 0.1 *sec* frame duration and a 0.2 *sec* analysis window for each channel. We use the first 7 cepstral coefficients along with their first and second derivatives. We add several energy terms which bring the total feature vector dimension to 26. Attempts to circumvent the feature extraction process by using a deep learning-based approach have not produced significantly better results than these model-based features.

A group of frames are classified into an event on a per-channel basis using a combination of deep learning networks. The deep learning system essentially looks across multiple epochs, which we refer to as temporal context, and multiple channels, which we refer to as spatial context, since each channel is associated with a location of an electrode on a patient's scalp. There are a wide variety of algorithms that can be used to produce a decision from these inputs. Even though seizures occur on a subset of the channels input to such a system, we focus on a single decision made across all channels at each point in time.

The five systems we included in this study were carefully selected because they represent a range of performance that is representative of state of the art on this task and because these systems exhibit different error modalities. The performance of these systems is sufficiently close so that the impact of these different scoring metrics becomes apparent. The systems selected are briefly described below.

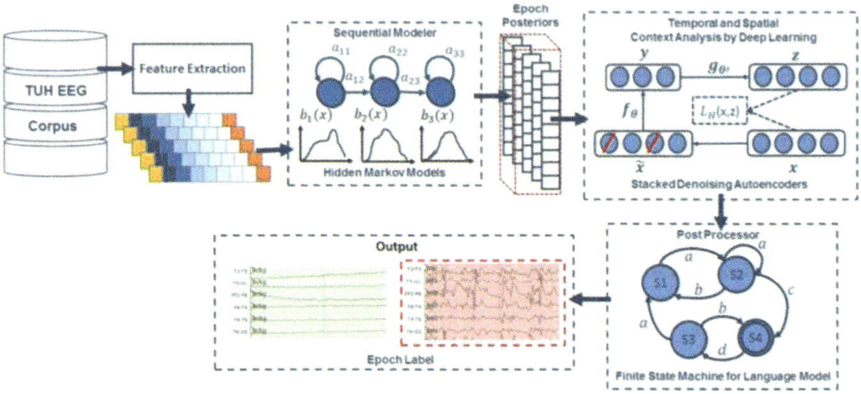

Fig. 8.10 A hybrid deep learning architecture that integrates temporal and spatial context

1. *HMM/SdA* (Golmohammadi et al. 2019)*:* a hybrid system consisting of a hidden Markov model (HMM) decoder and a postprocessor that uses a stacked denoising autoencoder (SdA). An N-channel EEG was transformed into N independent feature streams using a standard sliding window-based approach. The hypotheses generated by the HMMs were postprocessed using a second stage of processing that examines the temporal and spatial context. We apply a third pass of postprocessing that uses a stochastic language model to smooth hypotheses involving sequences of events so that we can suppress spurious outputs. This third stage of postprocessing provides a moderate reduction in the false alarm rate.

   Standard three state left-to-right HMMs with eight Gaussian mixture components per state were used for sequential decoding. We divide each channel of an EEG into 1 s epochs and further subdivide these epochs into a sequence of frames. Each epoch is classified using an HMM trained on the subdivided epoch, and then these epoch-based decisions are postprocessed by additional statistical models in a process similar to the language modeling component of a speech recognizer.

   The output of the epoch-based decisions was postprocessed by a deep learning system. The SdA network has three hidden layers with corruption levels of 0.3 for each layer. There are 800 nodes in the first layer, 500 nodes in the second layer, and 300 nodes in the third layer. The parameters for pre-training are learning rate =0.5, number of epochs =150, and batch size =300. The parameters for fine-tuning are learning rate =0.1, number of epochs =300, and batch size = 100. The overall result of the second stage is a probability vector of dimension two containing a likelihood that each label could have occurred in the epoch. A soft decision paradigm is used rather than a hard decision paradigm because this output is smoothed in the third stage of processing.
2. *HMM/LSTM* (Golmohammadi et al. 2019)*:* an HMM decoder postprocessed by a long short-term memory (LSTM) network. Like the HMM/SdA hybrid approach

previously described, the output of the HMM system is a vector of dimension: number of classes (2) × number of channels (22) × the window length (7) =308. Therefore, we also use principal components analysis (PCA) before LSTM in this approach to reduce the dimensionality of the data to 20. For this study, we used a window length of 41 for LSTM. This layer is composed of one hidden layer with 32 nodes. The output layer nodes in this LSTM level use a sigmoid activation function. The parameters of the models are optimized to minimize the error using a cross-entropy loss function. Adaptive Moment Estimation (Adam) is used in the optimization process.

3. *IPCA/LSTM (*Golmohammadi et al. 2019*):* a preprocessor based on incremental principal component analysis (IPCA) followed by an LSTM decoder. The EEG features are delivered to an IPCA layer for spatial context analysis and dimensionality reduction. A batch size of 50 is used in IPCA and the output dimension is 25. The output of IPCA is delivered to an LSTM for classification. We used a one-layer LSTM with a hidden layer size of 128. A batch size of 128 was used along with Adam optimization and a cross-entropy loss function.
4. *CNN/MLP (*Golmohammadi et al. 2020*):* a pure deep learning-based approach that uses a convolutional neural network (CNN) decoder and a multi-layer perceptron (MLP) postprocessor. The network contains six convolutional layers, three max pooling layers, and two fully connected layers. A rectified linear unit (ReLU) nonlinearity is applied to the output of every convolutional and fully connected layer.
5. *CNN/LSTM (*Golmohammadi et al. 2020*):* a pure deep learning-based architecture that uses a combination of CNN and LSTM networks. In this architecture, we integrate 2D CNNs, 1D CNNs, and LSTM networks to better exploit long-term dependencies. Exponential linear units (ELU) are used as the activation functions for the hidden layers. Adam is used in the optimization process along with a mean squared error loss function.

The details of these systems are not critical to this study. We selected these systems because we needed a range of typical system performance that would expose the differences in the scoring metrics. What is more important is how the range of performance is reflected in these metrics.

A comparison of the performance is presented in Table 8.2. For each scoring metric, we provide the measured sensitivity, specificity, and FA rate. For the ATWV metric, we also provide the ATWV score. Though the rankings of these systems vary as a function of the metric, the overall trends are accurately represented in Table 8.2. HMM/SdA generally performs the poorest of these systems, delivering a respectable sensitivity at a high FA rate. CNN/LSTM typically delivers the highest overall performance because it has a low FA rate, which is very important in this type of application.

Table 8.2 Performance vs. scoring metric

Metric	Measure	HMM/SdA	HMM/LSTM	IPCA/LSTM	CNN/MLP	CNN/LSTM
ATWV	Sensitivity	30.35%	26.73%	24.73%	29.52%	30.34%
	Specificity	61.38%	68.93%	64.51%	65.87%	93.15%
	FA/24 h	98.65	75.59	94.41	94.25	12.78
	ATWV	−0.8392	−0.8469	−0.4628	−0.7971	0.1737
DPALIGN	Sensitivity	44.11%	33.77%	35.77%	43.35%	32.46%
	Specificity	66.87%	72.99%	69.59%	71.49%	95.17%
	FA/24 h	86.15	66.98	81.17	77.67	10.19
EPOCH	Sensitivity	20.71%	50.46%	51.02%	65.03%	9.784%
	Specificity	98.22%	94.82%	94.09	91.55%	99.84%
	FA/24 h	1418.02	4133.34	4711.58	6738.82	125.79
OVLP	Sensitivity	35.35%	30.05%	32.97%	39.09%	30.83%
	Specificity	73.35%	80.53%	77.57%	76.84%	96.86%
	FA/24 h.	77.39	60.92	73.52	77.19	6.75
TAES	Sensitivity	17.29%	22.84%	22.12%	31.58%	12.48%
	Specificity	66.04%	70.41%	66.64%	64.75%	95.24%
	FA/24 h	82.26	68.31	83.01	91.53	7.54

8.5 Derived Measures

Most supervised machine learning algorithms are designed to classify labels with some type of bounded or unbounded confidence measure such as a posterior probability or a log-likelihood. Possible exceptions are nonparametric techniques such K-nearest neighbors and decision trees. These confidence measures allow algorithm designers to sweep through threshold values for the confidence measures and observe performance at different operating points. In this section, we analyze the performance of these systems using DET curves and derived measures such as AUC and F scores.

8.5.1 Detection Error Trade-off Analysis

Evaluating systems from a single operating point is always a bit tenuous. It is very difficult to compare the performance of various systems when only two values are reported (e.g., sensitivity and specificity) because these systems might simply be designed to balance the four basic error categories differently (e.g., using a different threshold to reject FPs). For example, in seizure detection, the a priori probability of a seizure is very low, which means assessment of background events dominate the error calculations. The degree to which a system is capable of producing a seizure hypothesis will greatly impact its specificity. Further, sensitivity varies significantly when the FA rate is very low. Therefore, comparing systems that differ significantly

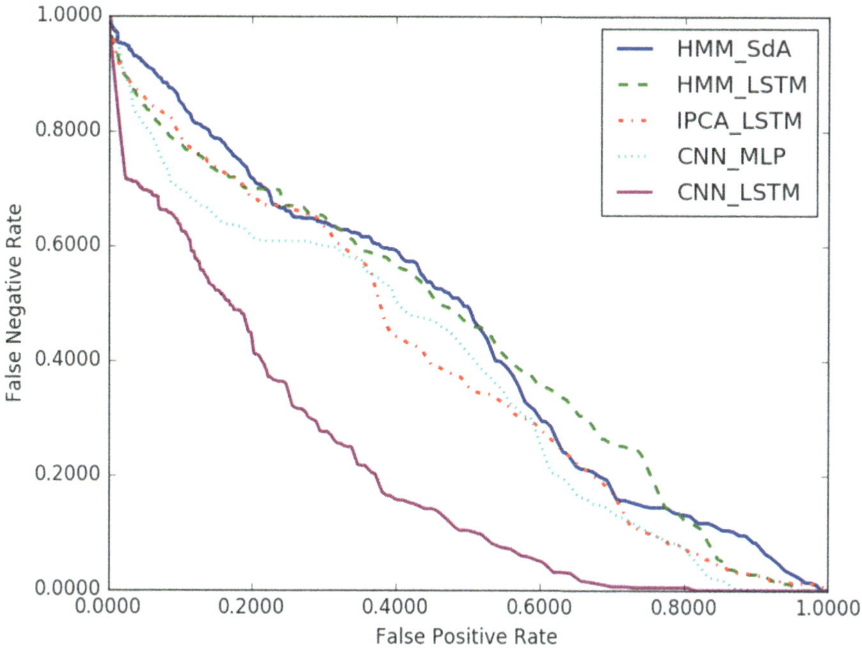

Fig. 8.11 A comparison of DET curves

in FA rate can be misleading. Often, we prefer a more holistic view of performance that is provided by a receiver operating characteristic (ROC) curve or a detection error trade-off (DET) curve. A ROC curve displays TP as a function of FP while a DET curve displays FN as a function of FP.

In Fig. 8.11, we provide DET curves for the systems presented in Table 8.2. We refer to this analysis as a derived measure because these curves require calculations of the four measures described in Sect. 8.2, which in turn requires the selection of a scoring metric. The DET curves in Fig. 8.11 were derived from output generated using the OVLP scoring metric. The shapes of the DET curves do not change significantly with the scoring metric though the absolute numbers vary similarly to what we see in Table 8.2.

From this data it is clear that CNN/LSTM performance is significantly different from the other systems. This is primarily because of its low FA rate. For this particular application, sensitivity drops rapidly as the FA rate is lowered. Therefore, comparing a single data point for each system is dangerous because the systems are most likely operating at different points on a DET curve if the sensitivities are significantly different. We find tuning these systems to have a comparable FA rate is important when comparing two systems only based on sensitivity.

The sensitivity for each metric is given in Table 8.2. For example, for HMM/SdA, we see the lowest sensitivities are produced by the TAES and EPOCH metrics, while the highest sensitivities are produced by OVLP and DPALIGN. This makes sense

Table 8.3 AUC comparison

Algorithm	AUC (OVLP)	AUC (TAES)
HMM/SdA	0.44	0.72
HMM/LSTM	0.44	0.71
IPCA/LSTM	0.39	0.72
CNN/MLP	0.38	0.65
CNN/LSTM	0.21	0.56

because OVLP and DPALIGN are very forgiving of time alignment errors, while TAES and EPOCH penalize time alignment errors heavily. We see similar trends for CNN/LSTM though the range of differences between the three highest scoring metrics is smaller. We also see that the five algorithms are ranked similarly by each scoring metric even though the scale of the numbers varies by metric. HMM/SdA consistently scores the lowest and CNN/LSTM consistently scores the highest. The other three systems are very similar in their performance.

The ATWV scores for all algorithms are extremely low. The ATWV scores are below 0.5 which indicates that overall performance is poor. However, the ATWV score for CNN/LSTM is significantly higher than the other four systems. ATWV attempts to reduce the information contained in a DET curve to a single number and does a good job reflecting the results shown in Fig. 8.11. The DET curves for HMM/LSTM and HMM/SdA overlap considerably for an FP rate between 0.25 and 1.0, and this is a primary reason why their ATWV scores are similar. However, for seizure detection we are primarily interested in the low FP rate region, and in that range, HMM/LSTM and IPCA/LSTM perform similarly.

When a single metric is preferred, the area under a DET or ROC curve (AUC) is also an effective way of comparing the performance. A random guessing approach to classification, assuming equal priors for each class, will give an AUC of 0.5, while a perfect classifier will give an AUC of 1.0. In Table 8.3 we provide AUCs for these DET curves calculated using OVLP and TAES for comparison. AUC values in Table 8.3 also follow a similar trend, but the differences are less pronounced than in Fig. 8.11 or in Table 8.2.

Note that the AUC value for the presumptive best system, CNN/LSTM, is significantly lower than the other four systems. If we examined the AUC in the FPR range of $[0.0, 0.2]$, which corresponds to a low FA rate, and is the region of greatest interest, CNN/LSTM is still significantly better than the other algorithms, but the margin of difference shrinks slightly. The difference in the FPR range of $[0.2, 0.8]$ is more pronounced. This is something we often see when evaluating new machine learning algorithms. They tend to deliver their best performance in the upper ranges of FPR but are not as impressive when the FPR rate is very low. This suggests the major issues an algorithm needs to address in the low FPR region are more related to auxiliary issues such as segmentation and noise rejection rather than optimal modeling of a complex decision surface. It is not uncommon that in machine learning applications involving real-world applications, such as clinical data, low-

Table 8.4 Accuracy vs. metric

Metric	HMM/SdA	HMM/LSTM	IPCA/LSTM	CNN/MLP	CNN/|LSTM
ATWV	54.0%	54.0%	52.1%	54.9%	70.7%
DPALIGN	61.5%	60.2%	59.2%	62.9%	73.6%
EPOCH	92.3%	91.5%	90.8%	89.5%	91.5%
OVLP	65.1%	66.5%	65.6%	66.9%	78.9%
TAES	56.6%	57.3%	55.4%	57.2%	69.7%

Table 8.5 F1 vs. metric

Metric	HMM/SdA	HMM/LSTM	IPCA/LSTM	CNN/MLP	CNN/LSTM
ATWV	0.24	0.28	0.24	0.28	0.42
DPALIGN	0.35	0.36	0.35	0.42	0.45
EPOCH	0.29	0.47	0.46	0.49	0.14
OVLP	0.31	0.33	0.34	0.38	0.45
TAES	0.16	0.26	0.24	0.31	0.19

level issues such as segmentation of the data, and robustness to spurious noises ultimately limit performance.

8.5.2 *Accuracy and Other Derived Scores*

A commonly used metric in the machine learning community that is somewhat intuitive is accuracy. The accuracies of the five systems are shown in Table 8.4. Accuracy places an equal weight on each type of error (though it is possible to apply heuristic weights in practice). This is acceptable if the dataset is balanced. However, for many bioengineering applications, such as seizure detection, the target class, or class of interest, occurs infrequently. According to the accuracies presented in Table 8.4, we see that CNN/LSTM is still significantly more accurate than the other four systems and the differences between the remaining four systems are minimal.

Another popular metric that attempts to aggregate performance into a single data point, and is popular in the information retrieval communities, is the F1 score. F1 scores for the five systems are shown in Table 8.5. We see there are significant variations between the systems, and the results don't completely correlate with Table 8.4. For example, for the TAES and EPOCH metrics, which emphasize time alignments, the best performing system is not CNN/LSTM. F1 scores weigh miss and false alarm errors equally. In our experience, changing the weight of these errors (e.g., F-score with beta value 0.2) does not adequately emphasize the FA rate for applications such as seizure detection where the classes are unbalanced.

The Matthews correlation coefficient (MCC) (Chicco and Jurman 2020) is an effective solution when a significant class imbalance exists. MCC is a contingency matrix method of calculating the Pearson product-moment correlation coefficient

Table 8.6 MCC vs. metric

Metric	HMM/SdA	HMM/LSTM	IPCA/LSTM	CNN/MLP	CNN/LSTM
ATWV	−0.07	−0.04	−0.11	−0.05	0.30
DPALIGN	0.01	0.07	0.05	0.15	0.35
EPOCH	0.28	0.43	0.41	0.45	0.23
OVLP	0.08	0.11	0.11	0.16	0.41
TAES	−0.16	−0.07	−0.12	−0.04	0.13

Table 8.7 Cohen's Kappa (κ) vs. metric

Metric	HMM/SdA	HMM/LSTM	IPCA/LSTM	CNN/MLP	CNN/LSTM
ATWV	−0.07	−0.04	−0.11	−0.05	0.26
DPALIGN	0.09	0.07	0.05	0.15	0.31
EPOCH	0.26	0.43	0.41	0.43	0.12
OVLP	0.08	0.11	0.11	0.16	0.35
TAES	−0.16	−0.07	−0.11	−0.04	0.09

(Powers 2011) between actual and predicted values. Recall (sensitivity) is the fraction of relevant samples that are correctly retrieved. Its dual metric, precision is the fraction of retrieved samples that are relevant. Meaningfully combining precision and recall generates alternative performance evaluation measures such as the F1 ratio, which combines these scores using a geometric mean. MCC takes into account all four values in the confusion matrix. A value close to 1.0 means that both classes are predicted well, even if one class is disproportionately represented. Since MCC is a correlation coefficient, it ranges from $[-1, 1]$. Perfect misclassification corresponds to a value of -1, perfect classification corresponds to a value of 1.0, and random guessing with equal priors corresponds to a value of 0.0. Since no class is more important than the other, MCC is symmetric.

In Table 8.6, we present MCC results for the five systems and the five metrics. It is interesting to note that for the overall best system CNN/LSTM, MCC produces higher correlations for the first three metrics (ATWV, DPALIGN, and OVLP). These metrics are based less on time alignments of the hypotheses. The latter two metrics (EPOCH and TAES) weigh the time alignments more heavily and generally produce lower scores because their matching criteria are more stringent.

Interrater agreement (IRA) is an extremely useful measure for the development of reference annotations. It is not uncommon that a team of annotators will be involved in the annotation of a large corpus. Individual annotators are evaluated and compared using IRA (Shah et al. 2020). Though there are numerous ways to measure IRA, Cohen's Kappa statistic, as shown in Eq. (8.14), is one of the most popular ways to compute IRA. In Table 8.7, we show IRA values for the five systems. Again, we observe that CNN/LSTM has higher IRA values than the other systems, except for the EPOCH metric. Both MCC and IRA report similar trends for CNN/LSTM versus the other four systems for the EPOCH metric.

8.5.3 *Additional Insight*

We generally prefer operating points where performance in terms of sensitivity, specificity, and FAs is balanced. The ATWV metric explicitly attempts to encourage balancing of these by assigning a reward to each correct detection and a penalty to each incorrect detection. None of the conventional metrics described here consider the fraction of a detected event that is correct. This is the inspiration behind the development of TAES scoring. TAES scoring requires the time alignments to match, which is a more stringent requirement than, for example, OVLP. Consequently, the sensitivity produced by the TAES and EPOCH metrics tends to be lower.

Comparing results across these five metrics can provide useful diagnostic information and provide insight into the system's behavior. For example, the IPCA/LSTM and HMM/LSTM systems have relatively higher sensitivities according to the EPOCH metric, indicating that these systems tend to detect longer seizure events. Conversely, since the CNN/LSTM system has relatively low sensitivities according to the TAES and EPOCH metrics, it can be inferred that this system misses longer seizure events. Similarly, if the sensitivity was relatively high for TAES and relatively low for EPOCH, it would indicate that the system tends to detect a majority of smaller to moderate events precisely regardless of the duration of an event. A comparison of ATWV scores with other metrics gives diagnostic information such as whether a system accurately detects the onset and end of an event or whether the system splits long events into multiple short events.

8.6 Statistical Analysis

To understand the pairwise statistical difference between these evaluation metrics and the hybrid deep learning systems, we have performed three tests: Kolmogorov-Smirnov (KS), Pearson's R (correlation coefficient), and *z*-test (Hammond et al. 2015). These tests were performed to evaluate results of these systems on the basis of sensitivity and specificity. Each individual patient from the TUSZ dataset was evaluated separately. Outliers were removed by rejecting all input values collected from patients which have no seizures and from those for which the systems detected no seizures.

8.6.1 *Kolmogorov-Smirnov and Pearson's R Tests*

Prior to performing statistical significance tests, it must first be determined whether or not the group sample, which in our case is the individual metric's score on per patient basis, is normally distributed. We performed KS tests on each separate evaluation metric and confirmed that the group distribution is indeed Gaussian. The

Table 8.8 Correlation of the scoring metrics based on sensitivity ($p < 0.001$)

Metric	ATWV	DPALIGN	EPOCH	OVLP	TAES
ATWV	–	0.87	0.50	0.92	0.71
DPALIGN		–	0.48	0.90	0.69
EPOCH			–	0.62	0.87
OVLP				–	0.78
TAES					–

Table 8.9 Correlation of the scoring metrics based on specificity ($p < 0.001$)

Metric	ATWV	DPALIGN	EPOCH	OVLP	TAES
ATWV	–	0.49	0.32	0.45	0.54
DPALIGN		–	0.38	0.94	0.89
EPOCH			–	0.44	0.56
OVLP				–	0.95
TAES					–

KS values range from 0.61 to 0.71 for sensitivity and 0.99 – 1.00 for specificity with the *p*-values equal to zero. We then evaluated the correlation coefficient (Pearson's R) between pairs of metrics.

Correlations for each pair of scoring metrics are shown in Table 8.8 (for sensitivity) and Table 8.9 (for specificity). It can be seen that the pairwise correlations between OVLP, ATWV, and DPALIGN are highest, while the pairs ATWV-EPOCH and DPALIGN-EPOCH have the lowest correlation (~0.5). The EPOCH method has a low correlation with all other metrics but TAES. This makes sense because the EPOCH method scores events on a constant time scale instead of on individual events. TAES takes into account the duration of the overlap, so it is the closest method to EPOCH in this regard.

Since OVLP and TAES both score overlapping events independently, we also expect these two methods to be correlated (sensitivity: 0.78; specificity: 0.95). ATWV on the other hand has fairly low correlations with the other metrics for specificity because of its stringent rules for FPs when there are multiple overlapping events. The overall highest correlation is between ATWV and OVLP for sensitivity and OVLP and TAES for specificity. All the correlation values (Pearson's R) collected in these tables are statistically significant with $p < 0.001$.

8.6.2 Z-Tests

To understand the statistical significance of each system, we perform two-tailed *z*-tests for sensitivity as shown in Table 8.10 and for specificity as shown in Table 8.11. Cells in these tables contain entries that consist of the sensitivity/specificity differences between the systems and a binary classification value (Yes/No) based on extracted *p*-values from the *z*-test with 95% confidence. (Due to space constraints, the five classification systems are represented using the abbreviations M1 to M5.) The data was prepared by scoring systems on individual patients. Prior to performing z-tests, the Gaussianity of each sample was evaluated using a KS test. All the samples were confirmed as normal with $p < 0.001$.

From Table 8.10, it can be observed that, aside from the EPOCH and TAES scoring metrics, the differences between the CNN-LSTM system and all the other systems are statistically significant (rejecting the null hypothesis with $p < 0.05$. On the other hand, the EPOCH and TAES metrics fail to reject the null hypothesis for CNN-LSTM. According to these metrics, the performance of HMM-SDA is statistically different from the other systems, confirming its poor performance. This can also be observed from EPOCH/TAES results shown in Table 8.2.

Table 8.11 shows a different trend than Table 8.10. The EPOCH metric fails to reject null hypothesis for all the systems. Since specificity is calculated from TN and FP values, for an evaluation set 167 h in duration and an epoch duration of 0.25 s, a few thousand seconds of FPs do not make any significant difference in terms of specificity. This can also be directly observed in Table 8.2, where the specificity of all systems according to the EPOCH metric is always greater than 90%. The huge difference between the duration of background and seizure events is the primary reason for such high specificities. However, the OVLP and TAES metrics completely agree with each other's z-test results for specificity.

8.7 Conclusions

Standardization of scoring metrics is an extremely important step for a research community to take in order to make progress on machine learning problems. There has been a lack of standardization in most bioengineering fields. Popular metrics such as sensitivity and specificity do not completely characterize the problem and neglect the importance that FA rate plays in achieving clinically acceptable solutions. In this chapter, we have compared several popular scoring metrics and demonstrated the value of considering the accuracy of time alignments in the overall assessment of a system. We have proposed the use of a new metric, TAES scoring, which is consistent with popular scoring approaches such as OVLP but provides more accurate assessments by producing fractional scores for recognition of events based on the degree of match in the time alignments. We have also demonstrated the efficacy of an existing metric, ATWV, that is popular in the speech recognition community.

We have not discussed the extent to which we can tune these metrics by weighting various types of errors based on feedback from clinicians and other customers of the technology. Optimization of the metric is a research problem in itself, since many considerations, including usability of the technology and a broad range of applications, must be involved in this process. Our informal attempts to optimize ATWV and OVLP for seizure detection have not yet produced significantly different results than what was presented here. Feedback from clinicians has been consistent that FA rate is perhaps the single most important measure once sensitivity is above

Table 8.10 Significance calculated using z-tests for α = 0.05 (for sensitivity)

ATWV (Abs. sensitivity difference (%), significant/non-significant)					
ML systems (Sens.)	**CNN-LSTM (M1)**	**CNN-MLP (M2)**	**HMM-LSTM (M3)**	**HMM-SDA (M4)**	**IPCA-LSTM (M5)**
M1 (30.34%)	–	(00.82%) Y	(03.61%) Y	(00.01%) Y	(05.61%) Y
M2 (29.52%)		–	(02.79%) N	(00.83%) N	(04.79%) N
M3 (26.73%)			–	(03.62%) N	(02.00%) N
M4 (30.35%)				–	(05.62%) N
M5 (24.73%)					–
DPALIGN (Abs. Sensitivity difference, significant/non-significant)					
ML systems (Sens.)	**CNN-LSTM (M1)**	**CNN-MLP (M2)**	**HMM-LSTM (M3)**	**HMM-SDA (M4)**	**IPCA-LSTM (M5)**
M1 (32.46%)	–	(10.89%) Y	(01.31%) Y	(11.65%) Y	(03.31%) Y
M2 (43.35%)		–	(09.58%) N	(00.76%) N	(07.58%) N
M3 (33.77%)			–	(10.34%) N	(02.00%) N
M4 (44.11%)				–	(08.34%) N
M5 (35.77%)					–
EPOCH (Abs. Sensitivity difference, significant/non-significant)					
ML systems (Sens.)	**CNN-LSTM (M1)**	**CNN-MLP (M2)**	**HMM-LSTM (M3)**	**HMM-SDA (M4)**	**IPCA-LSTM (M5)**
M1 (09.78%)	–	(55.25%) N	(40.68%) N	(10.93%) Y	(41.24%) N
M2 (65.03%)		–	(14.57%) Y	(44.32%) Y	(14.01%) N
M3 (50.46%)			–	(29.75%) Y	(00.56%) N
M4 (20.71%)				–	(30.31%) Y
M5 (51.02%)					–
OVLP (Abs. Sensitivity difference, significant/non-significant)					
ML systems (Sens.)	**CNN-LSTM (M1)**	**CNN-MLP (M2)**	**HMM-LSTM (M3)**	**HMM-SDA (M4)**	**IPCA-LSTM (M5)**
M1 (30.83%)	–	(08.26%) Y	(02.14%) Y	(04.52%) Y	(02.14%) Y
M2 (39.09%)		–	(09.04%) N	(03.74%) N	(06.12%) N
M3 (30.05%)			–	(05.30%) N	(02.92%) N
M4 (35.35%)				–	(02.38%) N
M5 (32.97%)					–
TAES (Abs. Sensitivity difference, significant/non-significant)					
ML systems (Sens.)	**CNN-LSTM (M1)**	**CNN-MLP (M2)**	**HMM-LSTM (M3)**	**HMM-SDA (M4)**	**IPCA-LSTM (M5)**
M1 (12.48%)	–	(19.10%) N	(10.36%) N	(04.81%) Y	(09.64%) N
M2 (31.58%)		–	(08.74%) N	(14.29%) Y	(09.46%) N
M3 (22.84%)			–	(05.55%) Y	(00.72%) N
M4 (17.29%)				–	(04.83%) Y
M5 (22.12%)					–

Table 8.11 Significance calculated using z-tests for $\alpha = 0.05$ (for specificity)

ATWV (Abs. specificity difference (%), significant/non-significant)					
ML systems (Spec.)	**CNN-LSTM (M1)**	**CNN-MLP (M2)**	**HMM-LSTM (M3)**	**HMM-SDA (M4)**	**IPCA-LSTM (M5)**
M1 (93.15%)	–	(27.28%) Y	(24.22%) Y	(31.77%) Y	(28.64%) Y
M2 (65.87%)		–	(03.06%) N	(04.49%) N	(01.36%) N
M3 (68.93%)			–	(07.55%) Y	(04.42%) N
M4 (61.38%)				–	(03.13%) N
M5 (64.51%)					–
DPALIGN (Abs. Specificity difference (%), significant/non-significant)					
ML systems (spec.)	**CNN-LSTM (M1)**	**CNN-MLP (M2)**	**HMM-LSTM (M3)**	**HMM-SDA (M4)**	**IPCA-LSTM (M5)**
M1 (95.17%)	–	(23.68%) Y	(22.18%) Y	(28.30%) Y	(25.58%) Y
M2 (71.49%)		–	(01.50%) N	(04.62%) Y	(01.90%) N
M3 (72.99%)			–	(06.12%) Y	(03.40%) N
M4 (66.87%)				–	(02.72%) Y
M5 (69.59%)					–
EPOCH (Abs. Specificity difference (%), significant/non-significant)					
ML systems (spec.)	**CNN-LSTM (M1)**	**CNN-MLP (M2)**	**HMM-LSTM (M3)**	**HMM-SDA (M4)**	**IPCA-LSTM (M5)**
M1 (99.84%)	–	(08.29%) N	(05.02%) N	(01.62%) N	(05.75%) N
M2 (91.55%)		–	(03.27%) N	(06.67%) N	(02.54%) N
M3 (94.82%)			–	(03.40%) N	(00.73%) N
M4 (98.22%)				–	(04.13%) N
M5 (94.09%)					–
OVLP (Abs. Specificity difference (%), significant/non-significant)					
ML systems (spec.)	**CNN-LSTM (M1)**	**CNN-MLP (M2)**	**HMM-LSTM (M3)**	**HMM-SDA (M4)**	**IPCA-LSTM (M5)**
M1 (96.86%)	–	(20.02%) Y	(16.33%) Y	(23.51%) Y	(19.29%) Y
M2 (76.84%)		–	(03.69%) N	(03.49%) Y	(00.73%) N
M3 (80.53%)			–	(07.18%) Y	(02.96%) N
M4 (73.35%)				–	(04.22%) Y
M5 (77.57%)					–
TAES (Abs. Specificity difference (%), significant/non-significant)					
ML systems (spec.)	**CNN-LSTM (M1)**	**CNN-MLP (M2)**	**HMM-LSTM (M3)**	**HMM-SDA (M4)**	**IPCA-LSTM (M5)**
M1 (95.24%)	–	(31.21%) Y	(24.83%) Y	(29.20%) Y	(28.60%) Y
M2 (64.03%)		–	(06.38%) N	(02.01%) Y	(02.61%) N
M3 (70.41%)			–	(04.37%) Y	(03.77%) N
M4 (66.04%)				–	(00.60%) Y
M5 (66.64%)					–

approximately 75%. As we move more technology into operational environments, we expect to have more to contribute to this research topic.

Finally, the Python implementation of these metrics is available at the project web site: https://www.isip.piconepress.com/projects/tuh_eeg/downloads/nedc_eval_eeg. This scoring software described here has been publicly available since late 2018. It has been used for two open-source evaluations (Kiral et al. 2019; Roy et al. 2020). Readers are encouraged to refer to the software for detailed questions about the specific implementations of these algorithms and the tunable parameters available.

Acknowledgments Research reported in this publication was most recently supported by the National Human Genome Research Institute of the National Institutes of Health under award number U01HG008468. The content is solely the responsibility of the authors and does not necessarily represent the official views of the National Institutes of Health. This material is also based in part upon work supported by the National Science Foundation under Grant No. IIP-1622765. Any opinions, findings, and conclusions or recommendations expressed in this material are those of the author(s) and do not necessarily reflect the views of the National Science Foundation. We are also grateful to our colleagues at IBM Research: Stefan Harrer, Jiri Navratil, and Subhrajit Roy. Their careful reading of early versions of this manuscript and valuable insights about the work were greatly appreciated. We also would like to acknowledge Seyedeh Saeedeh Khoshgoftar Ziyabari for her contributions to the initial portions of this work.

Conflict of Interest Statement Author Meysam Golmohammadi is employed by Internet Brands, El Segundo, California, USA. This work was completed at the Neural Engineering Data Consortium at Temple University prior to his employment at Internet Brands. All other authors declare no conflict of interest.

References

D.G. Altman, J.M. Bland, Diagnostic tests 1: Sensitivity and specificity. Br. Med. J. **308**(6943), 1552 (1994). https://doi.org/10.1136/bmj.308.6943.1552

S. Baldassano et al., A novel seizure detection algorithm informed by hidden Markov model event states. J. Neural Eng. **13**(3), 036011 (2016). https://doi.org/10.1016/j.clinph.2010.04.016

R. Banchs, A. Bonafonte, J. Perez, Acceptance testing of a spoken language translation system, in *Proceedings of the International Conference on Language Resources and Evaluation (LREC)*, (2006), p. 106. http://www.lrec-conf.org/proceedings/lrec2006/pdf/60_pdf.pdf

A.C. Bridi, T.Q. Louro, R.C.L. Da Silva, Clinical alarms in intensive care: Implications of alarm fatigue for the safety of patients. Rev. Lat. Am. Enfermagem **22**(6), 1034 (2014). https://doi.org/10.1590/0104-1169.3488.2513

D. Chicco, G. Jurman, The advantages of the Matthews correlation coefficient (MCC) over F1 score and accuracy in binary classification evaluation. BMC Genomics **21**(1), 6 (2020). https://doi.org/10.1186/s12864-019-6413-7

G.D. Clifford et al., False alarm reduction in critical care. Physiol. Meas. **37**(8), E5–E23 (2016). https://doi.org/10.1088/0967-3334/37/8/E5

Confusion matrix. [Online]. Available: https://en.wikipedia.org/wiki/Confusion_matrix. Accessed 31 Oct 2017.

A. Craik, Y. He, J.L. Contreras-Vidal, Deep learning for electroencephalogram (EEG) classification tasks: A review. J. Neural Eng. **16**(3), 031001 (2019). https://doi.org/10.1088/1741-2552/ab0ab5

M. Cvach Maria, Managing hospital alarms. Nurs. Crit. Care **9**(3), 13–27 (2014). https://doi.org/10.1097/01.CCN.0000446255.81392.b0

Y. Dodge, *The Concise Encyclopedia of Statistics*, 2008th edn. (Springer, 2008). https://doi.org/10.1007/978-0-387-32833-1

J.G. Fiscus, Overview of the NIST open keyword search 2013 evaluation workshop, in *IEEE Signal Processing Society – SLTC Newsletter*, (2013) https://www.nist.gov/publications/overview-nist-open-keyword-search-2013-evaluation-worksho

J.G. Fiscus, *Speech Recognition Scoring Toolkit* (National Instutue of Standards and Technology, 2017) [Online]. https://github.com/usnistgov/SCTK. Accessed 17 Oct 2017

J. Fiscus, J. Ajot, J. Garofolo, G. Doddingtion, Results of the 2006 Spoken Term Detection Evaluation, in *Proceedings of the ACM Special Interest Gruoup on Information Retrieval (SIGIR) Workshop "Searching Spontaneous Conversational Speech"*, (2007), pp. 45–50. https://www.nist.gov/publications/results-2006-spoken-term-detection-evaluation

M. Golmohammadi, A. Harati, S. de Diego, I. Obeid, J. Picone, Automatic Analysis of EEGs Using Big Data and Hybrid Deep Learning Architectures. Front. Hum. Neurosci. **13**, 76 (2019). https://doi.org/10.3389/fnhum.2019.00076

M. Golmohammadi, V. Shah, I. Obeid, J. Picone, Deep learning approaches for automatic seizure detection from scalp electroencephalograms, in *Signal Processing in Medicine and Biology: Emerging Trends in Research and Applications*, ed. by I. Obeid, I. Selesnick, J. Picone, 1st edn., (Sprínger, New York, 2020), pp. 233–274. https://doi.org/10.1007/978-3-030-36844-9

J. Gotman, Automatic recognition of epileptic seizures in the EEG. Electroencephalogr. Clin. Neurophysiol. **54**(5), 530–540 (1982). http://www.sciencedirect.com/science/article/pii/0013469482900384

J. Gotman, D. Flanagan, J. Zhang, B. Rosenblatt, Automatic seizure detection in the newborn: Methods and initial evaluation. Electroencephalogr. Clin. Neurophysiol. **103**(3), 356–362 (1997). https://doi.org/10.1016/S0013-4694(97)00003-9

K. Hajian-Tilaki, Receiver operating characteristic (ROC) curve analysis for medical diagnostic test evaluation. Casp. J. Intern. Med. **4**(2), 627–635 (2013) http://www.ncbi.nlm.nih.gov/pmc/articles/PMC3755824/

J.J. Halford et al., Inter-rater agreement on identification of electrographic seizures and periodic discharges in ICU EEG recordings. Clin. Neurophysiol. **126**(9), 1661–1669 (2015). https://doi.org/10.1016/j.clinph.2014.11.008

F. Hammond, J. Malec, R. Buschbacher, T. Nick, *Handbook for Clinical Research : Design, Statistics, and Implementation* (Demos Medical Publishing, New York City, 2015) https://www.springerpub.com/handbook-for-clinical-research-9781936287543.html

A. Harati, M. Golmohammadi, S. Lopez, I. Obeid, J. Picone, Improved EEG Event Classification Using Differential Energy, in *Proceedings of the IEEE Signal Processing in Medicine and Biology Symposium*, (2015), pp. 1–4. https://doi.org/10.1109/SPMB.2015.7405421

N. Japkowicz, M. Shah, *Evaluating Learning Algorithms: A Classification Perspective* (Cambridge University Press, New York City, 2014), p. 424. https://doi.org/10.1017/CBO9780511921803

K.M. Kelly et al., Assessment of a scalp EEG-based automated seizure detection system. Clin. Neurophysiol. **121**(11), 1832–1843 (2010). https://doi.org/10.1016/j.clinph.2010.04.016

R. Kemp, *European Data Format* (Department of Neurology, Leiden University Medical Centre, The Netherlands, 2013) [Online]. http://www.edfplus.info. Accessed 06 Jan 2013

I. Kiral et al., The Deep Learning Epilepsy Detection Challenge: Design, Implementation, and Test of a New Crowd-Sourced AI Challenge Ecosystem, presented at the Neural Information Processing Systems (NeurIPS) Workshop on Challenges in Machine Learning Competitions for All (CiML). https://isip.piconepress.com/publications/conference_presentations/2019/neurips_ciml/epilepsy_challenge/, (2019)

A. Liu, J.S. Hahn, G.P. Heldt, R.W. Coen, Detection of neonatal seizures through computerized EEG analysis. Electroencephalogr. Clin. Neurophysiol. **82**(2), 32–37 (1992). https://doi.org/10.1016/0013-4694(92)90179-L

A. Martin, G. Doddington, T. Kamm, M. Ordowski, M. Przybocki, The DET curve in assessment of detection task performance, in *Proceedings of the European Conference on Speech Commu-*

nication and Technology (Eurospeech), (1997), pp. 1895–1898. http://www.isca-speech.org/archive/eurospeech_1997/e97_1895.html

S.J. Mason, N.E. Graham, Areas beneath the relative operating characteristics (ROC) and relative operating levels (ROL) curves: Statistical significance and interpretation. Q. J. R. Meteorol. Soc. **128**(584), 2145–2166 (2002). https://doi.org/10.1256/003590002320603584

M.L. McHugh, Interrater reliability: The kappa statistic. Biochem. Med. **22**(3), 276–282 (2012). https://doi.org/10.11613/BM.2012.031

M. Michel, D. Joy, J.G. Fiscus, V. Manohar, J. Ajot, B. Barr, *Framework for Detection Evaluation (F4DE)* (National Institute of Standards and Technology, 2017) [Online]. [Accessed: 16-May-2017]. https://github.com/usnistgov/F4DE

D. Mostefa, O. Hamin, K. Choukri, Evaluation of automatic speech recognition and speech language translation within TC-STAR: Results from the first evaluation campaign, in *Proceedings of the International Conference on Language Resources and Evaluation (LREC)*, (2006), pp. 149–154. http://citeseerx.ist.psu.edu/viewdoc/summary?doi=10.1.1.323.5822&rank=4

M.A. Navakatikyan, P.B. Colditz, C.J. Burke, T.E. Inder, J. Richmond, C.E. Williams, Seizure detection algorithm for neonates based on wave-sequence analysis. Clin. Neurophysiol. **117**(6), 1190–1203 (2006). https://doi.org/10.1016/j.clinph.2006.02.016

I. Obeid, J. Picone, The Temple University Hospital EEG Data Corpus, in *Augmentation of Brain Function: Facts, Fiction and Controversy. Volume I: Brain-Machine Interfaces*, ed. by M. A. Lebedev, vol. 10, 1st edn., (Frontiers Media S.A., Lausanne, 2016), pp. 394–398. https://doi.org/10.3389/fnins.2016.00196

D. Ochal, S. Rahman, S. Ferrell, T. Elseify, I. Obeid, J. Picone, *The Temple University Hospital EEG Corpus: Annotation Guidelines* (Philadelphia, 2020) https://www.isip.piconepress.com/publications/reports/2020/tuh_eeg/annotations/

K. Papineni, S. Roukos, T. Ward, W.-J. Zhu, BLEU: A method for automatic evaluation of machine translation, in *Proceedings of the 40th Annual Meeting of the Association for Computational Linguistics (ACL)*, (2002), pp. 311–318. https://doi.org/10.3115/1073083.1073135

J. Picone, G. Doddington, D. Pallett, Phone-mediated word alignment for speech recognition evaluation. IEEE Trans. Acoust. Speech Signal Process. **38**(3), 559–562 (1990). https://doi.org/10.1109/29.106877

D.M.W. Powers, Evaluation: From precision, recall and f-factor to roc, informedness, markedness & correlation. J. Mach. Learn. Technol. **2**(1), 37–63 (2011) https://bioinfopublication.org/files/articles/2_1_1_JMLT.pdf

Y. Roy, H. Banville, I. Albuquerque, A. Gramfort, T.H. Falk, J. Faubert, Deep learning-based electroencephalography analysis: A systematic review. J. Neural. Eng. **16**(5), 37 (2019). https://doi.org/10.1088/1741-2552/ab260c

Y. Roy, R. Iskander, J. Picone, The Neureka(TM) 2020 Epilepsy Challenge. NeuroTechX (2020) [Online]. https://neureka-challenge.com/. Accessed 16 Apr 2020

V. Shah et al., The Temple University Hospital Seizure Detection Corpus. Front. Neuroinform. **12**, 1–6 (2018). https://doi.org/10.3389/fninf.2018.00083

V. Shah, E. von Weltin, T. Ahsan, I. Obeid, J. Picone, On the Use of Non-Experts for Generation of High-Quality Annotations of Seizure Events. J. Clin. Neurophysiol. (under review) (2020) https://www.isip.piconepress.com/publications/unpublished/journals/2019/elsevier_cn/ira/

P. von Goethem, B. Hambling, *User Acceptance Testing: A step-by-step guide* (BCS Learning & Development Limited, Swindon, 2013) https://www.oreilly.com/library/view/user-acceptance-testing/9781780171678/

Y.-Y. Wang, A. Acero, C. Chelba, Is word error rate a good indicator for spoken language understanding accuracy, in *Proceedings of the IEEE Workshop on Automatic Speech Recognition and Understanding (ASRU)*, (2003), pp. 577–582. https://doi.org/10.1109/ASRU.2003.1318504

S. Wegmann, A. Faria, A. Janin, K. Riedhammer, N. Morgan, The TAO of ATWV: Probing the mysteries of keyword search performance, in *Proceedings of the IEEE Workshop on Automatic Speech Recognition and Understanding (ASRU)*, (2013), pp. 192–197

S.B. Wilson, R. Emerson, Spike detection: A review and comparison of algorithms. Clin. Neurophysiol. **113**(12), 1873–1881 (2002). https://doi.org/10.1016/S1388-2457(02)00297-3

S.B. Wilson, M.L. Scheuer, C. Plummer, B. Young, S. Pacia, Seizure detection: Correlation of human experts. Clin. Neurophysiol. **114**(11), 2156–2164 (2003). https://doi.org/10.1016/S1388-2457(03)00212-8

M. Winterhalder, T. Maiwald, H.U. Voss, R. Aschenbrenner-Scheibe, J. Timmer, A. Schulze-Bonhage, The seizure prediction characteristic: A general framework to assess and compare seizure prediction methods. Epilepsy Behav. **4**(3), 318–325 (2003). https://doi.org/10.1016/S1525-5050(03)00105-7

J.M. Wozencraft, I.M. Jacobs, *Principles of Communication Engineering* (Wiley, New York City, 1965) https://books.google.com/books/about/Principles_of_communication_engineering.html?id=4ORSAAAAMAAJ

W. Xiong, L. Wu, F. Alleva, J. Droppo, X. Huang, A. Stolcke, The Microsoft 2017 Conversational Speech Recognition System, in *Proceedings of the IEEE International Conference on Acoustics, Speech, and Signal Processing (ICASSP)*, (2017), pp. 5255–5259. https://doi.org/10.1109/ICASSP.2018.8461870

T. Yamada, E. Meng, *Practical Guide for Clinical Neurophysiologic Testing: EEG* (Lippincott Williams & Wilkins, Philadelphia, 2017). https://doi.org/10.1111/j.1468-1331.2009.02936.x

Index

I. Obeid et al. (eds.), *Biomedical Signal Processing*,
https://doi.org/10.1007/978-3-030-67494-6

The manufacturer's authorised representative in the EU is Springer Nature Customer Service Centre GmbH, Europaplatz 3, 69115 Heidelberg, Germany. If you have any concerns regarding our products, please contact ProductSafety@springernature.com

Printed and bound by CPI Group (UK) Ltd, Croydon, CR0 4YY
28/09/2026
02224090-0012